AF335507

Speech Science

Recent Advances

Editor in chief, Speech, Language, and Hearing Science Series
Raymond G. Daniloff, PhD

SPEECH SCIENCE

Recent Advances

Edited by

Raymond G. Daniloff, PhD

Department of Speech Communication, Theater,
and Communication Disorders
Speech and Hearing Clinic
Louisiana State University
Baton Rouge, Louisiana

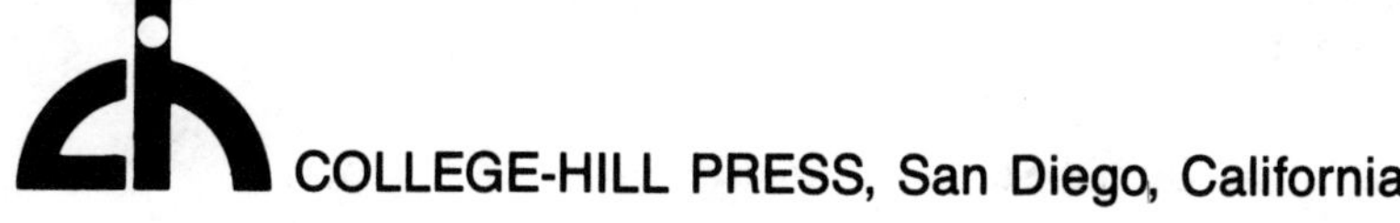

COLLEGE-HILL PRESS, San Diego, California

College-Hill Press
4284 41st Street
San Diego, California 92105

© 1985 College-Hill Press, Inc.

Library of Congress Cataloging in Publication Data

Main entry under title:

Speech science.

  Bibliography: p.
  Includes indexes.
  1. Speech—Physiological aspects. I. Daniloff, Raymond.
QP306.S67   1984   612'.78   84-23112
ISBN 0-933014-95-3

Printed in the United States of America

PUBLISHER'S NOTE

These volumes were developed under the supervision of a group of leading scientists charged with the responsibility of assessing the most critical book needs of the speech-language-hearing profession. In consultation with William H. Perkins and Raymond G. Daniloff, serving as editors in chief of the ensuing volumes on speech, language, and hearing disorders (Perkins) and speech, language, and hearing science (Daniloff), the publisher planned a series of nine mutually independent texts covering the entirety of state-of-the-art knowledge in these disciplines, with contributions by respected, productive, and current scholars known for their expertise as specialists in key areas.

Each contribution has been stringently refereed for content, pedagogy, and practical value for students and practitioners by the individual volume editors, Charles Berlin, Janis Costello, Raymond Daniloff, Audrey Holland, James Jerger, Rita Naremore, and their designated reviewers, in close consultation throughout with the editors in chief and the publisher. Users are thus assured that their needs for accurate, timely information, reflecting the highest standards of scholarship and professionalism, have been faithfully met.

On behalf of the speech-language-hearing profession, its researchers, teachers, practitioners, and students, present and future, the publisher thanks the more than 100 authors and editors who have given generously of their time and knowledge to produce this magnificent contribution to the literature.

Speech Science, edited by Raymond G. Daniloff, is one of nine state-of-the-art volumes comprising the College-Hill Press series covering the current body of knowledge in speech, language, and hearing.

Volume Titles:	**Editors:**
Speech Disorders in Children	Janis Costello
Speech Disorders in Adults	Janis Costello
Speech Science	Raymond Daniloff
Language Disorders in Children	Audrey Holland
Language Disorders in Adults	Audrey Holland
Language Science	Rita Naremore
Pediatric Audiology	James Jerger
Hearing Disorders in Adults	James Jerger
Hearing Science	Charles Berlin
Editor in chief, Speech, Language, and Hearing Disorders Series:	William H. Perkins
Editor in chief, Speech, Language, and Hearing Science Series:	Raymond G. Daniloff

CONTENTS

CONTRIBUTORS

James H. Abbs, PhD
Waisman Center on Mental Retardation
Speech Motor Control Laboratories
The University of Wisconsin-Madison
Madison, Wisconsin

Raymond G. Daniloff, PhD
Department of Speech Communication, Theater, and
Communication Disorders
Louisiana State University
Baton Rouge, Louisiana

Michael F. Dorman, PhD
Department of Speech and Hearing Science
Arizona State University
Tempe, Arizona

Carol A. Fowler, PhD
Dartmouth College
Hanover, New Hampshire, and
Haskins Laboratories
New Haven, Connecticut

Maureen T. Hannley, PhD
Department of Speech and Hearing Science
Arizona State University
Tempe, Arizona

Minoru Hirano, MD
Department of Otolaryngology
School of Medicine
Kurume University
Kurume, Japan

Paul R. Hoffman, PhD
Department of Speech Communication, Theater, and
Communication Disorders
Louisiana State University
Baton Rouge, Louisiana

Yuki Kakita, PhD
Department of Otolaryngology
School of Medicine
Kurume University
Kurume, Japan

Marcel A. Tatham
Languages and Linguistics
University of Essex
Essex, England

Herbert M. Teager, PhD
Evans Department of Clinical Investigation
Boston University Medical Center
Boston University
Boston, Massachusetts

Shushan M. Teager
Evans Department of Clinical Investigation
Boston University Medical Center
Boston University
Boston, Massachusetts

Gary Weismer, PhD
Waisman Center on Mental Retardation
Speech Motor Control Laboratories
The University of Wisconsin-Madison
Madison, Wisconsin

Carol Welt, PhD
Waisman Center on Mental Retardation
Speech Motor Control Laboratories
The University of Wisconsin-Madison
Madison, Wisconsin

PREFACE

The chapters in this textbook differ greatly in scope and purpose; there are general reviews, specific reviews, treatises on a single topic, and, in one case, an extensive investigation. This spread of topics reflects the increasing diversity of interests, both basic and applied, that characterize speech research in this decade. After a decade of intense experimental activity, reviews and model building reflect the stock-taking and synthesis needed to digest voluminous research.

Hirano and Kakita offer a summary of the elegant anatomical and biomechanical studies used to develop their "cover-body" model of vocal fold mechanical structure. This work had its roots in Hirano's massive clinical-anatomical tome, *Phonosurgery*, and reflects how anatomical, engineering, and phonetic talent mesh to provide a benchmark modeling of the laryngeal system that will guide and inform research in that area for the next decade.

Weismer's critical review of current research and modeling of respiratory function for speech has primarily a didactic purpose. Following an historical summary and critique of respiratory research, Weismer reviews physiological-anatomical and experimental factors that govern how such research is conducted, is interpreted, and has led to the current, popular model of speech breathing proposed by Mead and Hixon. The chapter concludes with a terse review of current research and predicts the topics and directions for research which will be the vanguard in this area for the coming decade.

Undoubtedly, Teager and Teager's chapter on vowel production is the most original and possibly the most controversial chapter within this volume. Based upon their own decade-long aerodynamic and acoustic studies of live and modeled vocal tracts, the authors *attack* the standard source-filter model of vowel production, which has been received wisdom since Fant's monumental "Acoustic Theory of Vowel Production." These authors argue strongly that the vocal tract is not a linear system in which a high impedance glottis injects air bursts that flow out the tract in a laminar fashion, but rather that eddies or vortices of turbulent air flow located at points other than the glottis are significant sources of intratract excitation. Whether or not their contentions ultimately are sustained by future research, this chapter should encourage investigators to assess the degree to which the vocal tract may depart from strictly linear acoustic behavior.

Dorman and Hannley offer a comprehensive and especially critical review of research in the area of speech and speechlike signal perception by the hearing impaired, in which their own research plays no small part.

Current research in the area is propelled by the desire to create better hearing aids, cochlear prostheses, and clinical management for the hearing impaired. Research has progressed from psychoacoustic studies of simple nonspeech to more speechlike signals in variously damaged ears, to current studies of synthetic speech perception. What is truly surprising about the research so cogently reviewed is that speech perception tested to date is relatively normal, despite some clear differences in the psychoacoustic performance of impaired ears on tasks involving temporal and frequency resolution. This chapter should serve as an effective review and entrée to this literature for some time to come.

Abbs and Welt provide perhaps the first modern, critical review of anatomical-physiological research on the function of the lateral, precentral, frontal cortex (which includes Broca's area) and its role in the control of human and nonhuman facial movement and vocalization. This was an arduous task, since most work is in the neuroanatomical literature, which the authors not only had to review but also had to reinterpret for an audience of speech scientists. What emerges from the review is that there are multiple areas of frontal cortex adjacent to the motor strip wherein separate representations of sensory and motor areas of the vocal tract exist. These areas are linked in functionally significant ways which reflect upon the dichotomy between the cognitive intentionality or planning for speech and the motoric processes of generating linear, coproduced streams of speech sound. The authors end their review by supporting, in principle, the notion of hierarchical coordinative neural circuits that entrain groups of motor subsystems into the synergistic wholes needed to produce articulate speech.

Fowler offers the reader perhaps the single most impressive and comprehensive review of models of speech production yet attempted. Her work is noteworthy for the inclusion of such higher level linguistic cognitive models of language encoding such as those of Garrett, Shattuck-Hufnagel, Dell, and Steinberg and colleagues, as well as lower level (phonetic) neurophysiological models such as those of Ohman, Lindblom, Perkell, and MacNeilage and associates. The researcher will be pleased with the inclusiveness of the survey—nothing much of importance is missed— whereas the student will be rewarded with Fowler's penetrating critique of strengths, weaknesses, and the explanatory niche of each model of production. It is difficult to imagine many workers today whose catholicity of interest would enable them to master the worlds of phonetics, linguistics, engineering, and physiology. The sole (and minor) shortcoming of the work is that the critique is not rich in linguistically motivated criticism. A particularly useful feature of her narrative is the use of mini-essays at the end of each section that "summarize, interpret, and reduce" the mass of the critical narrative. The second half of the review, which focuses on speech production, is issue oriented; questions such as the following are addressed: What *are* articulated segments? How are linguistic units realized-duration? What is coarticulation? What is the nature of specific vocal tract substem physiology? Her critique of coarticulation literature is, perhaps, the stepping stone to viewing the phenomena, in a new frame of reference, as "coproduction." The review ends by addressing the issue of the coordination of complex motor movement and the usefulness of "coordinative structure" models of motor organization. The narrative here meshes nicely with that of Abbs and Welt. The patient reader will be rewarded with a grand tour of speech encoding research, a tour rich with bias, but bias based upon long and critical thinking.

The chapter by Tatham, Daniloff, and Hoffman rounds out the volume by presenting results of a massive electromyographic study of the invariance of the lip-closing gesture for labial stops. In this study, the authors' strenuous attempts to control experimental and subject variability for surface electromyograms yields the relatively surprising finding that labial closure is a stereotyped (invariant) articulatory gesture, depending little upon voicing, syllabic position, stress, and even vowel context, inasmuch as no extensive, systematic perturbation of the EMG signal for lip closure was found in these various contexts. Efforts to control variability thus pay rich rewards in allowing phoneticians to make claims about the degree to which articulatory gestures are generally coproduced.

CHAPTER 1
Cover–Body Theory of Vocal Fold Vibration

Minoru Hirano
Yuki Kakita

From a phonatory point of view, the most important notion of the structure of the vocal fold is that the vocal fold consists of multiple layers, each having its own mechanical properties. In other words, the vocal fold is not a vibrator of uniform structure but a layer-structured vibrator.

Smith (1956) proposed the "membrane–cushion theory" with respect to vocal fold vibration. According to his theoretical model, the vocal fold is composed of the membrane (the mucous membrane) and the cushion (the vocalis muscle), which are coupled by the intervening vocal ligament. On the basis of his theory, Smith made mechanical models of rubber and demonstrated that vibration of the models resembled real vocal fold vibration. His models and their vibration were shown in a film. Unfortunately, this film has not been distributed on a worldwide basis and it was in 1980 when this author first saw the film at the 18th Congress of the International Association of Logopedics and Phoniatrics in Washington, DC. The membrane–cushion theory of Smith appears to be the earliest version of the cover-body theory developed by this author.

Schönhärl (1960), in his pioneering work on the modern stroboscopy of the larynx, emphasized that the vibratory movement of the vocal fold consisted of two different components: the movement of the base (Grundbewegung) and the shifting of the edge (Randkantenverschiebung). Although he did not specify which anatomical structures are involved in these two components of the vibratory movement, one can interpret the "base" as the muscle and the "edge" as the mucous membrane from his schemata.

Perelló (1962), on the basis of a literature review and his own clinical experiences, drew an inference that the vibratory movement of the vocal fold is the undulation of the mucous membrane.

Hiroto (1966) proposed the "mucoviscoelastic–aerodynamic theory" of the mechanism of vocal fold vibration. In contrast to the myoelastic-aerodynamic theory proposed by Van den Berg (1958) in which elasticity of the vocalis muscle and the Bernoulli effect were regarded as important components, Hiroto emphasized the importance of viscoelasticity of the mucous membrane for the vibratory movements.

All these investigators postulated that the outer part of the vocal fold moves differently from its inner part. This implies that they should have also postulated differences in the melchanical properties of these two parts of the vocal fold.

The senior author demonstrated the layer structure of a human vocal fold histologically and proposed the notion of cover–body complex (Hirano, 1972, 1974a). He inferred four different types of adjustment of the body–cover complex brought about by the activity of the cricothyroid and vocalis muscles. This was the beginning of a series of investigations on the structure, mechanical properties, adjustments, and vibratory behavior of the vocal fold conducted in the Department of Otolaryngology, Kurume University (Hirano, 1974a; Hirano, 1975; Hirano, 1977; Hirano, 1981; Hirano, Kakita, Kawasaki, and Matsushita, 1976; Hirano, Kakita, Ohmaru, and Kurita, 1982; Hirano, Koike, Hirose, and Kasuya, 1974; Hirano, Koike, Hirose, and Morio, 1973a; Hirano, Kurita, and Nagata, 1981a; Hirano, Kurita, and Nakashima, 1981b; Hirano, Kurita, and Toh, 1981c; Kakita, Hirano, Kawasaki, and Matsushita, 1976a, 1976b; Kakita, Hirano, and Ohmaru, 1981; Kasuya, 1976; Koike, Hirano, and Morio, 1976; Kurita, 1980; Mihashi, Okada, and Hirano, 1976; Mihashi, Okada, Kurita, Nagata, Oda, Hirano, and Nakashima, 1981; Morio, 1976; Ohmaru, 1981; Ohmaru, Kakita, and Hirano, 1981; Okada, 1978; Okada, Mihashi, Ito, and Hirano, 1978).

This paper describes several important aspects of our series of investigations conducted in this area.

MORPHOLOGICAL STRUCTURE OF THE HUMAN VOCAL FOLD CONSISTING OF A COVER–BODY COMPLEX

Histological Structure of the Adult Human Vocal Fold

Hirano, Koike, Hirose, and Morio (1973) investigated 10 normal male adult larynges histologically. They also drove excised human larynges with compressed air and investigated the vibratory behavior of three points marked on the vocal fold mucosa with the use of stroboscopic photography. The location of the points were histologically determined later and related to the structure. On the basis of their results, Hirano (1975) schematically presented an anatomical model of the layer structure of the vocal fold (Fig.

Figure 1–1. Histological structure of the adult human vocal fold. *A*, Frontal section of the middle of the membranous portion. *B*, A schematic representation of the cover–body complex. E, Epithelium; S, I, D, superficial, intermediate, and deep layers of the lamina propria; M, muscle. From Hirano, M. (1975). Phonosurgery: Basic and clinical investigations. *Otologia (Fukuoka)*, *21*, 239–440. Reprinted with permission.

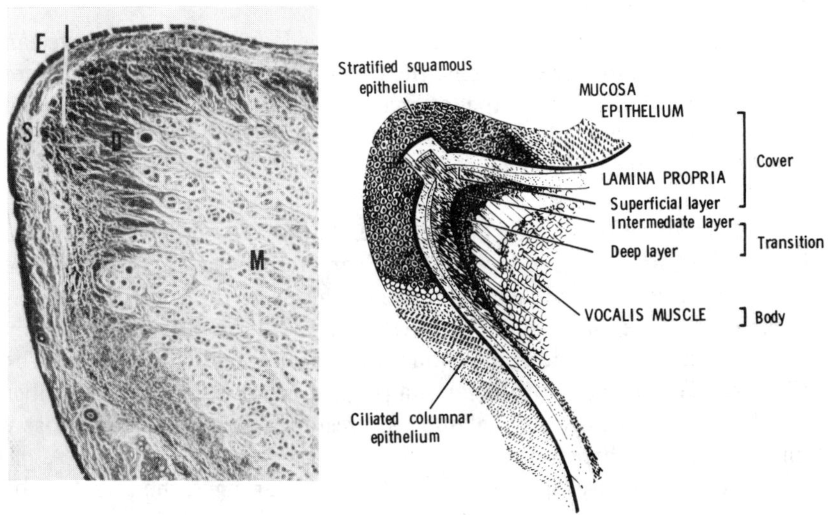

1–1). Since this notion is the keystone of the cover–body theory of vocal fold vibration, a detailed explanation is given here.

The vocal fold consists of the mucous membrane (mucosa) and the muscle. The mucosa, in turn, comprises the epithelium and the lamina propria. The epithelium is stratified squamous cell epithelium around the edge of the vocal fold. It can be regarded as a thin capsule of the vibrating structure. The lamina propria can be subdivided into three layers on the basis of the density of fibrous components, which are elastic and collagenous fibers: the superficial, intermediate, and deep layers. In the superficial layer, the fibrous components are loose. This layer is called Reinke's space. It is pliable and can be regarded as somewhat like a mass of soft gelatin. The intermediate layer consists chiefly of elastic fibers, which can be likened to soft rubber bands. The deep layer primarily consists of collagenous fibers, which are something like cotton thread. Thus there is a gradual increase in stiffness from the superficial to the deep layer. The portion that consists of the intermediate and deep layers of the lamina propria is referred to as the vocal ligament. The muscle, the vocalis muscle, constitutes the main body of the vocal fold and can be likened to stiff rubber bands.

Anatomically, it is controversial to assign the vocal ligament to the lamina propria of the mucosa or to the tela submucosa. We consider the vocal ligament to be a part of the lamina propria, but we do not necessarily insist on this conception. Since this issue is not the focus of this article, we do not go into it further.

From a mechanical point of view, the five layers described above can be reclassified into three sections: the *cover,* consisting of the epithelium and the superficial layer of the lamina propria; the *transition,* consisting of the intermediate and deep layers of the lamina propria; and the *body,* which constitutes the vocalis muscle, as shown in Figure 1–1*B*.

The superficial layer of the lamina propria is clearly delineated from the intermediate layer, but, on the other hand, the border between the intermediate and the deep layers is not clear. In the vocal ligament, elastic fibers decrease while collagenous fibers increase as the vocalis muscle is approached. The intermediate and deep layers can be differentiated only when the elastic and the collagenous fibers are individually stained. The fibers of the deep layer of the lamina propria insert into the muscle fiber bundles of the vocalis muscle, and as a result the two layers are closely linked to each other morphologically.

In our early investigation of 10 adult male larynges, the thickness of the cover measured 0.3 mm on the average, with the range from 0.2 to 0.5 mm, that of the transition 0.8 mm on the average, with the range from 0.5 to 1.1 mm, and that of the entire mucosa 1.1 mm on the average, with the range from 0.9 to 1.3 mm (Hirano et al., 1973a). The thickness of each layer varies according to age and sex, as will be described later in this article.

The collagenous and elastic fibers in the lamina propria, as well as the muscle fibers in the vocalis muscle, run roughly parallel to the edge of the vocal fold as shown in Figure 1–2 (Hirano, 1975; Hirano, 1977; Hirano, 1981a; Hirano et al., 1973a; Kurita, 1980). In other words, the fibers run at a right angle to the direction of the airflow. This orientation of the fibers is well suited for the resulting vibration. The direction of the fibers also indicates that the elastic property of the vocal fold tissue is orthotropic, as will be discussed in the section on Mechanical Properties of the Vocal Fold Tissue.

Fine Structure of the Collagenous and Elastic Fibers

To discuss vibratory behavior of the vocal fold, it is important to understand the fine structure of the collagenous and elastic fibers. Hirano

Figure 1–2. Histological sections showing the direction of elastic (*A*, single arrow), collagenous (*B*, single arrow), and muscle fibers (double arrows) in the vocal fold. From Hirano, M. (1981a). Structure of the vocal fold in normal and disease states. Anatomical and physical studies. *ASHA Report, 11,* 11–27. Reprinted with permission.

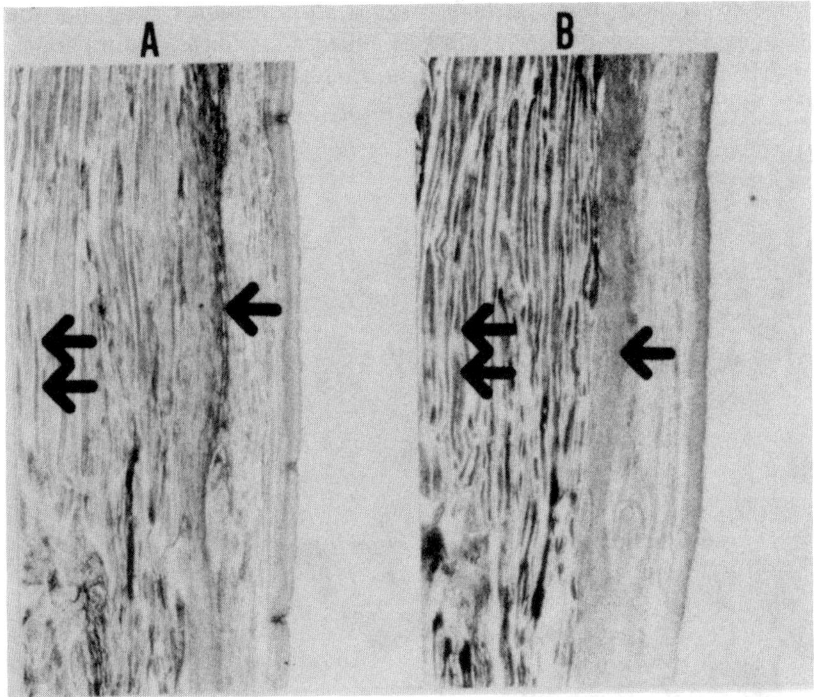

(1975, 1977, 1981) reported the results of an electron microscopic investigation of human vocal folds. In his reports, the specimens for electron microscopic observations were obtained from the middle of the membranous portion of intact vocal folds of 12 larynges that were surgically removed because of carcinoma. Both transmission (TEM) and scanning electron (SEM) microscopy was conducted.

Figure 1–3 presents electron microscopic pictures of each layer of the lamina propria of the vocal fold. In the superficial layer of the lamina propria, extremely thin collagenous fibrils, 0.05 to 0.07 μm in diameter, are tangled loosely like cotton fibers (Fig. 1–3*A*). A few elastic fibers are also found. These networks of thin fibers appear to give an elasticity to what we have called the mass of soft gelatin. In the intermediate layer of the lamina propria, there are bundles of elastic fibers; these fibers are 0.5 to 1.5 μm in diameter. They are not straight fibers; rather, they branch and

Figure 1–3. Electron micrographs of the human vocal fold tissue. *A*, The superficial layer of the lamina propria (SEM). *B*, Longitudinal section of the intermediate layer demonstrating the branching and the anastomosing of elastic fibers (TEM). *C*, Longitudinal section of the deep layer of the lamina propria demonstrating the twisting of collagen fibers (SEM). *D*, Some collagenous fibers at high magnification demonstrating that the collagen fibers consist of a number of collagenous fibrils. From Hirano, M. (1975). Phonosurgery: Basic and clinical investigations. *Otologia (Fukuoka), 21*, 239–440. Reprinted with permission.

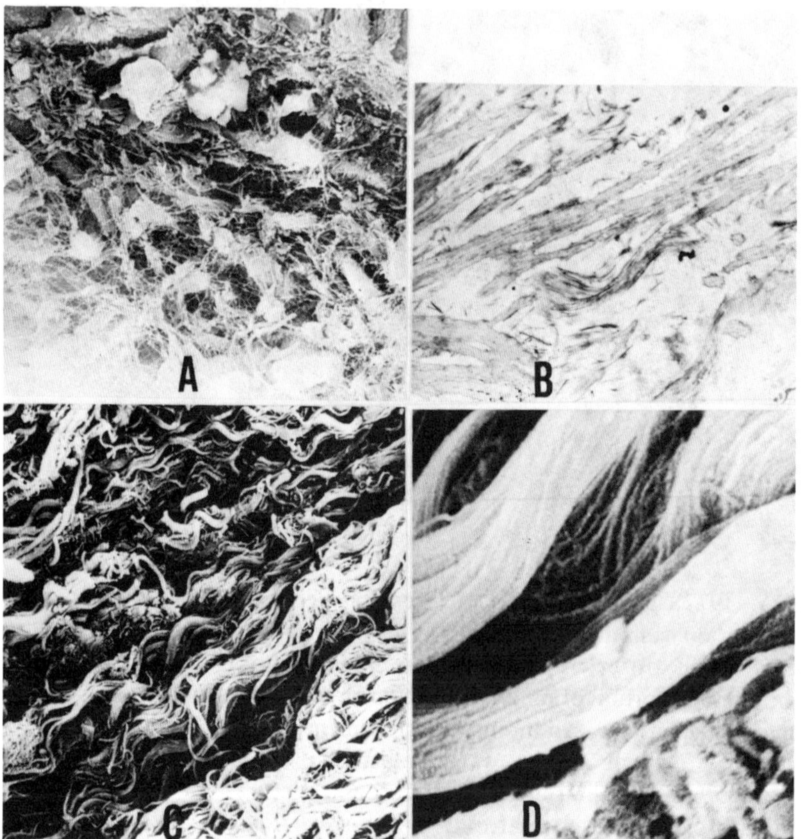

then anastomose (Fig. 1–3*B*). This appears to give them greater extensibility. A few collagenous fibers are found between the elastic fibers. In the deep layer of the lamina propria, there are densely crowded collagen fibers running roughly parallel to the edge of the vocal fold. They are not straight but rather present a twisting, spiral-like structure (Fig. 1–3*C*). The collagenous fibrils which make up the collagenous fibers themselves are also slightly twisted (Fig. 1–3*D*). This twisting of the collagenous fibrils and fibers appears to give a certain extensibility to the fibers.

Variation of the Structure along the Length of the Vocal Fold

The layer structure of the vocal fold varies along its length. Hirano, Kurita, and their co-workers have elaborated on this (Hirano, 1981; Hirano et al., 198b1; Hirano et al. 1982; Kurita, 1980). The following is a detailed explanation of this phenomenon.

There are unique structures at the anterior and posterior ends of the membranous portion of the vocal folds where the membranous vocal folds are connected to the cartilaginous framework (Fig. 1–4). At the anterior end of the vocal fold, there is a mass of elastic fibers called the anterior macula flava. It is coupled to a mass of collagenous fibers referred to as the anterior commissure tendon. The anterior commissure tendon is connected to the thyroid cartilage anteriorly. Thus, there are gradual changes in stiffness of the structure from the stiff cartilage to the pliable mucosa. At the posterior end of the membranous vocal fold, there is a mass of elastic fibers called the posterior macula flava. It is connected to the arytenoid cartilage, again, presenting gradual changes in stiffness. The anterior and posterior maculae flavae are continuations of the intermediate layer of the lamina propria, whereas the collagenous fibers in the anterior commissure tendon are connected to the deep layer of the lamina propria.

Hirano (1975) interpreted these facts as variations of the layer structure of the vibrator, that is, the vocal fold. He concluded that the maculae flavae have a function to protect the ends of the membranous portion of the vocal fold from mechanical damage possibly caused by vibration.

Kurita, Hirano, and their co-workers measured the thickness of each layer that varies along the length. They examined histologically five larynges of each of the following groups: (1) males in their 20s, (2) females in their 20s, (3) males in their 50s, and (4) females in their 50s. The larynges were obtained from autopsy cases. Frontal sections of each vocal fold were made at five locations shown in Figure 1–4: *A,* at the anterior macula flava; *C,* at the midpoint of the membranous portion; *E,* at the posterior macula flava; *B,* at the midpoint between *A* and *C;* and *D,* at the midpoint between *C* and *E.* With a light microscope, the thickness of the cover, of the intermediate layer of the lamina propria, and of the deep layer of the lamina propria were measured at the edge.

Figure 1–4. Histological structure of a horizontal section of the adult human vocal fold. From Hirano, M., Kurita, S., and Nakashima, T. (1983). Growth, development, and aging of the vocal fold. In D. M. Bless and J. Abbs (Eds.), *Vocal fold physiology* **(pp. 22–43). San Diego: College-Hill Press.**

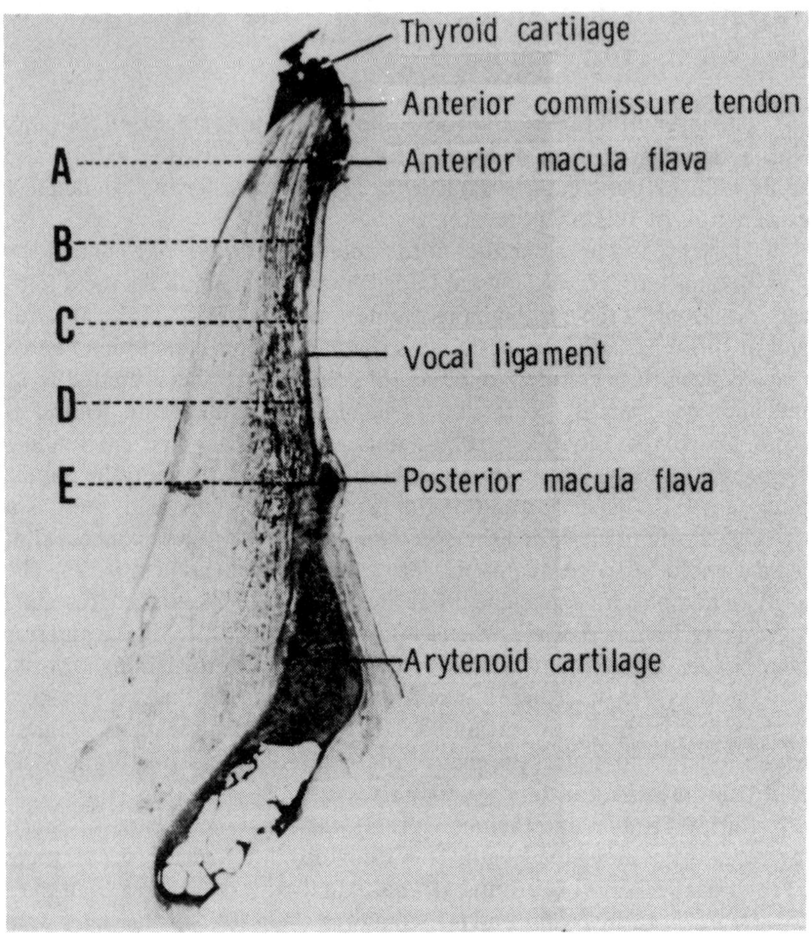

As described earlier, the superficial layer of the lamina propria is clearly delineated from the intermediate layer. However, the border between the intermediate and deep layers of the lamina propria is not clear. We arbitrarily defined the intermediate layer as the portion where the ratio of the density of elastic fibers to that of collagenous fibers is 2:1 or greater.

Table 1–1 and Figure 1–5 show the results. In Figure 1–5, the values averaged over the five larynges in each group are graphed. In all four groups,

Table 1–1.
Thickness of the Cover, Intermedial Layer, and Deep Layer of the Lamina Propria at Five Locations

Layer	Location	Male		Female	
		20s	50s	20s	50s
Cover	A	0.15(.10− .20)	0.17(.15− .20)	0.12(.10− .15)	0.15(.10− .20)
	B	0.28(.20− .30)	0.41(.25− .55)	0.31(.20− .40)	0.29(.25− .30)
	C	0.41(.35− .50)	0.51(.35− .75)	0.35(.30− .45)	0.39(.30− .55)
	D	0.31(.20− .50)	0.36(.20− .70)	0.25(.20− .35)	0.29(.20− .45)
	E	0.22(.15− .30)	0.21(.15− .30)	0.15(.10− .20)	0.15(.10− .20)
Intermediate layer	A	1.03(.85− 1.20)	1.11(.65− 1.40)	0.93(.85− 1.15)	1.08(.95− 1.35)
	B	0.45(.30− .70)	0.28(.20− .40)	0.43(.35− .45)	0.52(.45− .55)
	C	0.33(.30− .40)	0.25(.20− .35)	0.35(.30− .40)	0.36(.25− .45)
	D	0.31(.20− .50)	0.31(.25− .40)	0.46(.40− .55)	0.43(.30− .55)
	E	0.22(.15− .30)	0.83(.75− .90)	0.78(.70− .85)	0.80(.75− .85)
Deep layer	A	0.24(.20− .30)	0.52(.30− .65)	0.18(.15− .25)	0.24(.10− .30)
	B	0.32(.20− .35)	0.53(.30− .65)	0.23(.20− .25)	0.25(.20− .30)
	C	0.34(.25− .45)	0.47(.30− .70)	0.17(.15− .20)	0.19(.15− .30)
	D	0.33(.20− .50)	0.63(.35− .90)	0.24(.15− .35)	0.24(.20− .35)
	E	0.71(.55− 1.00)	0.92(.75− 1.05)	0.37(.30− .45)	0.37(.30− .45)

From Hirano, M., Kakita, Y., Ohmaru, K., and Kurita, S. (1982) Structure and mechanical properties of the vocal fold. *Speech and Language, 7,* 271–297. Reprinted with permission.

Figure 1–5. Variations of the thickness of the cover, intermediate layer of the lamina propria, and deep layer of the lamina propria along the length of the vocal fold. *A*, Males in their 20s. *B*, Females in their 20s. *C*, Males in their 50s. *D*, Females in their 50s. From Hirano, M., Kakita, Y., Ohmaru, K., and Kurita, S. (1982). Structure and mechanical properties of the vocal fold. *Speech and Language, 7,* 271–297. Reprinted with permission.

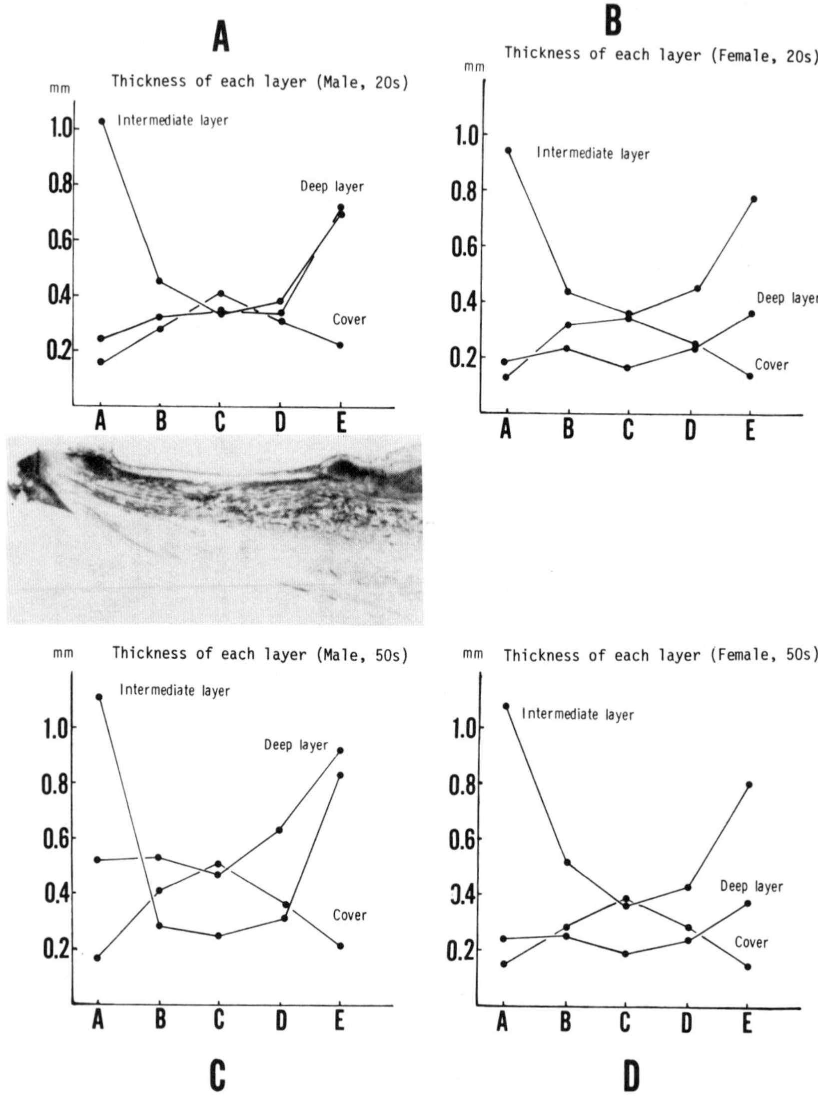

the cover is the thickest at the midportion and becomes thinner toward the anterior and posterior ends of the membranous vocal fold. The intermediate layer of the lamina propria is the thinnest at the midportion and becomes very thick near the ends, forming two masses of elastic fibers, that is, the anterior and posterior maculae flavae. The deep layer of the lamina propria is the thickest in the posterior portion. The cover is the most pliable layer in the vocal fold. The variations of the layer structure described above indicate that the membranous vocal fold is structurally the most pliant at the midportion.

The body, that is, the vocalis muscle, is much thicker than the mucosa. Its thickness was not actually measured. However, it is clearly evident in Figure 1–4 that the body is the thinnest at the anterior end and becomes thicker toward the posterior end.

Changes in the Structure with Age

Hirano and co-workers investigated structural changes of the vocal fold with age (Hirano, 1981a; Hirano et al., 1981c; Hirano et al., 1983).

They histologically investigated 88 normal larynges obtained from autopsy cases. Of these, 48 cases were males and 40 cases were females. The age ranges was from newborn to 69 years. A frontal section was made through the middle of the membranous portion of the vocal fold. In addition, a horizontal section was made with the other vocal fold in some cases. The following is a detailed description of their results.

Development of the Vocal Fold Structure. From birth to age 20, no significant changes in the epithelium were observed. The lamina propria of the mucosa, on the other hand, presented marked changes with growth.

In newborns (Fig. 1–6*A, B*), the mucosa is very thick relative to the length and there is no ligamentous structure. The entire lamina propria appears fairly uniform and seems pliable in structure. It resembles the superficial layer of the lamina propria in adults. Only near the ends of the membranous portion are the fibrous components slightly dense. These fibrous structures seem to be the origins of the maculae flavae; some fibers appear to be extending toward the middle portion from these structures. In newborns, the structure of the cover–body complex is rather simple compared to that in adults: The body, which is the muscle, is directly mantled with the cover, which consists of the entire mucosa.

Between the ages of one and four years, an immature vocal ligament, a bundle of fibers that runs from the anterior to the posterior end of the membranous portion of the vocal fold, appears. Figure 1–6*C* and *D* shows vocal folds of a 4 year old boy that demonstrate an immature vocal

Figure 1-6. Histological sections demonstrating the structure of the vocal folds of a newborn male infant (*A, B*) and a 4 year old boy (*C, D*). *A, C,* Frontal sections. *B, D,* Horizontal sections. AMF, Origin of anterior macula flava; PMF, origin of posterior macula flava; VL, immature vocal ligament. From Hirano, M. (1981a). Structure of the vocal fold in normal and disease states. Anatomical and physical studies. *ASHA Report, 11,* 11-27. From Hirano, M., Kurita, S., and Nakashima, T. (1981b). The structure of the vocal folds. In K. N. Stevens and M. Hirano (Eds.), *Vocal fold physiology* (pp. 33-41). Tokyo: University of Tokyo Press. Reprinted with permission.

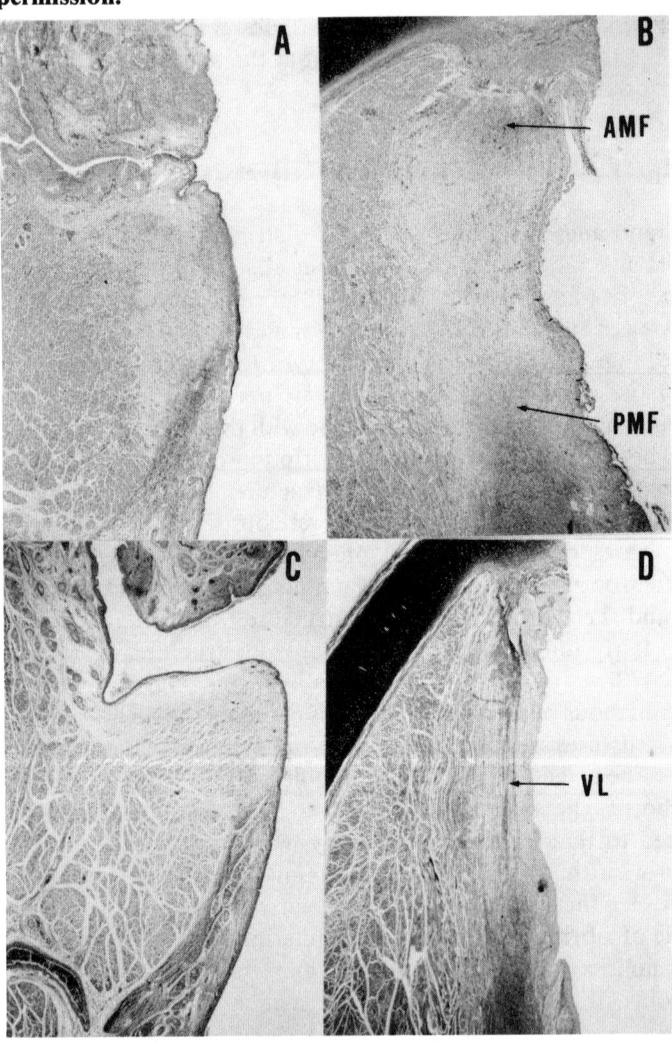

ligament. In this stage, however, there is no differentiation of the layer of elastic fibers from that of collagenous fibers. In other words, the intermediate and deep layers of the lamina propria are not differentiated. Differentiation of these two layers begins at the ages 6 to 12 years. The mucosa is relatively thinner than in newborns, but thicker than in adults. After the age of 15, a clear differentiation of the two layers is consistently observed. Before the age of 20, however, the vocal ligament is occasionally thinner or the fibers in the ligament are occasionally looser compared with those of adults. Thus, maturation of the layer structure of the vocal fold appears to take place near the end of adolescence.

Aging of the Vocal Fold Structure. Changes in the vocal fold structure with aging vary significantly from individual to individual. Figures 1–7 to 1–9 illustrate schematically the changes in the three layers of the mucosa. The thickness of the layers shown in these figures was measured under a microscope. The rating scales for various parameters shown in these figures were obtained in the following way. A larynx typical of a 27 year old male was assigned an arbitrary value for each of the parameters of interest. The vocal folds of all other subjects were then compared to these standard values and scored on a 5 point equal-appearing interval scale for most parameters. In cases of judgments of abnormal conditions, a 6 point equal-appearing interval scale was used with 0 equaling no abnormality and 5 equaling maximum deviation. The findings are summarized as follows.

1. Changes in the cover:

a. The cover tends to become thicker with age. Since there is no systematic change in the thickness of the epithelium with aging, the increase in the thickness of the cover implies an increase in the thickness of the superficial layer of the lamina propria.

b. The density of fibroblasts, collagenous fibers, and elastic fibers tends to decrease with aging.

c. The superficial layer tends to become edematous with aging.

d. These tendencies are more marked in males than in females.

2. Changes in the intermediate layer of the lamina propria:

a. The thickness of the intermediate layer decreases with aging in males.

b. Elastic fibers tend to become looser with aging. This is especially marked in males aged 40 years or older.

c. Elastic fibers become atrophied in males after 40 years of age.

d. In males, the contour of the intermediate layer becomes deteriorated after 40 years of age. This seems to be caused chiefly by a fibrotic change in the deep layer of the lamina propria. Deterioration of the contour of

Figure 1–7. Schematic representation of changes in the cover of the vocal fold with aging. From Hirano, M., Kurita, S., and Nakashima, T. (1983). Growth, development, and aging of human vocal folds. In D. M. Bless and J. H. Abbs (Eds.) , *Vocal fold physiology* (pp. 22–43). San Diego: College–Hill Press.

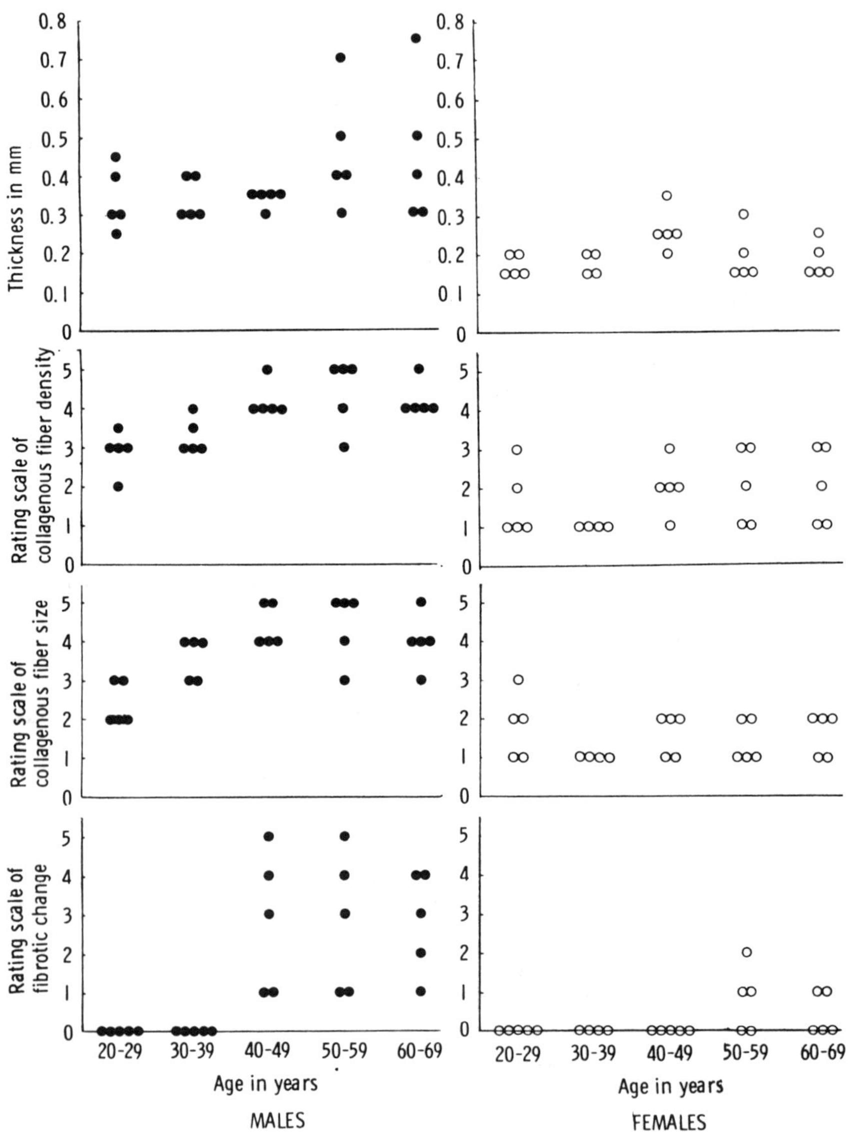

Figure 1–8. Schematic representation of changes in the intermediate layer of the lamina propria with aging. From Hirano, M., Kurita, S., and Nakashima, T. (1983). Growth, development, and aging of human vocal folds. In D. M. Bless and J. H. Abbs (Eds.), *Vocal fold physiology* (pp. 22–43). San Diego: College–Hill Press.

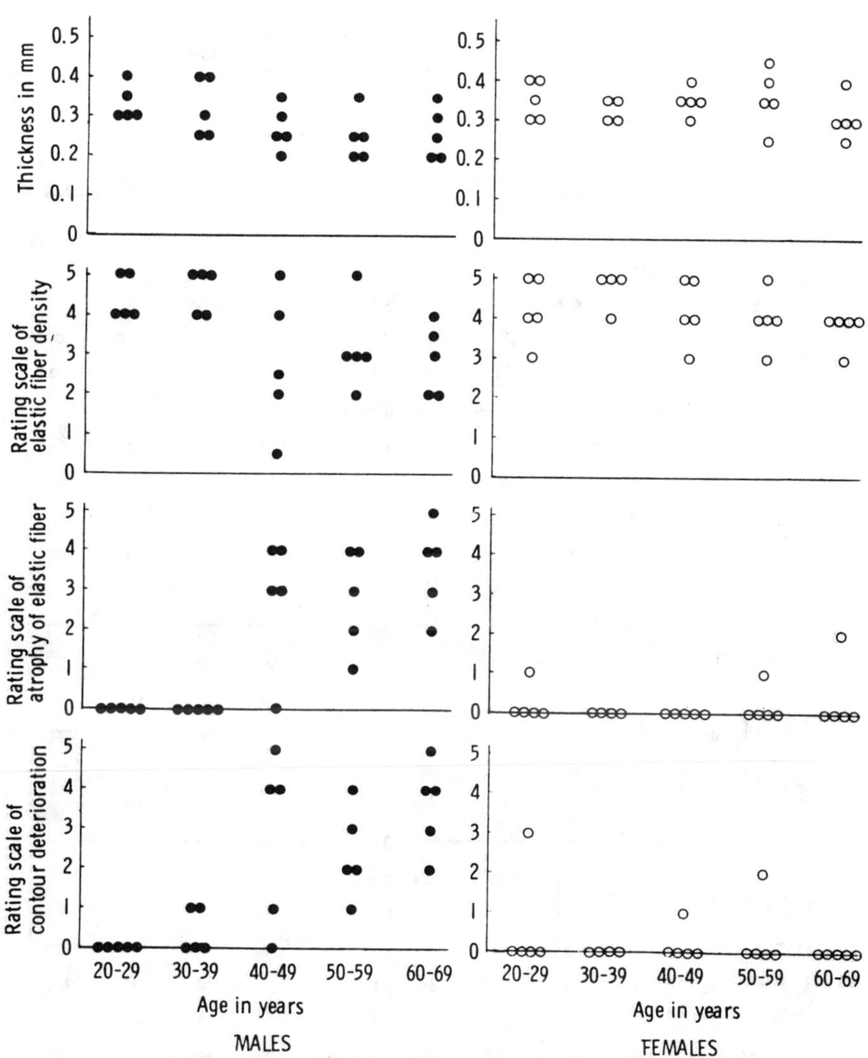

Figure 1-9. Schematic representation of changes in the deep layer of the lamina propria with aging. From Hirano, M., Kurita, S., and Nakashima, T. (1983). Growth, development, and aging of human vocal folds. In D. M. Bless and J. H. Abbs (Eds.), *Vocal fold physiology* **(pp. 22-43). San Diego: College-Hill Press.**

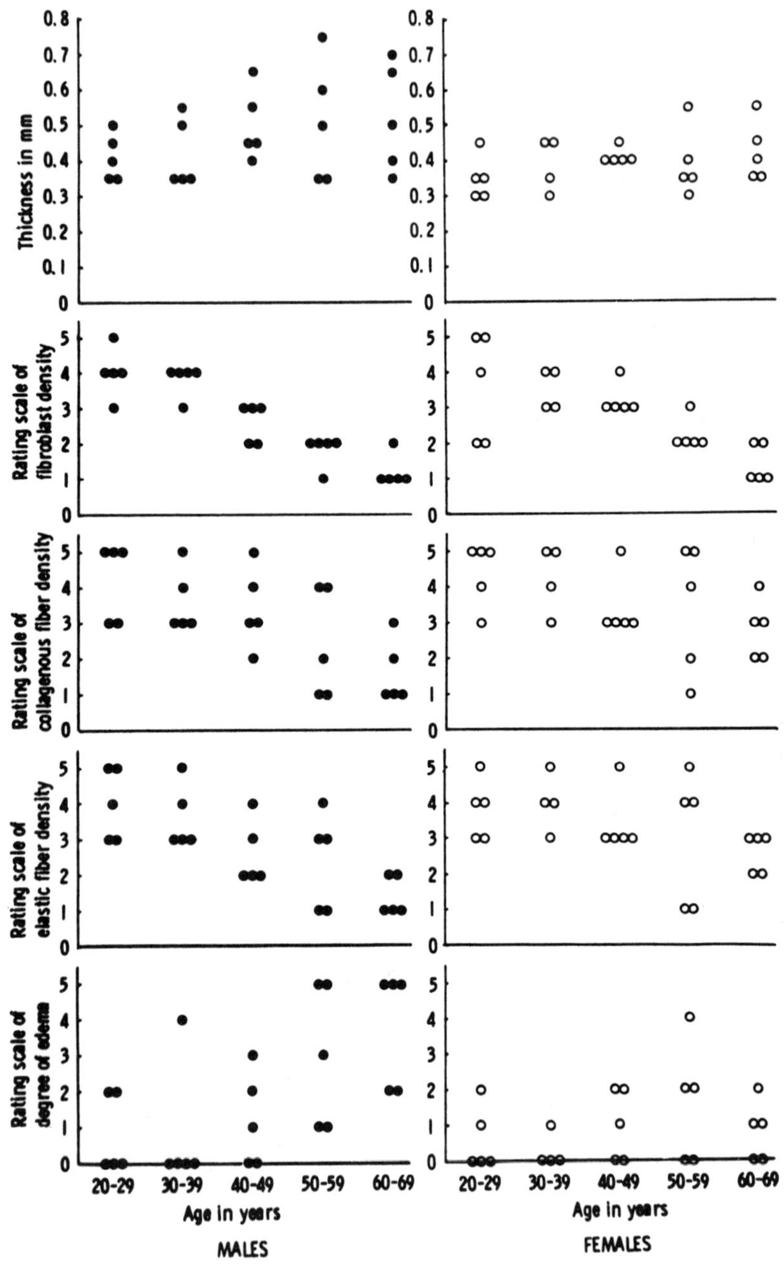

the intermediate layer is not marked in females.

3. Changes in the deep layer of the lamina propria:

a. In males, the deep layer tends to become thicker after 50 years of age.
b. Collagenous fibers tend to become thicker and denser with aging. This tendency is not marked in females.
c. In some males of 40 years of age or older, collagenous fibers increase locally and run in varying directions, a condition called fibrosis.

COVER-BODY COMPLEX IN ANIMALS

Larynges of various animals are often used in experimental research of the larynx and phonation. It is not clear, however, whether or not animal larynges are sufficiently similar to human larynges to draw any meaningful analogies with respect to phonatory behavior. Comparative studies of the laryngeal structure are important from several points of view: (1) They are useful for elucidating the evolution of phonatory function; (2) differences tell us more about the mechanism of phonation; (3) they are useful in helping researchers determine the most appropriate animal for their experimental study of phonation; and (4) they are useful for researchers in interpreting the results obtained from animal experiments.

Differences in the laryngeal structure among different animals have been well documented in gross anatomy by Negus (1949) in his monumental study. Toyozumi (1979) investigated differences in the muscle bundle configuration among seven species of mammals and related it to phonatory function. Hirano (1975) first pointed out that the layer structure of the canine vocal fold is different from that of the human vocal fold. Nagata (1982) and Kurita, Nagata, and Hirano (1983) compared the layer structure of the vocal fold of 11 different species of mammals and related the structure to phonatory function. The results of investigations by Hirano (1975), Nagata (1982), and Kurita, Nagata, and Hirano (1983) on three species, dogs, monkeys, and cats, which are used in experimental studies of laryngeal physiology more frequently than other animals, are described below. The epithelium that lines the vocal fold edge is stratified squamous cell epithelium in all three species. Mechanical properties of the muscular tissue are presumed not to differ significantly between species. Therefore, the discussion in the following sections focuses on the lamina propria.

Dog

Figure 1–10 shows light micrographic histological sections of the vocal folds of dogs.

Figure 1-10. Histological sections of the vocal fold of dogs. *A*, Frontal section. *B*, Frontal section at higher magnification. *C*, Horizontal section. *D*, Anterior portion at higher magnification. *E*, Posterior portion at higher magnification, SLP, Superficial layer of the lamina propria; DLP, deep layer of the lamina propria; M, muscle; CE, conus elasticus; ACT, anterior commissure tendon; AMF, anterior macula flava; PMF, posterior macula flava. From Nagata, K. (1982). A comparative study of the layer structure of the vocal fold. A morphological investigation of 11 mammalian species. *Otologia (Fukuoka), 28*, 699-738. Reprinted with permission.

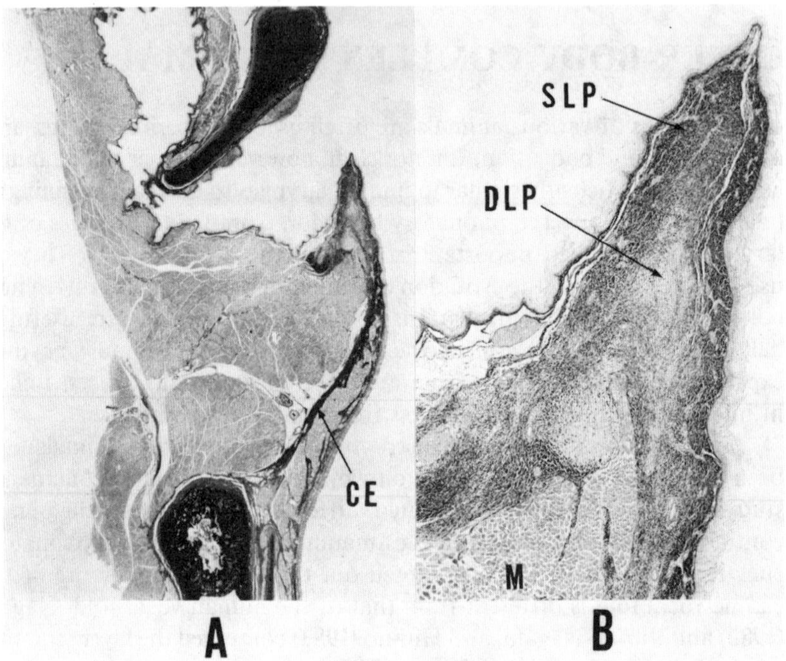

Illustration continued on opposite page.

The lamina propria of the mucosa around the vocal fold edge consists of two layers, as opposed to three layers in the human vocal fold: the superficial layer and the deep layer. The former is comparatively dense in collagenous and elastic fibers, whereas the latter is very loose in structure. There is no clear boundary between the two layers. The collagenous and elastic fibers in the superficial layer gradually decrease in density and form the deep layer. Some fat tissue occurs sporadically in the deep layer. Along the border line of the vocalis muscle, collagenous fibers intermesh with the muscle bundles, but, unlike the human vocal fold, the connection is loose. In dogs, there is no structure that is likened to the vocal ligament

Figure 1–10 (continued). See legend on opposite page.

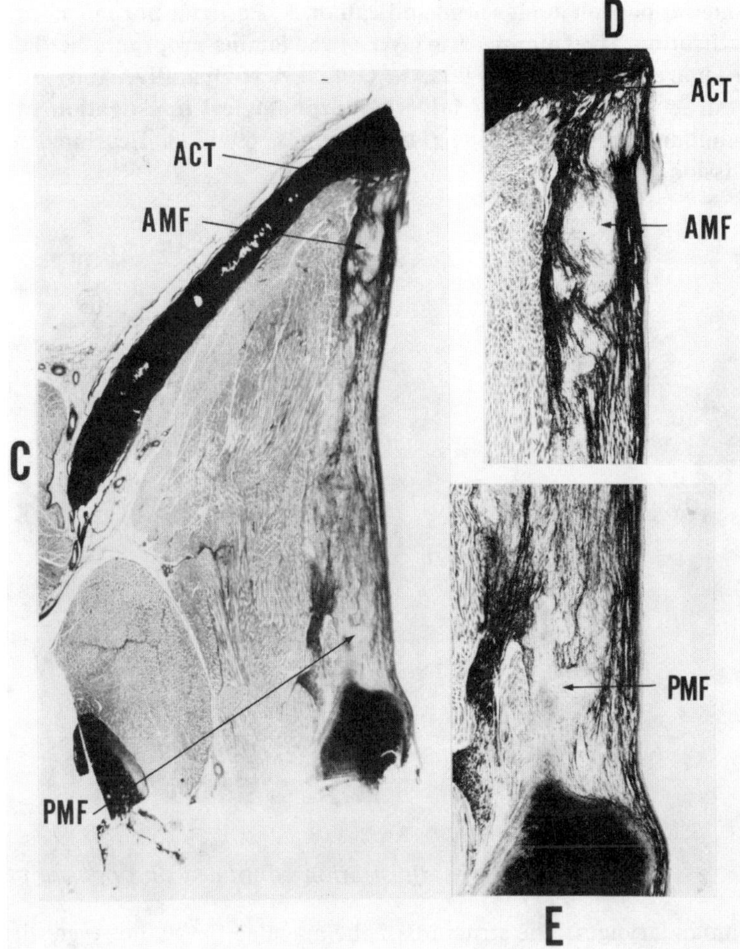

of human vocal fold. The conus elasticus is connected to the fibers in the superficial layer of the lamina propria, without forming a ligamentous structure. The thickness of the mucosa is approximately 3 mm at the vocal fold edge.

At the anterior end of the vocal fold, there is the anterior commissure tendon and the anterior macula flava. At the posterior end of the membranous portion of the vocal fold is the posterior macula flava. The anterior commissure tendon consists primarily of collagenous fibers, as

Figure 1–11. Histological sections of the vocal fold of monkeys. *A*, Frontal section. *B*, Frontal section at higher magnification. *C*, Horizontal section. *D*, Anterior portion at higher magnification. *E*, Posterior portion at higher magnification. IIP, Intermediate layer of the lamina propria; other labels as in Figure 1–10. From Nagata, K. (1982). A comparative study of the layer structure of the vocal fold. A morphological investigation of 11 mammalian species. *Otologia (Fukuoka), 28,* 699–738. Reprinted with permission.

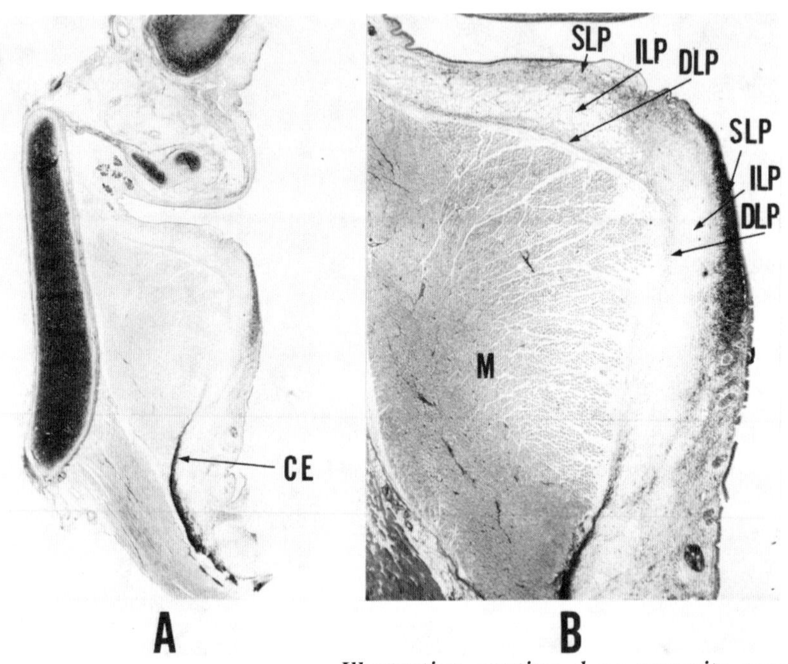

Illustration continued on opposite page.

in human larynges. The structure of the maculae flavae, however, differs significantly in dogs from that of human beings. The maculae flavae are poor in fibrous components and consist chiefly of amorphous substance, in contrast to the human maculae flavae, which are primarily composed of elastic fibers. The length of the maculae flavae relative to that of the membranous portion of the vocal fold is longer in dogs than in human beings.

Most elastic and collagenous fibers in the lamina propria run roughly parallel to the edge of the vocal fold. Most elastic fibers in the superficial layer of the lamina propria are connected to the anterior and the posterior maculae flavae, whereas most collagenous fibers in the same layer are connected to the anterior commissure tendon anteriorly and to the arytenoid perichondrium posteriorly.

Figure 1–11 (Continued). See legend on opposite page.

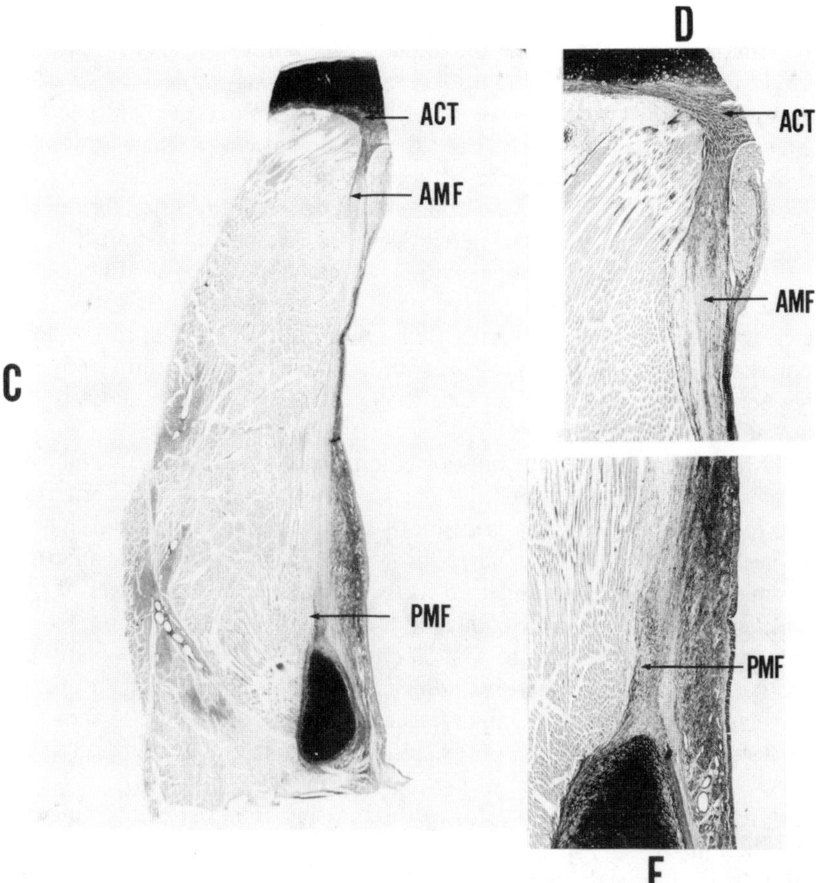

In summary, the vocal fold of dogs consists of the mucosa and the muscle: the former being the *cover* and the latter, the *body*. Unlike the human vocal fold, the stiffness of the tissue in the cover decreases as the body is approached. At the anterior and posterior ends, there are gradational changes in stiffness between the stiff cartilage and the pliable mucosa.

Monkey

Figure 1–11 depicts histological sections of the vocal folds of monkeys.

The structure of the lamina propria differs significantly between the upper and the lower parts of the vocal fold. At the upper part, the lamina propria can be divided into three layers. The superficial and deep layers consist of loose networks of elastic and collagenous fibers. The intermediate layer is composed primarily of fat tissue, which is a unique feature compared to the larynx of other mammals. The lamina propria of the lower part of the vocal fold can also be divided into three layers. The superficial layer is very dense with collagenous fibers. These fibers run not parallel to but oblique or perpendicular to the vocal fold edge. The orientation of the fibers is not conducive to vibration. The intermediate layer consists chiefly of fat tissue. Fibrous components are loose in this layer. The deep layer is thin and composed of networks of elastic and collagenous fibers.

In monkeys, there is no structure comparable to the vocal ligament of the human larynx. The conus elasticus is connected to the fibers in the deep layer of the lamina propria. It becomes, however, thinner and less remarkable as the vocal fold edge is approached instead of forming a thick, ligamentous structure. The average thickness of the entire mucosa is 1.1 mm at the vocal fold edge.

Monkeys also have the anterior commissure tendon and the anterior and posterior maculae flavae. Like in other mammals, the anterior commissure tendon is composed chiefly of collagenous fibers and tightly connected to the thyroid cartilage. Most collagenous fibers of the anterior commissure tendon are connected to those in the superficial layer of the lamina propria, while some collagenous fibers are coupled to those in the deep layer of the lamina propria. The maculae flavae consist chiefly of elastic fibers, although there are some collagenous fibers and fibroblasts. The elastic fibers in the maculae flavae are mostly connected to those in the deep layer of the lamina propria and partly to those in the superficial layer.

In summary, the vocal folds of monkeys also consist of the mucosa and the muscle. The structure of the mucosa, however, differs markedly from that of human beings. The mucosa appears fairly stiff and, therefore, it is hard to postulate a cover-body complex in which a stiff body is mantled with a pliable cover. The lack of variety in voice control in monkeys can be attributed, at least partly, to the unique layer structure of the vocal fold. Along the longitudinal axis, there are gradational changes in stiffness between the firm cartilage and the relatively soft mucosa.

Cat

Figure 1–12 presents histological sections of the vocal folds of cats.

It should be noted that, in cats, the ventricular and vocal folds are not separated and, therefore, there is no laryngeal ventricle. In other words, there is only one fold on the lateral wall of the larynx. When one drives excised larynges of cats, the lower portion of this fold vibrates (Hirano, personal communication). Therefore, we assume this portion to be the structural equivalent of the vocal fold. It is also interesting to note that the thyroarytenoid muscle is composed of two portions, as if the upper portion corresponded to the ventricular fold and the lower portion to the vocal fold. The lamina propria of the mucosa exists as if it occupied the ventricle.

Although elastic fibers become slightly denser as one moves toward the middle of the lamina propria and collagenous fibers slightly increase as the muscle is approached, the entire lamina propria appears rather uniform and pliable in structure. Most fibers of the conus elasticus disappear in the lower surface of the vocal fold, and, therefore, do not form a ligamentous structure. The average thickness of the mucosa is 1.4 mm.

The anterior commissure tendon and the anterior and posterior maculae flavae also occur in cats. The anterior commissure tendon is composed of collagenous fibers and is connected to the thyroid cartilage anteriorly. The maculae flavae are not as distinguished as those of humans, dogs, and monkeys. Elastic and collagenous fibers are a little denser in the maculae flavae than in the middle portion of the vocal fold. Most collagenous fibers in the lamina propria are connected to the anterior commissure tendon anteriorly and to the arytenoid perichondrium posteriorly. They run roughly parallel to the vocal fold edge. Most elastic fibers, on the other hand, are connected to the anterior and posterior maculae flavae and they also run roughly parallel to the edge.

In summary, the vocal fold of cats consists of the mucosa and the muscle, the former being a pliable *cover* and the latter, an elastic *body*. The cover is rather uniform in structure, resembling that of human newborns. The auditory resemblance of baby cry and cat cry may be attributed, at least partly, to the similarity in the structure of the cover-body complex. Along the longitudinal direction, there are gradual changes in stiffness between the firm cartilage and the pliable mucosa.

It should be emphasized that only the adult human vocal fold has the vocal ligament. This appears to account, at least partly, for the remarkable versatility in sound production which only adult human beings have.

MECHANICAL PROPERTIES OF THE VOCAL FOLD TISSUE

Kakita, Hirano, and Ohmaru conducted a series of studies on the mechanical properties of the vocal fold tissue (Hirano, 1981a; Hirano et

Figure 1-12. Histological sections of the vocal fold of cats. *A*, Frontal section. *B*, Frontal section at higher magnification. *C*, Horizontal section. *D*, Anterior portion at higher magnification. *E*, Posterior portion at higher magnification. LP, Lamina propria; other labels as in Figure 1-10. Arrow indicates the portion equivalent to the vocal fold edge. From Nagata, K. (1982). A comparative study of the layer structure of the vocal fold. A morphological investigation of 11 mammalian species. *Otologia (Fukuoka), 28,* 699-738. Reprinted with permission.

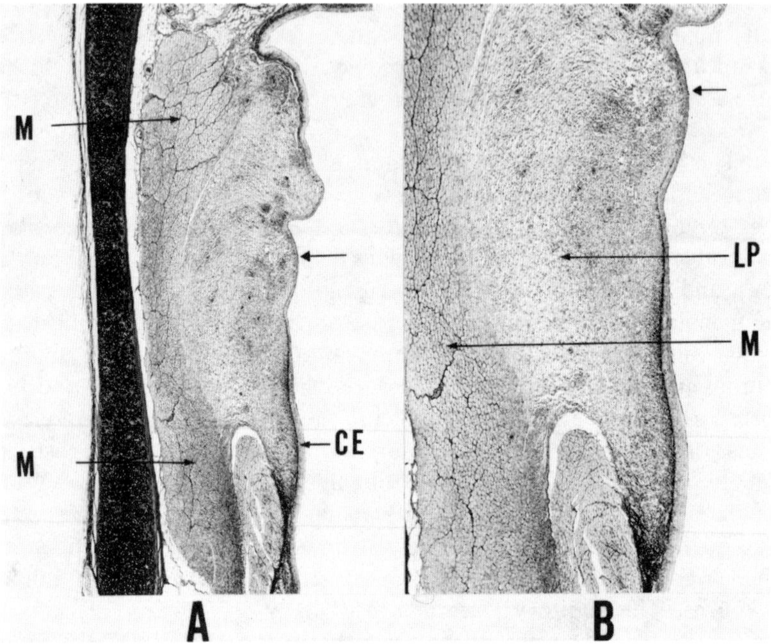

Illustration continued on opposite page.

al., 1982; Kakita et al., 1981; Ohmaru 1981). The important results of these studies are described below.

Measurements of Mechanical Properties of Each Layer of the Canine Vocal Fold

Kakita, Hirano, and Ohmaru determined viscoelastic properties of the epithelium, lamina propria and muscle of canine vocal folds (Hirano, 1981; Hirano et al., 1982; Kakita et al., 1981; Ohmaru, 1981). Following are their results.

Young's Modulus. Excised canine larynges were trimmed so that only the single layer of the vocal fold tissue to be investigated was left between

Figure 1–12 (continued). See legend on opposite page.

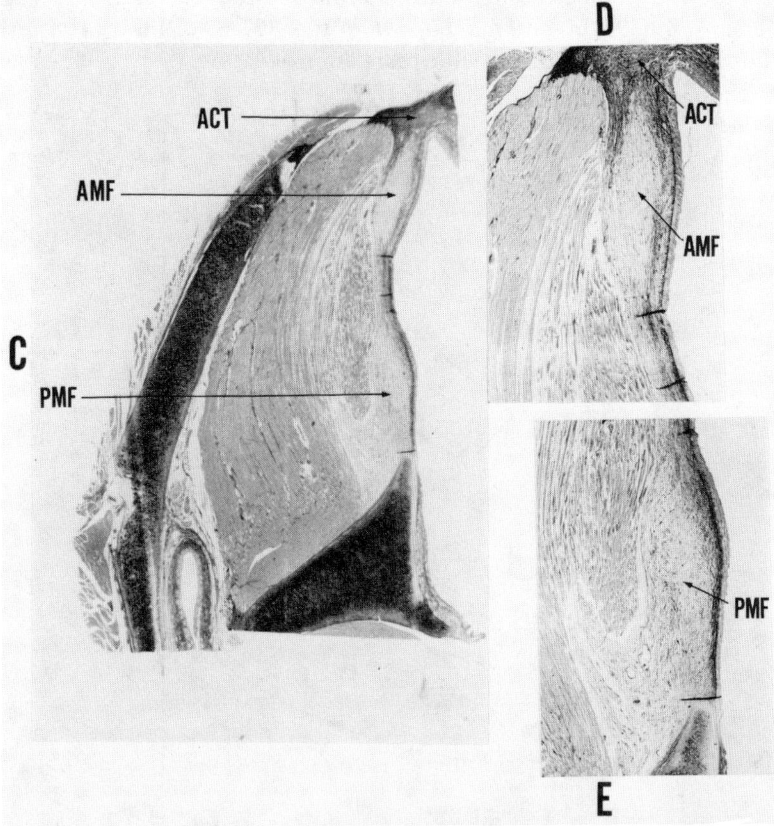

the arytenoid carilage and the anterior portion of the thyroid ala, keeping
a portion of these cartilages attached at each end. The specimen was fixed
at the thyroid cartilage and was hung vertically. They applied various
weights to the arytenoid cartilage and measured the elongation of the tissue
with a microscope. The specimen was kept moist by dripping saline solution
during the experiment. Young's modulus was calculated from the formula,
$E = \sigma/\varepsilon$, where $\sigma = $ stress (T/S), $\varepsilon = $ strain $(\Delta L/L)$, T tension, S
$= $ cross-sectional area, $\Delta L = $ elongation, and $L = $ original length (at no
load).

Figure 1–13 shows Young's modulus in the longitudinal direction of
each layer. The areas labeled E, L, and M show the ranges of the values
obtained from about 10 specimens for the epithelium, the lamina propria
of the mucosa, and the muscle, respectively. For elongation ranging from
10 to 50% of the original length (at no load) of the specimen, Young's
modulus for the epithelium, E_E, is larger than the modulus for the lamina

Figure 1-13. Range of values for Young's modulus for each layer of the canine vocal fold as a function of elongation. E, Epithelium; L, lamina propria of the mucosa; M, muscle. From Kakita, Y., Hirano, M., and Ohmaru, K. (1981). *Vocal fold physiology* (pp. 377–396). Tokyo: University of Tokyo Press. Reprinted with permission.

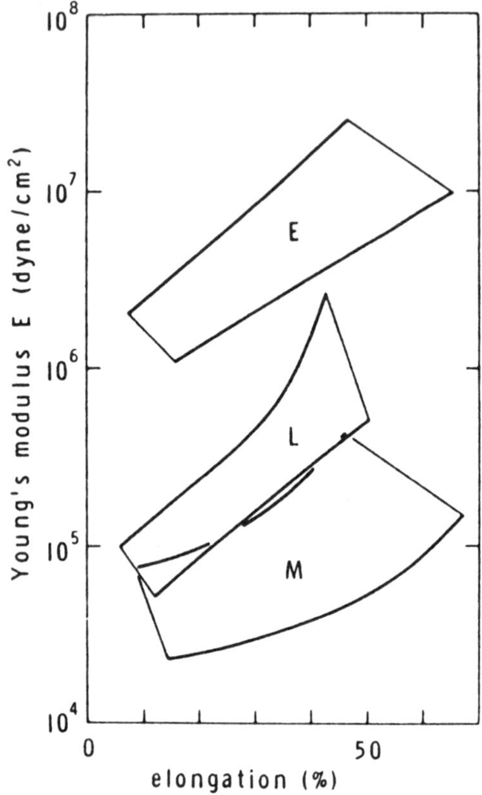

propria, E_L, by about one order of magnitude. E_L is larger than E_M, the modulus for muscle, by one third to one order of magnitude as the elongation increases. Thus, the tensile stiffness becomes smaller in the order of the epithelium, the lamina propria, and the muscle.

Differential Young's Modulus. The vocal fold tissue, like other biological tissue, has a nonlinear stress–strain relation, as shown in Figure 1-14. Young's modulus, $E = \sigma/\epsilon$, presented in the preceding section, is graphed geometrically as the slope of the dashed line. On the other hand, elongation of the vocal fold tissue caused by vibration is very small relative to the original length. Young's modulus is, therefore, not relevant in discussing vibratory behavior of the cover–body complex. Generally speaking, when the variation of elongation is small compared with the total

Figure 1-14. Schematic representation of stress-strain relationships showing the Young's modulus (secant modulus, dashed line) and the differential Young's modulus (tangent modulus, straight solid line). From Kakita, Y., Hirano, M., and Ohmaru, K. (1981). Physical properties of the vocal fold tissue: Measurement on excised larynges. In K. N. Stevens and M. Hirano (Eds.) *Vocal fold physiology* (pp. 377–396). Tokyo: University of Tokyo Press. Reprinted with permission.

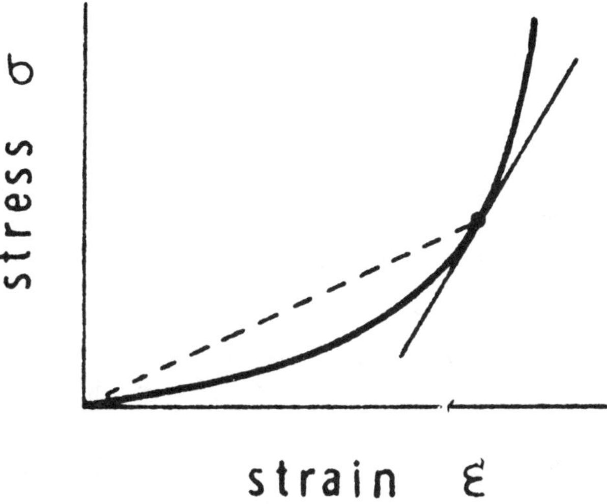

length, the differential Young's modulus, $\xi = d\sigma/d\epsilon$, becomes more useful. The modulus, ξ is geometrically depicted as the slope of the solid tangent line in Figure 1-14. The differential Young's modulus, ξ, is called "the tangent modulus," whereas Young's modulus, E, is referred to as " the secant modulus."

Figure 1-15 shows the range of the values of ξ for each layer. Abbreviations E, L, and M are the same as those in Figure 1-13. Two additional moduli for the lamina propria were determined. One was the modulus for the superficial layer only (LS in Figure 1-15). As described earlier in this article, this layer is denser with elastic and collagenous fibers, and therefore is considered to be stiffer than the deep layer. The other was the modulus under the tension in a transverse direction (LT in Figure 1-15). The latter was measured in the following way. A piece of the tissue was obtained from the middle portion in the longitudinal direction. A short wire was attached with a quick-setting glue to each of the medial and the lateral edges of the piece. The wire of one edge was fixed and the specimen was hung. Weights were applied on the wire glued to the other edge of the tissue piece.

Figure 1-15. Range of values for differential Young's modulus for each layer of the canine vocal fold as a function of elongation. E, Epithelium; L, lamina propria; LS, superficial layer of the lamina propria; M, muscle; LT, moduli for lamina propria in a transverse direction. From Kakita, Y., Hirano, M., and Ohmaru, K. (1981). Physical properties of the vocal fold tissue: Measurement on excised larynges. In K. N. Stevens and M. Hirano (Eds.), *Vocal fold physiology* (pp. 377-396). Tokyo: University of Tokyo Press. Reprinted with permission.

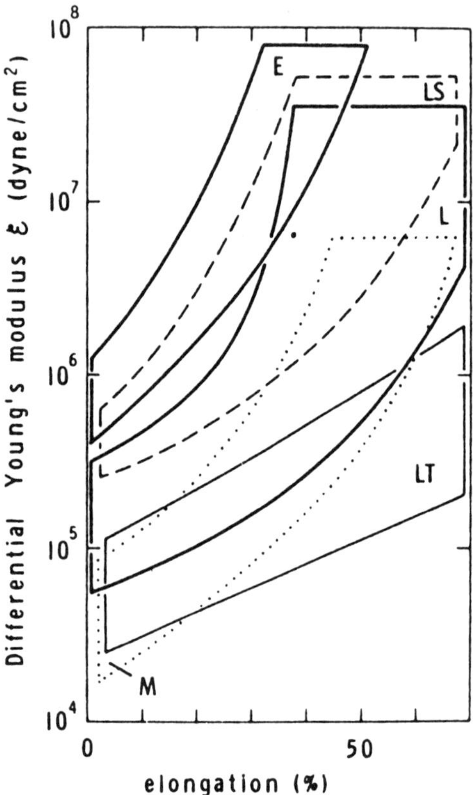

The results shown in Figure 1-15 seem to support the following conclusions:

1. The values of the differential Young's modulus become smaller in the order of the epithelium ξ_E, the superficial layer of the lamina propria ξ_{LS}, the entire lamina propria ξ_L, and the muscle ξ_M. This relative relation is the same as for Young's modulus E.

2. The modulus ξ_E is larger than ξ_{LS} by about a half order of magnitude; ξ_{LS} is larger than ξ_L by about a half order of magnitude; and ξ_L is larger than ξ_M by about a half order of magnitude.

3. The moduli ξ_E, ξ_{LS}, ξ_L, and ξ_M all show a saturation effect with respect to elongation in the range between 30 and 70%.

4. The moduli for the lamina propria along a transverse direction ξ_{LT} are much smaller than those along a longitudinal direction ξ_L. The modulus ξ_{LT} is smaller than ξ_L by about a half order of magnitude at elongations of less than 10% and by about one order of magnitude at elongations of around 40%. Under a transverse tension the tissue of the lamina propria is stretched up to 200–300% of its original length, without presenting any significant saturation effect, and then the tissue is torn.

Shear Modulus and Viscous Constant. The shear modulus and the viscosity for the lamina propria and the muscle were obtained by the method of free rotational damped oscillation. Figure 1–16 shows the experimental preparation. The tissue of the vocal fold was trimmed in the same way as for the measurement of Young's modulus (Fig. 1–16*A, B*). The specially made disk shown in Figure 1–16*C* is tightly attached to the arytenoid cartilage of the specimen. The disk is twisted from the resting position, then released to bring it into a twisting oscillation. The twisting angle of oscillation gradually gets smaller and finally the disk stops. The rotational angle of the damped oscillation is determined in the following way. An incident light beam, from a He–Ne laser light source, is reflected by a small mirror placed at the center of the shaft attached to the rotating disk (Fig. 1–16*C*). The reflected light beam is projected onto a screen placed at a fixed distance from the mirror. The light spot on the screen moves as the disk rotates. This oscillatory movement of the light spot is recorded on a film with the use of a continuous recording camera.

The shear modulus G and the shear viscosity η are calculated from the angular frequency, the attenuation constant, the moment of inertia of the disk, and the form factor of the specimen. The details of the calculation are described elsewhere (Kakita et al., 1981).

Figure 1–17 shows the data for one specimen for each of the laminae propriae and the muscle. A solid circle and a solid square indicate the shear modulus G, whereas an open circle and an open square indicate the viscosity η. Squares indicate the muscle and circles the lamina propria. This distinction is conveyed also by the subscripts M and L. Each data point represents an average of two successive measurements for the same condition. Letters *a* and *b* indicate the distinction between two different longitudinal tensions: the tension was approximately 40% larger for case *b* than for case *a*. For reference, the values of Young's moduli (E_M and

Figure 1-16. Schematic representation of the experimental preparation for measuring shear viscoelastic properties. (From Kakita, Y., Hirano, M., and Ohmaru, K. (1981). Physical properties of the vocal fold tissue: Measurement on excised larynges. In K. N. Stevens and M. Hirano (Eds.), *Vocal fold physiology* (pp. 377-396). Tokyo: University of Tokyo Press. Reprinted with permission.

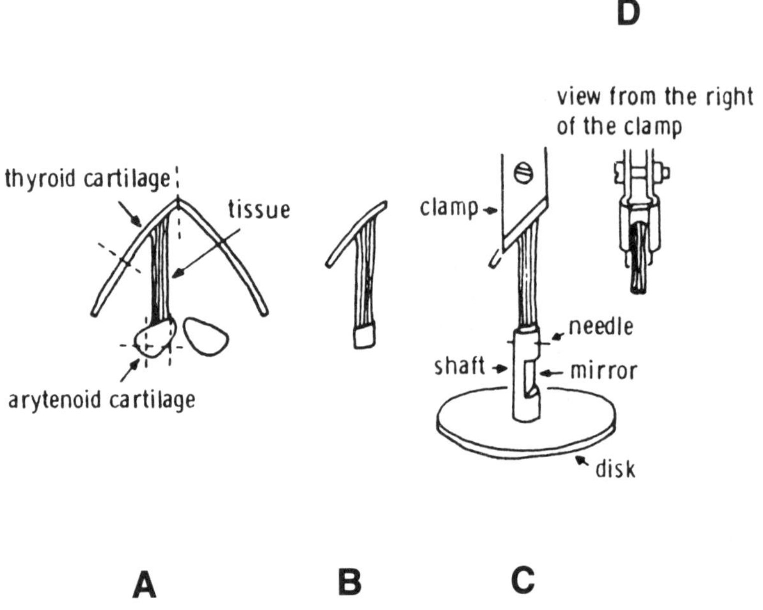

E_L shown in dashed line segments) and the differential Young's moduli (ξ_M and ξ_L shown in solid line segments) for this specimen are also shown.

From the results shown in Figure 1-17, Kakita, Hirano, and Ohmaru made the following points:

1. The shear modulus is almost the same for the lamina propria (G_L) and for the muscle (G_M), being 2 to 3 X 10^5 dyne/cm^2.

2. The shear viscosity for the muscle (η_M) is twice to three times as large as that for the lamina propria (η_L), and is of the order of 10^4 poise (P).

3. The shear modulus and viscosity become larger with increasing longitudinal tension.

Figure 1-17. Shear moduli (G, solid symbols) and viscosities (η, open symbols) for muscle (M) and lamina propria (L). Two different longitudinal tensions are indicated by *a* and *b*. Value of Young's moduli (E_M and E_L) and those of differential Young's moduli (ξ_M and ξ_L) are shown for reference. From Kakita, Y., Hirano, M., and Ohmaru, K. (1981). Physical properties of the vocal fold tissue: Measurement on excised larynges. In K. N. Stevens and M. Hirano (Eds.), *Vocal fold physiology* (pp. 377–396). Tokyo: University of Tokyo Press. Reprinted with permission.

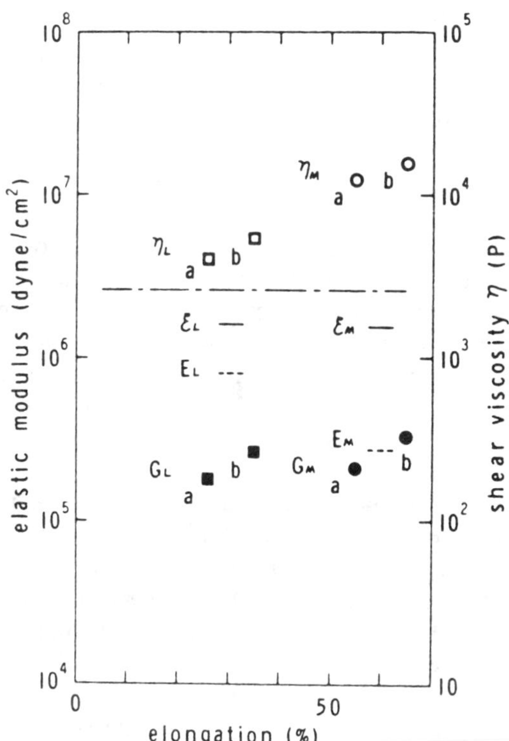

4. The value of the differential Young's modulus is almost the same for the muscle (ξ_M) as for the lamina propria (ξ_L), being close to the values in the saturated region in Figure 1-15.

5. The ratio of ξ_M to G_M and that of ξ_L to G_L are almost the same, being 5:1 to 8:1.

Interpretation and Implications

The majority of the description in this section is based on the article by Kakita, Hirano, and Ohmaru (1981).

Orthotropy of the Vocal Fold Tissue. When the mechanical characteristics of a given material are the same for any orientation, the material is said to be isotropic. If the mechanical characteristics vary for different orientations, the material is referred to as being anisotropic. There is a special type of anisotropy referred to as orthotropy. In an orthotropic material, mechanical characteristics for one axis, called "the axis of symmetry," are different from those for two other axes, which are perpendicular to the first axis. Mechanical characteristics for the latter two axes are the same. A plane formed by the latter two axes is called "the plane of isotropy." Therefore, we use "uniaxial anisotropy" and "orthotropy" synonymously.

Titze (1976) assumed vocal fold tissue to be orthotropic in his modeling. On the basis of the histological structure described in the preceding two sections in this article, his assumption appears to be justifiable for the vocal fold of humans, dogs, and cats, at least as a first approximation. Figure 1–18 depicts schematically a vocal fold as an orthotropic composition. The y-axis, which lies in the anteroposterior direction, is called the longitudinal axis, whereas the x- and the z-axes are called the transverse axes. The y-axis is the axis of symmetry and the plane formed by the x- and the z-axes (indicated by dots in Fig. 1–18) is the plane of isotropy.

To specify an orthotropic medium, given that the medium is incompressible, the following three independent parameters must be determined: Young's modulus along the axis of symmetry (E_a), Young's modulus in the plane of isotropy (E_i), and shear modulus along the axis of symmetry (G_a). It was also assumed by Titze (1976) that the vocal fold tissue was incompressible. Shear moduli in the plane of isotropy (G_i) are determined from the formula $E_i = 3G_i$. On the other hand, there is no functional relationship between E_a and G_a because of the anisotropy with respect to the longitudinal and transverse orientations. Among the data presented in the preceding section, the moduli measured under the longitudinal tension correspond to E_a, whereas those measured under the transverse tension correspond to E_i. The shear moduli measured with a rotation around the longitudinal axis correspond to G_a. Approximate values of these moduli are shown in Table 1–2. The values of E_a and E_i are the differential Young's moduli taken from the same region of elongation in which G_as were measured. In Table 1–2, there are some estimated data, such as G_i and the data for contracting muscle, in addition to actually measured data.

Figure 1–18. Schematic drawing of the left vocal fold as an orthotropic composition. The face of the small cube (dotted) embedded in the vocal fold is the plane of isotropy. From Kakita, Y., Hirano, M., and Ohmaru, K. (1981). Physical properties of the vocal fold: Measurement on excised larynges. In K. N. Stevens and M. Hirano (Eds.), *Vocal fold physiology* (pp. 377–396). Tokyo: University of Tokyo Press. Reprinted with permission.

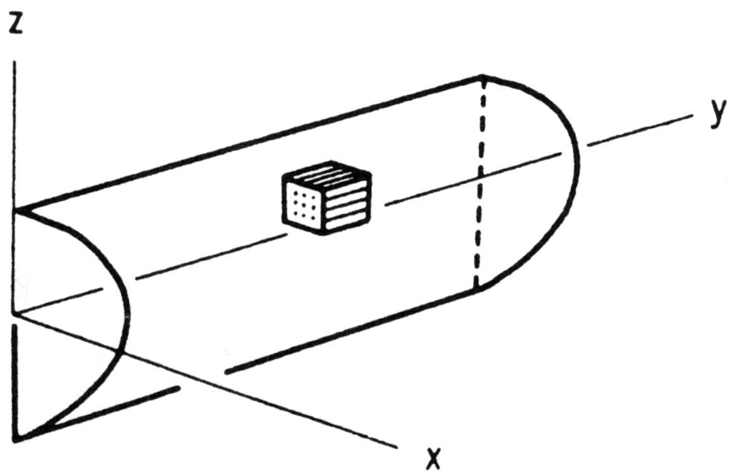

Results in Table 1–2 show the following findings:

1. For the lamina propria, E_a is larger than E_i by more than 10 times. This indicates that the medium is anisotropic with respect to the tensile deformation between the longitudinal and transverse (lateral) directions, and that the tissue is much stiffer in a longitudinal direction than in a transverse direction. G_a is also much larger than G_i.

2. For the lamina propria and the muscle, E_a is larger than G_a not by three times but by approximately 10 times. This also shows that the medium is anisotropic with respect to the deformation in a plane parallel to the longitudinal axis. (For an isotropic and incompressible material, $E = 3G$.)

Since we have not actually compared the tensile modulus E_i in the "vertical" direction (along the z-axis in Figure 1–18), we cannot specifically check the isotropy in the transverse plane. However, we believe, on the basis of histological structure, that E_is for those two orientations do not differ significantly within the same layer of the vocal fold tissue. Therefore, the assumption of orthotropy seems quite reasonable, at least as a first approximation.

Table 1-2.
Elastic Moduli Relevant to the Modeling of the Vocal Folds

	Epithelium	Lamina propria	Muscle (resting)	Muscle (contracting)
E_i	—	$5 \times 10^4 - 10^5$	—	—
G_i	—	$(1.5-3) \times 10^4$*	—	—
E_a	10^7†	10^6†	10^6†	10^7‡
G_a	—	10^5	10^5	10^6‡

* Calculated by a functional relation $G_i = E_i/3$ based on the assumption of isotropy in the frontal plane.

† Values shown are read from Figure 15 at approximately a working length (130% of the length with no load) during the rotational experiment for obtaining values of G_a.

‡ Estimated on the basis of what has been described in the literature (Hill, 1970). These values are simply 10 times those for a resting muscle.

From Kakita, Y., Hirano, M., and Ohmaru, K. (1981). Physical properties of the vocal fold tissue: Measurement on exercised larynges. In K. N. Stevens and M. Hirano (Eds.), *Vocal fold physiology* (pp. 377-396). Tokyo: University of Tokyo Press. Reprinted with permission.

The only exception may be the epithelium. Structurally, the epithelium also appears to be orthotropic. However, the axis of symmetry lies in a direction perpendicular to the surface of the epithelium and the plane of isotropy lies in the plane parallel to the surface. When we discuss the mechanical properties of the epithelium in relation to vibratory behavior, however, we do not need to take the orthotropic property of the epithelium into consideration for the following reason. The epithelium is very thin relative to the entire structure, being 0.05 to 0.08 mm in thickness. Furthermore, it is much stiffer than the other portion of the vocal fold, as shown in Figures 1-13 and 1-15 and Table 1-2. Therefore, deformation within the epithelium caused by vibratory movement is minimal and negligible. The significance of the epithelium for the vocal fold as a vibrator is discussed later.

Estimation of the Tissue Properties During Vibration In Vivo A biological tissue is a highly polymeric material. It is composed of many networked molecules with large molecular weights. Viscoelastic properties of highly polymeric materials vary, depending on the frequency of mechanical vibration and the temperature to which the material is exposed. The frequency and the temperature during the measurement of shear viscoelasticity were about 0.1 Hz and 19 °C, respectively. When we discuss vocal fold vibrations in vivo, the relevant frequency is of the order of 100 Hz and the temperature is approximately 36 °C.

Generally, the elastic moduli increase (tissues become more rigid) as the frequency increases, whereas they decrease as the temperature increases. The viscous constant decreases (tissues flow more easily) as either the frequency or the temperature increases. The effect of temperature changes on the viscoelastic properties is larger than the effect of frequency changes. Due to this dependency, the behavior of the viscoelastic material is classified into three regions: rubbery, transition, and glassy regions (Ferry, 1960). The material is relatively soft in the rubbery region, whereas it is hard in the glassy region. For the transition region that lies between the rubbery and the glassy regions, a transition frequency is specific for a material, provided that the temperature is fixed. Also, transition temperature is specific for a particular frequency.

No specific data on transition frequency and temperature have been documented, except that the transition frequency for shear viscosity of muscle was 400 kHz (Dunn, 1962) at an unknown temperature. If this experiment was conducted at room temperature (approximately 20 °C), 400 kHz is high enough for us to assume that the muscle tissue is in the rubbery region at both 0.1 and 100 Hz. We assume that the tissue is also in the rubbery region at both 19 °C and 36 °C if the frequency is lower than 100 Hz, since the tissue presents "soft" texture.

On the basis of the data reported in some literature, approximate values of the change in the shear modulus and the shear viscous constant were estimated for the vocal fold tissue (for a detailed explanation, see Kakita et al., 1981). At a frequency of 100 Hz and a body temperature of 36 °C, the viscosity decreases considerably and is reduced to 0.5% of its value at 0.1 Hz and 19 °C, whereas the elastic modulus increases by about 10%. Consequently, at a frequency of 100 Hz and 36 °C, the shear modulus of the muscle is estimated to be approximately 2.5×10^5 dyne/cm^2 at rest and the viscosity about 50 P. The shear modulus of the muscle in contraction is estimated to be approximately 2.5×10^6 dyne/cm^2. If the same change can be applied for the lamina propria, the shear modulus would be approximately 2×10^5 dyne/cm^2 and the viscosity 25 P. Glycerine has viscosity of about 15 P at the room temperature of 20 °C. Therefore, at a frequency of 100 Hz and a temperature of 36 °C the viscous property of the lamina propria appears similar to that of an oily liquid.

Another relevant factor is the hardening of muscle tissue after death (rigor mortis). According to Bendall (1960), tissue properties, extensibility in this case, remain almost unchanged for a certain period of time, generally a couple of hours. After that, the hardening starts and extensibility is easily reduced by one order of magnitude within several hours. The initiation of hardening, however, depends on the temperature and the condition of the animal before death. Hardening starts earlier and proceeds faster when the temperature is higher or when the animal is more poorly fed or more exhausted before death. In our experiment on shear properties the measurement was started within a half hour and was completed before 2 hr after death. The temperature, 19 °C, was not too high. Therefore, the effect of the death rigor was presumably minimized.

Generally speaking, the effect of rigor mortis is avoided if the experiment is carried out either (1) within a short time, when the tissue temperature is at in vivo conditions, or (2) at a sufficiently low temperature, when longer time for experimentation is needed. In the latter case the measured data must be corrected in order to obtain the measurement of the property at in vivo temperature. We can reasonably estimate the property at a different temperature, however, when we combine measured data with theoretical considerations, as we have shown by example in this section.

ADJUSTMENTS OF THE COVER–BODY COMPLEX

Notion

Hirano (1977, 1981b) emphasized that human beings can produce vocal sounds within a wide range of fundamental frequencies and intensities with a great variety of tonal qualities by use of only one sound generator, a single pair of vocal folds. This is in contrast to many other musical instruments that have multiple sound generators in order to cover varieties of tone. In other words, the vocal folds can become vibrators with many different properties. This remarkable versatility in sound production is possible because of two features of the vocal folds: (1) Their structure is layered as desribed in the previous section. The layered structure is advantageous over a uniform structure in terms of variability. (2) The vocal folds are subject to fine-grained and delicate muscular control. In the following section, these two features are explained.

Function of the Laryngeal Muscles in Adjusting the Vocal Fold

There are five intrinsic laryngeal muscles that are very important in adjusting the vocal folds: the cricothyroid (CT), thyroarytenoid or vocalis (VOC), lateral cricoarytenoid (LCA), interarytenoid (IA), and posterior cricoarytenoid (PCA) muscles. In the living human, many combinations in the degree of contraction of these muscles take place during speech and singing. To understand the function of each muscle, however, it is useful to investigate the position, shape, and structure of the vocal fold when a given single muscle is activated.

Hirano and co-workers conducted investigations in which each laryngeal muscle of excised canine larynges was electrically stimulated (Hirano, 1975; Koike et al., 1976; Morio, 1976). They photographed the vocal folds from above and from the inner side before and during electrical stimulation of each muscle. They then determined the changes in the position and shape of the vocal fold caused by the electrical stimulation as shown on photographs. They also froze the larynges in 100% alcohol solution at $-30\,^\circ$C while electrically stimulating them; then they examined the vocal folds histologically. Table 1–3 summarizes their results with application to the human vocal fold. Figure 1–19 schematically presents the action of each laryngeal muscle on important laryngeal structures (Hirano, 1974b). The function of each muscle is explained in the following paragraphs.

The Cricothyroid Muscle (CT). When CT is activated, the vocal fold is located in a paramedian position. More precisely, the vocal fold edge is located along the line between the anterior commissure and the posterior cricoarytenoid ligament. CT lowers the vocal fold within the larynx. It markedly elongates and thins the vocal fold. The edge of the vocal fold is sharpened. All the layers, the cover, transition, and body, are markedly stiffened.

The Vocalis Muscle (VOC). The VOC adducts the vocal fold chiefly at the membranous portion. It also lowers the vocal fold. It markedly shortens and thickens the vocal fold. The vocal fold edge is rounded by VOC. When VOC is activated, the body is actively stiffened whereas the cover and the transition are passively slackened. In other words, VOC adjusts the cover and the body in different directions.

Table 1–3.
Characteristic Functions of the Laryngeal Muscles in Vocal Fold Adjustments

	CT	VOC	LCA	IA	PCA
Position	Paramed	*Adduct*	*Adduct*	*Adduct*	*Abduct*
Level	Lower	Lower	*Lower*	0	*Elevate*
Length	*Elongate*	*Shorten*	Elongate	(Shorten)	*Elongate*
Thickness	*Thin*	*Thicken*	Thin	(Thicken)	Thin
Edge	*Sharpen*	*Round*	Sharpen	0	Round
Muscle (body)	*Stiffen*	*Stiffen*	Stiffen	(Slacken)	Stiffen
Mucosa (cover and transition)	*Stiffen*	*Slacken*	Stiffen	(Slacken)	Stiffen

0: no effect;   parentheses: slightly;   italics: markedly.
CT: the cricothyroid muscle, VOC: the vocalis muscle, LCA: the lateral cricoarytenoid muscle, IA: the interarytenoid muscle, PCA: the posterior cricoarytenoid muscle.

The Lateral Cricoarytenoid Muscle (LCA). The LCA adducts the entire vocal fold. It also lowers the vocal fold at the tip of the vocal process of the arytenoid cartilage. LCA elongates and thins the vocal fold to some extent. The vocal fold edge is sharpened by LCA. All the layers are stiffened to some extent.

The Interarytenoid Muscle (IA). The IA adducts the vocal fold chiefly at the cartilaginous portion. It does not affect the shape and structure of the vocal fold significantly. It slightly shortens, thickens, and slackens the vocal fold.

The Posterior Cricoarytenoid Muscle (PCA). The PCA markedly abducts the entire vocal fold. It also elevates the vocal fold at the tip of the vocal process. PCA elongates and thins the vocal fold. The vocal fold edge, however, is rounded by PCA. The PCA stiffens all the layers of the vocal fold.

It is important to note that the mechanical properties of the cover and transition of the cover–body complex are always adjusted passively by the laryngeal muscles, whereas those of the body (i.e., the vocalis muscle) are controlled actively by its own contractions as well as passively by the other laryngeal muscles. This fact partly explains the reason the layered structure is advantageous over a uniform structure with respect to variability of the mechanical properties.

Effects of Longitudinal Tension upon Each Component of the Cover–Body Complex

It should be noted that the effects of longitudinal tension, brought about chiefly by CT, upon different components of the vocal fold tissue

Figure 1–19. Schematic representation of the function of the laryngeal muscles. The left column shows the location of the cartilages an the edge of the vocal folds when the laryngeal muscles are activated individually. Arrows indicate the direction of the force exerted. *1*, Thyroid cartilage. *2*, Cricoid cartilage. *3*, Arytenoid cartilage. *4*, Vocal ligament. *5*, Posterior cricoarytenoid ligament. The middle colum illustrates the view from above. The right column presents contours of frontal sections at the middle of the membranous portion of the vocal fold; the dotted line shows a control in which no muscle is activated. CT, Cricothyroid muscle; VOC, vocalis muscle; LCA, lateral cricoarytenoid muscle; IA, interarytenoid muscle; PCA, posterior cricoarytenoid muscle. From Hirano, M. (1974b). Standard patterns of vocal fold movements. *Journal of Otolaryngology of Japan, 77*, 108–111.

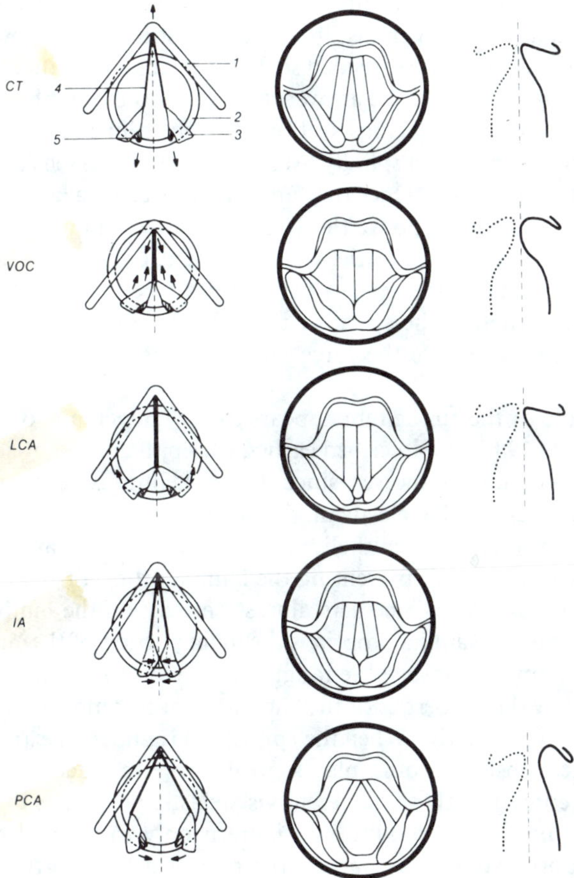

varies depending on the degree of the tension and on the tissue components.

Van den Berg and Tan (1959) measured the extensibilities of excised human vocal folds. The results indicated that the extensibilities of the entire vocal folds were practically the same as those of the corresponding ligaments. The load–extension curves for the vocal ligaments were close to those for the tendon that was nearly pure collagenous tissue. Therefore, they concluded that the longitudinal behavior of the vocal ligament is determined mainly by the collagenous fibers. Later, Van den Berg (1963) reported that at small elongations, only the elastic fibers oppose the stretching force whereas, at large elongations, the collagenous fibers become stretched and allow no further elongation. He related the elongations of the vocal folds to the vocal registers, as shown in Figure 1-20.

The notion proposed by Van den Berg appears to be, at least partly, reasonable. According to Fields and Dunn (1973), Young's modulus of the collagenous fibers is as high as 10^9 dyne/cm^2, whereas that of elastic fibers is of the order of 10^6 dyne/cm^2. Thus, the elastic fibers are much more extensible than the collagenous fibers. The question then follows as to why the collagenous fibers are extended so easily at small longitudinal tensions, as shown in Figure 1-20. The answer rests with structural phenomena that were described in the previous section. As shown in Figure 1-3C and D, the collagenous fibers run spirally. At small longitudinal tensions, the spiral is rather easily extended. Once they are straightened by a large longitudinal tension, they strongly oppose the stretching force, allowing little further elongation. Elastic fibers in the vocal ligament branch and anastomose, forming longitudinally extended nets, as described earlier. It is difficult to determine whether the spiral of the collagenous fibers or the nets of the elastic fibers oppose the force more dominantly at small stretching forces.

The role of the epithelium appears to vary depending on the tension (Kakita et al., 1981). As described earlier, the epithelium shows high values of Young's modulus. However, since the epithelium is very thin, unless it receives tension, the high elastic modulus will not play its proper role. This suggests that when the epithelium is loosened, it behaves just like a "protective cover sheet" preventing the lamina propria from being blown off, and that extrinsic force acts almost entirely on the lamina propria. In other words, the lamina propria is the main portion of the "cover" when the epithelium is loosened enough. The vibratory modes are thus determined by the properties of the lamina propria combined with the state of the underlying "body." When the epithelium is under an extreme tension, the "surface tension" would play a greater role in reacting to the outer force, and consequently the inherent viscoelastic properties of the lamina propria would affect the vibration pattern only to a small extent. The lamina propria would play, rather, the role of a "supporting element."

Figure 1–20. Elongation of the vocal ligaments versus longitudinal tension per square millimeter cross-sectional area in excised larynges. The dotted lines show the elongations used in the main registers. From Van den Berg, Jw. (1963). Vocal ligaments versus register. *NATS Bulletin*, December, pp. 16–21. Reprinted with permission.

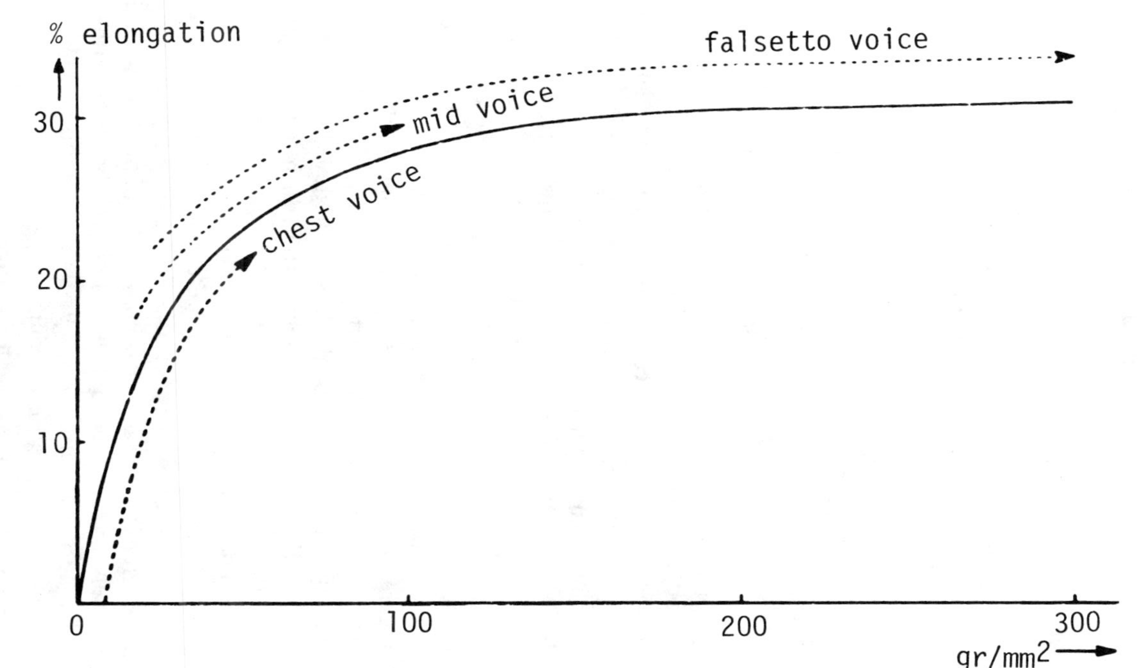

Adjustments Versus Variations of Vibratory Pattern of the Cover–Body Complex

On the basis of histological findings regarding the vocal fold, electromyographic data from the laryngeal muscles, and ultra-high-speed cinematographic analyses of vocal fold vibration, Hirano (1972, 1974a, 1975) proposed four typical laryngeal adjustments, as shown in Figure 1–21, in terms of the relationship between the cover and the body. In earlier publications, the vocal ligament was regarded as a part of the body. Later, he postulated the ligament to be a transitional structure between the body and the cover and called it the transition. In the model shown in Figure 1–21, the transition is left out. Substantially most of the transition should be included in the cover in this abbreviated model.

Parts *a, b,* and *c* of Figure 1–21 represent conditions of heavy or modal register. There is a marked wavy movement of the cover. Two ripples in these pictures represent the so-called upper and lower lips, respectively.

In Figure 1–21*a*, contraction of both the vocalis and the cricothyroid muscles is very weak. This occurs in soft phonation at low pitch levels. The stiffness of both the cover and the body is small, since there is little tension in or on the vocal fold. Both the body and the cover are very flexible, and are almost equally involved in the deformation caused by vibration.

In Figure 1–21*b*, the vocalis muscle contracts much more powerfully than the cricothyroid. This probably happens in loud, heavy voices at medium pitch levels. The body is stiff, whereas the cover is slackened. Deformation during vibration occurs mainly in the cover; the wavy movement, especially, involves only the cover.

Figure 1–21*c* represents a set of conditions in which contraction of the vocalis muscle is a little more dominant than that of the cricothyroid, that is, conditions transitional between Figure 1–21*a* and *b*. This is supposedly the case with most phonations in heavy or modal register. Deformation of the vocal fold, especially the wavy movement, involves both the body and the cover, but more markedly the cover.

The last part, Figure 1–21*d*, represents conditions for light register or falsetto. The vocalis muscle is not active or only slightly active, whereas the cricothyroid muscle contracts powerfully. Both the body and the cover are passively stretched, being tense. In this condition, deformation of the vocal fold during vibration is smaller than in the modal register, and little wavy movement occurs on the mucosa.

Needless to say, the expiratory force is one of the most important factors that determine the mode of vibratory behavior. Figure 1–21 shows conditions where the expiratory force is at its optimum.

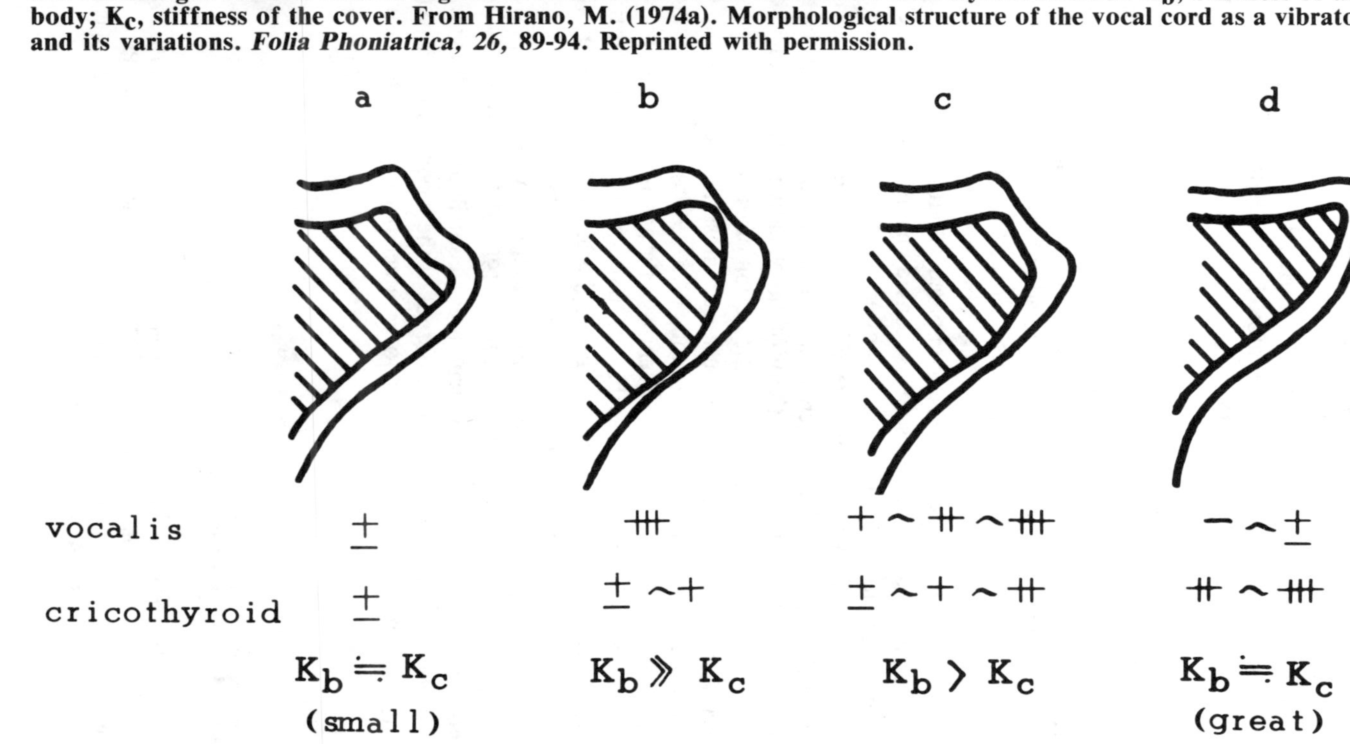

Figure 1–21. Schematic drawings (exaggerated) of cross-sectional structure of the body (shaded) and the cover. Plus and minus signs indicate relative degrees of contraction of the vocalis and cricothyroid muscles. K_b, Stiffness of the body; K_c, stiffness of the cover. From Hirano, M. (1974a). Morphological structure of the vocal cord as a vibrator and its variations. *Folia Phoniatrica, 26*, 89-94. Reprinted with permission.

CONCLUDING REMARKS

This chapter has emphasized the significance of the concept that the vocal fold is a layer-structured vibrator. In voice physiology and voice science, this notion is particularly important in investigating the vibratory behavior of the vocal fold and in modeling vocal fold vibration. The structure, consisting of a stiff *body* covered with a pliable *cover*, presents unique vibratory movements: the body and the cover move with a certain phase difference. In addition, there are also phase differences between different points on the cover along the vertical dimension. The remarkable versatility in voice production specific to adult human beings is attributed, in part, to the unique layer structure of the vocal fold in humans.

Studies of vocal fold vibration using models involve vocal fold structures more or less simplified as compared with reality. This is inevitable, or rather, necessary, when the study is focused on any selected parameters(s) in voice production. There are, however, some instances when an oversimplified model is inadequate. For example, the notion of the *cover-body complex* should be taken into consideration, especially in those modeling studies where the activity of the vocalis muscle is of interest.

From a clinical point of view, the notion of the layer structure of the vocal fold is extremely important because almost all diseases of the vocal fold originate in a given layer (Hirano, 1975, 1981a). This is reflected in the vibratory behavior and, consequently, in the acoustic output—the voice. Analysis of unique vocal fold vibration patterns as well as acoustic and psychoacoustic analyses of the resulting glottal source, therefore, will all prove to be useful for diagnostic purposes. The recognition of the layer(s) involved in a given disease is also essential when one performs phonosurgical treatment (Hirano, 1975, 1981a). Therefore, a working knowledge of the unique layer structures's contribution to the vibratory characteristics subsequent acoustic output of the larynx allows us to make rational diagnostic decisions and to conduct reasonable phonosurgical treatment.

REFERENCES

Bendall, J. R. (1960). Post mortem changes in muscle. In G. H. Bourne (Ed.), *The structure and function of muscle* (Vol. 3., pp. 227–272). New York: Academic Press.
Dunn, F. (1962). Temperature and amplitude dependence of acoustic absorption in tissue. *Journal of the Acoustical Society of America, 34,* 1545–1547.

Ferry, J. D. (1960). *Viscoelastic properties of polymers.* New York: J. Wiley.

Fields, S., and Dunn F. (1973). Correlation of echographic visualizability of tissue with biological composition and physiological state. *Journal of the Acoustical Society of America, 54,* 809–812.

Hill, A. V. (1970). *First and last experiments in muscle mechanics.* Cambridge: Cambridge Univ. Press.

Hirano, M. (1972). The vocal fold during phonation. *Igaku-no-ayumi, 80,* 622–627.

Hirano, M. (1974a). Morphological structure of the vocal cord as a vibrator and its variations. *Folia Phoniatrica, 26,* 89–94.

Hirano, M. (1974b). Standard patterns of vocal fold movements. *Journal of Otolaryngology of Japan, 77,* 108–111.

Hirano, M. (1975). Phonosurgery. Basic and clinical investigations. *Otologia (Fukuoka), 21,* 239–440.

Hirano, M. (1977). Structure and vibratory behavior of the vocal folds. In M. Sawashima and F. S. Cooper (Eds.), *Dynamic aspects of speech production* (pp. 13–30). Tokyo: University of Tokyo Press.

Hirano, M. (1981a). Structure of the vocal fold in normal and disease states. Anatomical and physical studies. *ASHA Report, 11,* 11–27.

Hirano, M. (1981b). The laryngeal examination. In J. K. Darby (Ed.), *Speech evaluation in medicine* (pp. 47–75). New York: Grune & Stratton.

Hirano, M., Kakita, Y., Kawasaki, H., and Matsushita, H. (1976). Vocal cord vibration. Behavior of the layer-structured vibrator in normal and pathological conditions. 16-mm film. Department of Otolaryngology, Kurume University, Kurume, Japan.

Hirano, M., Kakita, Y., Ohmaru, K., and Kurita, S. (1982). Structure and mechanical properties of the vocal fold. *Speech and Language, 7,* 271–297.

Hirano, M., Koike, Y., Hirose, S., and Kasuya, T. (1974). An electron microscopic investigation of the human vocal cord mucosa. *Journal of Otolaryngology of Japan, 77,* 650–656.

Hirano, M., Koike, Y., Hirose, S., and Morio, M. (1973a). Structure of the vocal cord as a vibrator. *Journal of Otolaryngology of Japan 76,* 1341–1348.

Hirano, M., Kurita, S., and Nagata, K. (1981a). Layer structure of the vocal fold and its vibratory behavior. *Japanese Journal of Logopedics and Phoniatrics, 22,* 224–229.

Hirano, M., Kurita, S., and Nakashima, T. (1981b). The structure of the vocal folds. In K. N. Stevens and M. Hirano (Eds.), *Vocal fold physiology* (pp. 33–41). Tokyo: University of Tokyo Press.

Hirano, M., Kurita, S., and Nakashima, T. (1983). Growth, development, and aging of human vocal folds. In D. M. Bless and J. H. Abbs (Eds.) *Vocal Fold physiology* (pp. 22–43). San Diego: College–Hill Press.

Hirano, M., Kurita, S., and Toh, Y. (1981c). Growth, development and aging of the vocal fold. *Practice of Otolaryngology of Kyoto, 74,* 1791–1802.

Hiroto, I. (1966). The mechanism of phonation. Pathophysiological aspects of the larynx. *Practice of Otolaryngology of Kyoto, 39,* 229–291.

Kakita, Y., Hirano, M., Kawasaki, H., and Matsushita, H. (1976a). Schematical presentation of vibration of the vocal cord as a layer-structured vibrator. Normal larynges. *Journal of Otolaryngology of Japan, 79,* 1333–1340.

Kakita, Y., Hirano, M., Kawasaki, H., and Matsushita, H. (1976b). Schematical presentation of vibration of pathological vocal cords. *Journal of Otolaryngology of Japan, 79,* 1533–1548.

Kakita, Y., Hirano, M., and Ohmaru, K. (1981). Physical properties of the vocal fold tissue: Measurement on excised larynges. In K. N. Stevens and M. Hirano (Eds.), *Vocal fold physiology* (pp. 377–396). Tokyo: University of Tokyo Press.

Koike, Y. Hirano, M., and Morio M. (1976). Function of the laryngeal muscles on position and shape of the vocal cord. In E. Loebell (Ed.), *Proceedings of the 16th international congress of logopedics and phoniatrics* (pp. 257–263). Basel: Karger.

Kurita, S. (1980). Layer structure of the human vocal fold. A morphological investigation. *Otologia Fukuoka, 26,* 973–997.

Kurita, S., Nagata, K., and Hirano, M. (1983). A comparative study of the layer structure of the vocal fold. D. M. Bless and J. H. Abbs (Eds.), *Vocal fold physiology* (pp. 3–21). San Diego: College–Hill Press.

Mihashi, S., Okada, M., and Hirano, M. (1976). Distribution and direction of the blood vessel in the canine vocal cord. An X-ray investigation. *Journal of Otolaryngology of Japan, 79,* 435–438.

Mihashi, S., Okada, M., Kurita, S., Nagata, K., Oda, M., Hirano, M., and Nakashima, T. (1981). Vascular network of the vocal fold. In K. N. Stevens and M. Hirano (Eds.), *Vocal fold physiology* (pp. 45–58). Tokyo: University of Tokyo Press.

Morio, M. (1976). Experimental investigations of the function of the intrinsic laryngeal muscles upon the position and shape of the vocal cord. *Otologia (Fukuoka), 22,* 143–179.

Nagata, K. (1982). A comparative study of the layer structure of the vocal fold. A morphological investigation of 11 mammalian species. *Otologia (Fukuoka), 28,* 699–738.

Negus, V. E. (1949). *The comparative anatomy and physiology of the larynx.* New York/London: Hafner.

Ohmaru, K. (1981). An experimental study of the visco–elastic properties of canine vocal fold tissue. *Otologia (Fukuoka), 27,* 530–554.

Ohmaru, K., Kakita, Y., and Hirano, M. (1981). Elastic structure of the lamina propria of the vocal fold. *Otologia (Fukuoka), 27,* 434–440.

Okada, M. (1978). An investigation of the blood vessels of the vocal fold. *Otologia (Fukuoka), 24,* 974–994.

Okada, M., Mihashi, S., Ito, T., and Hirano, M. (1978). Distribution and direction of the blood vessel in the canine vocal cord. A histological investigation with Indian ink injection method. *Otologia (Fukuoka), 24,* 225–232.

Perello, J. (1962). La theorie muco-ondulatoire de la phonation. *Annales d'Oto-Laryngologie, 79,* 722–725.

Schonharl, E. (1960). *Die Stroboscopie in der Praktischen Laryngologie.* Stuttgart: Georg Thieme Verlag.

Smith, S. (1956). Membran-Polster-Theorie der Stimmlippen. *Archiv fur Ohren-Nasen-Kehlkopfheilkunde, 169,* 485.

Titze, I. (1976). On the mechanics of vocal fold vibration. *Journal of the Acoustical Society of America, 60,* 1366–1380.

Toyozumi, Y. (1979). Structure of the vocal fold viewed in frontal section. A comparative anatomical investigation of some selected mammals. *Otologia (Fukuoka), 25,* 53–62.

Van den Berg, Jw. (1958). Myoelastic-aerodynamic theory of voice production. *Journal of Speech and Hearing Research, 1,* 227–244.

Van den Berg, Jw. (1963). Vocal ligaments versus register. *NATS Bulletin,* December, 16–21.

Van den Berg. Jw., and Tan, T. S. (1959). Results of experiments with human larynxes. *Practical Otorhinolaryngology, 21,* 425–450.

CHAPTER 2

Speech Breathing: Contemporary Views and Findings

Gary Weismer

For many years, research on respiratory function for speech has been somewhat less popular than research on laryngeal and supralaryngeal function for speech. To the extent that the perceived importance of any area is crudely proportional to the quantity of relevant research, two explanations of the perceived *un*importance of work on speech breathing can be offered here. First, the role of respiration in speech production has often been regarded as rather uninteresting, characterized by gross and straightforward physiological principles. For example, one recent textbook (Daniloff, Schuckers, and Feth, 1980, p. 144) has offered the opinion that speech breathing and breathing for life are not fundamentally different. As far as the exchange of carbon dioxide and oxygen is concerned, this may be an appropriate statement, but comparison of the muscular work of breathing for speech and life support suggests that it is not. The latter position is best supported by observations of speech breathing difficulties in certain persons with disordered speech who have no difficulty with vegetative breathing (see below, Recent Studies of Speech Breathing). As Hixon (1973) has pointed out, the process of speech breathing is a relatively complex phenomenon which requires a thorough understanding of the relationship of respiratory physiology to the task of maintaining relatively constant alveolar pressures for speech production. Second, the main issues associated with speech breathing have been regarded as settled by the findings reported in a series of publications by Draper and his associates (Draper, Ladefoged, and Whitteridge, 1959, 1960; Ladefoged, Draper, and Whitteridge, 1958; see also Ladefoged, 1960, 1962, 1964, 1967, 1974). The general results of these investigations, or a well-known summary figure from Draper and co-workers (1959, p. 20, Figure 2), have been included in almost every speech physiology textbook published in the last 15 years (see, for example, Borden and Harris, 1980, pp. 70–72; Hardcastle, 1976, pp. 59–61; Hixon, 1973, p. 107; Lieberman, 1977, pp. 73–74; Zemlin, 1968, p. 103; see Dickson and Maue-Dickson, 1982, for an exception). In addition, several review chapters (MacNeilage, 1972, pp. 2–5; Warren, 1976, p. 117) described the data from Draper and colleagues as the accepted account of speech breathing physiology.

The publications by Draper and co-workers reported data based on a combined electromyographic-aerodynamic investigation of speech breathing. Whereas the general methodological approach had some merit, Draper and colleagues apparently did not realize that the pressure-generating capabilities of the chest wall parts—the thorax and diaphragm-abdomen—could not be assessed adequately with a limited electromyographic (EMG) sampling of muscular sites. This probably explains, at least in part, why more recent work by Hixon and colleagues (Hixon, Goldman, and Mead, 1973; Hixon, Mead, and Goldman, 1976) suggested a view of speech breathing physiology that is inconsistent with most details of the work by Draper and associates. Hixon and co-workers (1973, 1976) used techniques that do not allow the determination of exactly which muscles are contributing to the generation of alveolar pressures, but do provide a precise analysis of the overall (net) muscular effort of each chest wall part in generating alveolar pressures. Thus, for example, limited EMG sampling might not include a muscle important for speech breathing, but the kinematics and dynamics analysis employed by Hixon and colleagues could not miss the *effect* of that muscle's action.

The general strategy of the kinematics and dynamics analyses, as used by Hixon and co-authors (1973, 1976), is quite straightforward. If the chest wall configuration (kinematics) or pressures exerted by individual chest wall parts (dynamics) can be recorded throughout the lung volume range when a subject is *relaxing* his or her respiratory muscles, then deviations from the "relaxation" configurations or pressures during speech must be produced by muscular action. By carefully comparing the pressure deviations (pleural pressure for thorax, and abdominal pressure for diaphragm–abdomen) to the configuration deviations, one can make fairly precise statements about the *net* muscular contribution of a chest wall part to a speech breathing event. Draper and co-workers (1959, 1960) did not have the benefit of this global view of respiratory function for speech, and based their inferences of chest wall muscular effort on a technique that could give them only partial information on the muscular activity of chest wall parts (see later section on Future Directions). These considerations suggest that the account of speech breathing proposed by Hixon and colleagues—the "contemporary" account—is to be preferred over the "classic" account by Draper and associates. Complete details of the experimental techniques employed by Draper and colleagues and Hixon and colleagues are given in the publications cited earlier.

Apart from these methodological considerations, several details of the "classic" account of speech breathing physiology can be called into question on logical grounds alone. The first section of this chapter contrasts the "classic" and "contemporary" views of speech breathing physiology by considering how *efficiently* the mechanism would function under the respective accounts. The notion of biological efficiency has often served as a guiding principle in studies of respiratory physiology (see review in Daubenspeck, 1981; and also Bishop, 1974; Roussos and Macklem, 1982). When this notion is extended to consideration of respiratory function for speech, the classic view does not appear to be reasonable. Because there is no textbook chapter that reviews the work of Hixon and associates (1973, 1976) and compares it to that of Draper and co-workers (1959, 1960), this section is written in a pedagogical fashion. A much more detailed account of problems with the studies by Draper and co-authors, was reported by Hixon, Weismer, and Putnam (1979) and is the subject of a forthcoming publication by the same authors.

The second section of the chapter reviews recent studies of both normal and disordered speech breathing. The review is designed to give the reader a survey of current investigations in the area of speech breathing, and does not provide in-depth critical assessment of each cited study. The final section of the chapter describes selected directions for future research, with specific suggestions as to methodological and theoretical approaches to studies of speech breathing physiology.

SPEECH BREATHING AS AN EFFICIENT PROCESS

Biological systems are generally characterized by functional properties that allow them to operate most efficiently. In other words, a biological system may be able to achieve a goal in several different ways, yet it often functions in a manner that yields the greatest efficiency. The notion of *efficiency* is one in which the output of a biological system is related to the *energy expended* by the system to produce that output. A high-efficiency system produces a large output with a minimum expenditure of energy; conversely, a low-efficiency system has to work very hard to produce a similar output. It is often the case, as shall be seen below, that the functional difference between a normal and pathological respiratory system can be thought of in part as a difference between a high-efficiency and low-efficiency system.

Like other biological systems, the normal respiratory system during speech production can be shown to function in a highly efficient manner. Hixon and colleagues have demonstrated that (1) speech is typically produced within a range of lung volumes that allows a substantial output (that is, alveolar or subglottal pressure) with minimal expenditure of energy, (2) the abdominal muscles are contracted constantly throughout speech production, as a result of which both the expiratory and inspiratory phases of speech breathing are highly efficient, and (3) the respiratory system is always under some type of muscular control during speech production and so does not require sudden contractions of muscles that may be needed to contribute to the regulation of a sustained or briefly incremented subglottal pressure. Each of these points is discussed separately below.

The Restricted Lung Volume Range for Speech Production

In Hixon's work, speakers typically initiated conversational speech at approximately 60% of the vital capacity, continued speaking until they exhaled to approximately 35% to 40% vital capacity (VC) (the resting expiratory level [REL], or elastic rest position of the respiratory structures), and then refilled their lungs back to approximately 60% VC to begin the next utterance. These lung volume measurements were derived from volume-calibrated displacement transducers (magnetometers) located on the rib cage and abdomen, and so were not contaminated by airway loading and dead-space effects associated with respirometers and facemasks (see below). At first glance, it might seem odd that speakers used only about *one fifth* of their vital capacity during speech production. After all, it could be argued that the use of a greater lung volume range during speech production would reduce the number of inspiratory "interruptions" during speech production, and so result in a more connected speech message. However, consideration of several characteristics of the respiratory system suggests that the advantage of a more connected speech message could be gained only at greater cost to the mechanical efficiency of the system.

The subglottal pressure (Ps) demand for an utterance is met by a combination of forces generated by respiratory structures. One of these forces is passive, and is associated with the elastic recoil characteristics of the respiratory structures (Agostoni, 1970b). The other forces are generated actively, by contraction of the respiratory muscles. In the absence of any muscular activity, the passive forces of the respiratory system will generate Ps, which increases as lung volume increases, and vice versa. It is important to remember that these passive pressures, or relaxation pressures (Pr), are due strictly to the *structural characteristics* of the respiratory system. They are *not* produced by muscular force, and are not under the speaker's control. Thus, if we asked a subject to inspire from resting expiratory level (REL) to 80% VC and measured a relaxation pressure of 22 cm H_2O at that lung volume, we could be sure that, for this subject, the relaxation pressure is *always* 22 cm H_2O at 80% VC. Subglottal pressures that result from active muscular contraction are referred to as *muscular pressures* (Pmus). Pmus can be defined more precisely as the amount of Ps that is generated by muscular forces alone, independent of Pr. For example, if a Ps of 13 cm H_2O is measured at a lung volume where the Pr is known to be 10 cm H_2O, Pmus must equal 3 cm H_2O. In other words, the measured Ps can be considered as the sum of relaxation (Pr) and muscular (Pmus) pressures (Hixon, 1973). Pmus is under a speaker's control and is variable at any lung volume within a range determined by the maximum expiratory and inspiratory muscular force that can be generated by the respiratory muscles. The range of Pmus required for speech production is much smaller than the maximum Pmus capabilities of the respiratory system.

Now consider that the "average" magnitude of Ps during conversational speech production by adults is approximately 10 cm H_2O (Lieberman, 1967, 1977). In principle, conversational speech could be initiated at a lung volume well above REL (say, 80% VC), slightly above REL (say, 60% VC), or below REL (about 30% VC). Examination of the consequences for respiratory function of beginning conversational speech at each of these three lung volumes indicates why normal speech occurs within a relatively narrow range of lung volumes. For example, if a speaker initiated conversational speech at 80%, VC his or her respiratory system would generate a relaxation pressure more than double the desired Ps of 10 cm H_2O. Since the elastic characteristics of the respiratory system cannot be adjusted by the speaker, he or she would have to resort to active muscle contraction to produce a Ps of 10 cm H_2O at 80% VC. In this case, the net muscular effort would have to be inspiratory, because the compression of the lungs caused by the inward recoil forces would have to be partly offset by an expanding force. Thus, this situation would demand that active (muscular) and passive (elastic) forces be pitted against each other.

The same general situation would arise if conversational speech were initiated at 30% VC. At this lung volume the passive characteristics of the respiratory system exert an inspiratory force (outward recoil), but the Ps demand is positive. The negative alveolar pressure that results from the passive recoil in an inspiratory direction at 30% VC must therefore be offset by an expiratory muscular effort. Here the speaker is again faced with a situation in which his passive and active respiratory forces must work against each other to produce the Ps required for conversational speech.

Opposing respiratory forces are typically not required when conversational speech is initiated at approximately 60% VC. The relaxation pressure at this lung volume is nearly 10 cm H_2O, so the expiratory muscles need to exert only small forces at the beginning of speech to achieve the desired Ps. As the utterance proceeds on a decreasing lung volume, the available relaxation pressure also decreases and a steadily increasing force from the expiratory muscles is required to maintain a constant Ps. Thus, if a speaker begins an utterance at 60% VC and does not continue into lung volumes below REL, the respiratory system is not required to use opposing forces at any time to achieve the magnitudes of Ps which are typical of conversational speech. Stated otherwise, speaking throughout the 60%-REL lung volume range will involve active and passive forces working in the same direction to produce the desired Ps, a situation which seems to be more efficient than the case where the respective forces are opposed. One implication of using a lung volume range for speech in which active and passive forces work in the same direction is that unusually large amounts of muscular effort are not required. The required amount of supplemental muscular pressure ($Pmus$) will, as described earlier, increase as utterance proceeds (i.e., as lung volume decreases). By confining conversational speech production to the 60%-REL lung volume range, however, the *greatest* $Pmus$ required would rarely exceed 10 cm H_2O. Moreover, in the 60%-REL lung volume range the greatest $Pmus$ would be required only at the *end* of an expiratory phrase. In contrast, conversational speech initiated at either 80% or 30% VC would, assuming a Ps demand of 10 cm H_2O, require larger absolute amounts of $Pmus$ (greater than 10 cm H_2O) at the *beginning* of an utterance.

The 60%-REL lung volume range is thus an efficient one for conversational speech production because it permits the active and passive respiratory forces to work in the same direction, a circumstance that means that excessive muscular pressures are not required to meet the subglottal pressure demand. This style of efficiency appears to be adaptable to situations that deviate from "conversational" speech production. For example if a speaker wants to produce very loud speech, he or she must generate a Ps in excess of that used in conversational speech. Suppose this speaker produced speech with a subglottal pressure of 15 cm H_2O, which would result in very loud phonation—what range of lung volumes would be used? It would seem as if the starting lung volume for conversational speech loudness (i.e., approximately 60% VC) would not be maximally efficient, because the speaker would have to immediately generate relatively substantial $Pmus$ (5 cm H_2O) to achieve the Ps demand of 15 cm H_2O. If the situation in conversational speech is taken as a "model" of efficiency, it might be predicted that the most efficient way to produce this loud speech would be to initiate utterance at a lung volume where the available relaxation pressure is nearly 15 cm H_2O. This prediction is upheld by the research by Hixon and colleagues (1973), which shows that as speakers increase their speech loudness (i.e., as they increase their Ps), they tend to initiate speech at higher lung volumes. In a sense, speakers recognize that louder speech demands higher Ps, and therefore adjust their starting lung volumes to get the relaxation pressure which is the best "match" to the Ps demand. They also end above REL, perhaps to avoid expending the large amounts of $Pmus$ which would be required if utterance was extended to REL.

Another manifestation of the adaptability of a "most efficient lung volume range" is the change in lung volumes used for speech in different postures. The best example of this is the supine posture, which because of gravitational effects on the abdominal contents has an REL of approximately 20% VC, rather than the 35% to 40% VC associated with the upright posture (Agostoni, 1970b). Since REL is defined as the point in lung volume where the net passive force exerted on the lungs by chest wall structures is zero, the lower zero point in the supine, as compared to upright, posture implies that for equivalent lung volumes in the two postures the available relaxation pressure (Pr) is always *more positive in the supine posture.* Thus, if speech were initiated at 60% VC in the supine posture, the available Pr would probably exceed the Ps demand, and negative muscular pressures would have to be used to offset the "overpressure" due to the elastic characteristics of the respiratory system. Note that this is similar to the inefficient situation described above for speech initiated at 80% VC in the upright posture. Hixon and colleagues (1973) have shown that in the supine posture conversational speech takes place between roughly 40% and 20% VC, which is exactly the range that would be expected for the efficiency reasons described above, if speech production were tied to certain parts of the relaxation pressure function. As the relaxation pressure function is modified with changes in posture, so is the range of lung volumes used for speech production.

Apparently not all speakers use the lung volume range for speech which seems most efficient a priori. Three of the eight speakers studied by Wilder (1983) initiated some utterances within the tidal volume or *below* REL, and Bless (personal communication) reports similar observations for a small number of subjects. In addition, data obtained by Hoshiko (1965) indicated that phonation is typically initiated at lung volumes close to the end of rest inspiration, a finding clearly at odds with observations by Hixon and co-workers (1973). Hoshiko's (1965) study should be interpreted with caution, however, because his "speech" task was phonation of the vowel /a/ and the reported tidal volumes are much larger than expected (see Agostoni, 1970a, p. 96). In addition, Hoshiko's (1965) subjects were breathing through a facemask-respirometer apparatus that introduces dead space and resistance to airflow, both of which are likely to induce inspiratory muscle fatigue (Roussos and Macklem, 1982). The observations of Wilder and Bless are probably valid, but are likely to represent no more than an infrequent departure from the "best" lung volume strategy. It might be argued that the subjects studied by Hixon and associates (1973) did not provide representative data because they are all respiratory physiologists and may have performed in accordance with certain scientific expectations; however, many of the persons with disordered speech studied by Hixon and colleagues (see later section, Recent Studies of Speech Breathing) used the same lung volume ranges for speech as did the original normal, more sophisticated subjects.

Perhaps some speakers choose to continue speaking below REL to reduce the frequency of inspiration during discourse. It might even be argued that limiting the end of utterance to REL is an inefficient way to breathe for speech because of the more frequent demand for inspiration and the respiratory work associated with it. However, the efficiency gained by continuing speech below REL and therefore reducing the frequency of inspiration would be more than offset by (1) the need to use expiratory muscular force against inspiratory recoil force, as discussed above, and (2) the possible displacement of the diaphragm from its rest position, which is discussed in detail below. The latter point is particularly relevant because it suggests that the "advantages" of reducing the frequency of inspiration can be gained only at the expense of the efficiency of the muscular mechanisms that produce the inspirations.

Abdominal Activity During Speech Production

The muscular activities of the chest wall which have been shown to occur during conversational speech production can be summarized as follows: (1) during the utterance (i.e., during speech expiration) there is *expiratory* muscle activity in *both* the thorax and abdomen; and (2) during the inspiratory "refills" which separate consecutive utterances, there is some *expiratory* muscular activity in both the thorax and abdomen, but the net inspiratory effort of the chest wall is provided by rapid and forceful contraction of the diaphragm (Hixon et al., 1976, p. 350). It is interesting to note that these observations on abdominal muscular activity during conversational speech, which come from relatively recent research efforts (Hixon et al., 1973, 1976), are in conflict with the classic account of respiratory function for speech production (Ladefoged et al., 1958; Draper et al., 1959, 1960). The latter view of speech breathing held that the abdominal muscles were rarely, if ever, active during conversational speech production. Thus the classic and contemporary views of speech breathing are characterized by opposite accounts of the role of the abdominal muscles in conversational speech production. One way to evaluate the relative merits of these two views is to ask if one or the other appears to provide for more efficient speech breathing.

Consider first the expiratory side of speech breathing. As stated earlier, there is a clear need for an increasingly positive muscular effort to maintain a constant Ps as an utterance proceeds (as lung volume decreases). Assuming the abdominal muscles were *not* active for conversational speech, this increasingly positive muscular effort would have to be generated by muscles of the rib cage alone. As positive muscular effort increases, so does the pleural pressure (Ppl) (Kunze, 1964). In the absence of abdominal muscular activity, the increasing Ppl would tend to drive the diaphragm caudally and therefore displace the abdominal contents outward. This means, then, that the diaphragm–abdomen would be driven in the *inspiratory* direction, even though the muscles of the rib cage were attempting to develop expiratory force. Thus, the downward motion of the diaphragm would compromise the compressive effort of the rib cage, making it relatively difficult for the thoracic muscles to develop and maintain a constant Ps.

How would respiratory function for speech differ if the abdominal muscles were active? Contraction of the abdominal muscles would displace the diaphragm rostrally, and so compress the thorax. One result of abdominal activity during compressive efforts of the rib cage, therefore, is that the positive Ppl is not applied to a passive diaphragm–abdomen. Rather, the active abdominal muscles oppose caudal displacement of the diaphragm, and thus allow compressive efforts of the thorax to contribute to the Ps demand without losses due to a caudally moving diaphragm. This suggests that it may be more efficient for the abdominal muscles to be active, as compared to inactive, during conversational speech production.

It could be argued, of course, that the gain in efficiency for thoracic muscular activity is made only at the expense of additional muscular effort in another part of the chest wall, that is, the abdomen. To provide a clearer picture of whether speech breathing is more efficient with or without abdominal activity, it may be useful to explore the relative efficiency of these two views for a different aspect of speech breathing, the need to refill the lungs between successive utterances.

Once again, assume initially that the abdominal muscles are largely inactive during utterance. As described above, the positive (expiratory) effort of the internal intercostals would drive the diaphragm caudally, and more so as utterance proceeds and the magnitude of the positive effort increases. This positive rib cage drive would affect the *shape* of the diaphragm, distorting the muscle from its typical domed shape to a more flattened configuration as it is displaced caudally. The domed shape of the diaphragm is observed when this muscle is in an uncontracted state, that is, at its *physiological rest length.* It is known that, generally, muscles are capable of generating maximal contractile force when a contraction is initiated from the physiological rest length, as compared to any other length (Newsom Davis, 1970). Thus, diaphragmatic contraction for the purpose of inspiratory refill between utterances should be most forceful (and probably most rapid) when the contraction is initiated from the domed configuration (see Hixon et al., 1976; Loring and Mead, 1982).

The assumption of inactive abdominal muscles during conversational speech production, however, implies that the diaphragm will be in a less than favorable configuration for producing efficient inspiratory refills. At the end of the utterance, Ppl would be at its greatest magnitude compared to all other points within the utterance, and the resulting caudal displacement of the diaphragm would cause a substantial flattening of the muscle. The diaphragm would then be far from the configuration that allows maximum contractile force, and it seems reasonable to conclude that the inspiratory side of speech breathing might be controlled by a somewhat less than efficient mechanism.

The respiratory system can prevent the caudal displacement and consequent flattening of the diaphragm during speech simply by contracting the abdominal muscles. If the magnitude of abdominal muscular effort balances the expiratory muscle effort of the thorax, the diaphragm will be maintained roughly at its physiological rest configuration, and can generate forceful contractions for the utterance refills. An assumption of this discussion has been that it is the diaphragm that is responsible for inspiratory refills during speech breathing. One could assume, however, that the external intercostals play a major role in speech inspiration, because certain regions of this muscular sheet are known to be active during *rest* breathing (Campbell and Newson Davis, 1970). Although the results of previous research (Hixon et al., 1976) indicate that the external intercostals do *not* play a major role in speech inspiration, it may be useful to consider the implications for speech breathing efficiency if they did. Assuming that the *internal* intercostals were providing their maximum expiratory effort at the end of an utterance, the use of the *external* intercostals for speech inspiration would require a rapid shift in rib cage muscular control from expiratory to inspiratory. Moreover, muscular control of the rib cage would have to be reversed again—back to expiratory effort—for the next utterance. This cyclic reversal of rib cage effort, from expiratory to inspiratory, and vice versa, is avoided if the diaphragm alone provides the muscular effort needed for inspiratory refills. In fact, Hixon and colleagues (1976) found that a small *expiratory* effort of the rib cage may be maintained during diaphragmatic contraction for speech inspiration. Because of the relative force of the diaphragmatic contraction, the small expiratory forces generated by the internal intercostals are overcome, and the net effect is expansion of the thorax and thus the lungs. Hixon and colleagues (1976, pp. 349–350) have summarized this argument by stating that activity of abdominal muscles during speech "tunes" the diaphragm to an optimal configuration for generating contractile force.[1]

The small expiratory force generated by rib cage muscles during inspiration could be regarded as another manifestation of speech breathing efficiency. This small muscular force may anticipate, during inspiration, the small positive muscular effort required at the beginning of the next utterance.

To summarize, it appears that the contemporary view of the role played by the abdominal muscles during speech breathing describes a more efficient respiratory mechanism than does the classic view. Specifically, if the abdominal muscles are assumed to be active throughout conversational speech production (the contemporary view), the respiratory system can (1) develop positive alveolar pressures without "losses" due to inspiratory movements of the diaphragm–abdomen and (2) "tune" the diaphragm to a configuration which allows maximum contractile forces for inspiration (Hixon et al., 1976). When the abdominal muscles are assumed to be *inactive* during conversational speech production (the classic view), the former and latter advantages are lost. In addition, other aspects of respiratory function for speech production can be shown to be most efficient when the abdominal muscles are active.

Muscular Control of the Chest Wall

In some speaking situations the net muscular effort of the chest wall will be inspiratory at the onset of utterance, and expiratory later in the utterance.[2] This pattern of respiratory muscular activity occurs when the available Pr at the starting lung volume for speech exceeds the Ps demand of the utterance. To "offset" the excess Pr at the starting lung volume, a net inspiratory muscular effort is required of the chest wall, the magnitude of which is determined by the difference between the Pr and the Ps demand. As utterance proceeds, of course, the available Pr decreases in magnitude and eventually becomes less than the required Ps. This latter situation demands a net expiratory muscular effort from the chest wall to "add" to the available Pr. The amount of "added" expiratory muscular effort is simply equal to the difference between the available Pr and the Ps demand (Hixon, 1973).

In this type of utterance the Pr and Ps demand must be equal at some point. It would seem that when this point is reached, a speaker may choose one of two ways to control the Ps. One way would be to "turn off" all muscular activity and let the Ps demand be met by the available Pr. In this case it could be said that the chest wall is controlled for an instant by *passive forces alone.* An alternate approach would be to have simultaneous inspiratory and expiratory muscular effort *of the same magnitude* at the point where Pr equals the Ps demand. Under these conditions, the muscular efforts will cancel completely and the pressure remaining in the lungs will be that provided by passive forces, but with a net muscular pressure of zero.

At first glance it might seem as if the first of these possibilities, in which all muscles are "turned off" for an instant, would allow the respiratory system to function more efficiently than the case in which the inspiratory and expiratory muscles are simultaneously active. Further consideration reveals, however, that allowing passive forces alone to control the chest wall for the instant when Pr equals the Ps demand may make speech breathing less efficient in other respects. For example, it is obvious that as lung volume decreases from this instant of passive control of the chest wall, there must be a net expiratory muscular effort of the respiratory system to supplement the declining Pr. If the expiratory muscles are inactive at the lung volume at which $Pr = Ps$ demand, they must be activated—that is, contracted from their physiological rest length—to provide the expiratory force required to meet the Ps demand at lower lung volumes. This contraction, however, cannot occur instantaneously. The mechanical properties of muscle impose a delay between the time the muscle is instructed by the central nervous system to contract and the time the actual contraction develops a substantial force. In human intercostal muscle, this delay may be as long as one tenth of a second (100 ms) (Hofman, Alston, and Rowe, 1966), a duration which is as long as many speech sounds in conversational speech. Thus, by turning off all muscles when $Pr = Ps$ demand, a speaker may temporarily *lose* some control of speech breathing. This follows from the fact that Pr will fall below the Ps demand as utterance proceeds but cannot be supplemented immediately (i.e., for a period on the order of 0.1 s) by expiratory muscle contraction. One way to conceptualize this is that the delay in muscle contraction introduces what might be called a "dead spot" in the control of the respiratory system during speech production (Hixon et al., 1979). This "dead spot" is where muscular effort is needed, but not available, to supplement the Pr.

Another apparent difficulty with the notion that the respiratory system is controlled solely by passive forces when $Pr = Ps$ demand concerns *linguistic stress.* The physiological phenomena associated with stress are not fully understood, but it does seem fairly clear that greater stress is produced in part by a brief increase of Ps relative to the roughly constant Ps throughout the rest of an utterance (Ladefoged, 1967; Lieberman, 1967).

This physiological aspect of stress has certain implications for the interaction of passive and active forces during speech breathing. The demand for a roughly constant Ps during speech production requires a constantly changing balance of muscular effort and passive forces as utterance proceeds. Since the passive forces are not under a subject's control, the goal of developing a constant Ps must be met by adjustments of respiratory muscle activity. The continuous change in muscular effort through utterance, which is directed specifically at maintaining a constant Ps, may be viewed as the *volume solution* of the respiratory system during speech production (Hixon, 1973). It is called the "volume solution" because it describes how the respiratory muscles *compensate* for the change in Pr which occurs as a function of lung volume.

When a speaker wants to stress a syllable during an utterance—and therefore produce a brief increase of the otherwise constant Ps—there must be some modification of the volume solution. In a sense, what is needed is a positive muscular effort which is momentarily in excess of that required by the volume solution. This excess muscular effort will produce a brief, extra compression of the lungs and so raise the Ps. When this excess effort is removed, the remaining muscular activity will be that needed to maintain the overall Ps demand of the utterance (i.e., it will provide the volume solution for the utterance). These brief expiratory muscular efforts are part of the *pulsatile solution* of speech breathing (Hixon, 1973). The pulsatile solution can be thought of as being superimposed on the volume solution during any speech production task. It is not nearly as predictable as the volume solution, for it may occur anywhere throughout the course of an utterance. That is, linguistic stress is not tied to specific positions-in-utterance, and in fact may recur several times throughout an utterance. The question can now be asked, how would a speaker stress a syllable at that point in lung volume where $Pr = Ps$ demand if all respiratory muscles are "turned off"? If the respiratory system was controlled by passive forces alone at this point, it is obvious that the pulsatile solution—a muscular solution—would be momentarily unavailable for stressing a syllable. It could be argued, perhaps, that the brain plans utterances in such a way as to avoid stressed syllables at the point where $Pr = Ps$ demand, but this would place enormous memory and organization demands on the central nervous system, given the variability of stress placement and utterance-initiating conditions.

The problems that occur when the respiratory system is assumed to be controlled momentarily by passive forces alone can be avoided if there is some muscular activity at the point where $Pr = Ps$ demand. The *net* muscular effort at this point must be zero, because Pr is already meeting the Ps demand, but this is easily achieved when both inspiratory and expiratory muscles are active simultaneously and generating the *same amount of muscular pressure*.

There is an advantage to be gained by having simultaneous activity of the inspiratory and expiratory muscles even though their effects cancel each other. First, there is no "dead spot" associated with lung volume events for speech; this means that the stress-related, positive muscular increments to the volume solution do not have to be achieved by contracting the expiratory muscles from their rest positions. Rather, these increments can be generated by slight adjustments in the *balance* of expiratory and inspiratory muscle activity. The "grading" of opposing forces for fine respiratory control has been discussed previously by Sears (1971). Secondly, the absence of a "dead spot" in the volume history of speech utterances frees the central nervous system from the potential constraint of avoiding stress placements at certain points in lung volume. Thus, utterances do not have to be planned around a point in lung volume that involves passive control only.

RECENT STUDIES OF SPEECH BREATHING

Studies of Normal Speakers

The results of several recent studies (Bless, Hixon, and Miller, unpublished manuscript[3]; Conrad and Schonle, 1979; Grosjean and Collins, 1979; Horii and Cooke, 1978) suggest that respiratory function for speech production is guided by the grammatical structure of utterances. In continuous speech tasks such as *reading,* inspiratory refills typically occur at major constituent and sentence boundaries; some inspiratory refills do occur at minor constituent boundaries, but they tend to be shorter in duration than refills at major constituent boundaries and are selectively eliminated as speaking rate increases (Grosjean and Collins, 1979). Inspiratory refills seem to be tied so closely to grammatical structure that a certain amount of mechanical efficiency will be sacrificed (such as continuing utterance below resting expiratory level) to coordinate inspiration with constituent boundaries (Bless et al., unpublished manuscript). This orderly relationship between constituent boundaries and inspiratory pauses, however, may not hold under all speech production conditions. Goldman Eisler's (1968) studies of speech breathing included an examination of inspiratory pauses in both reading situations and spontaneous speech. She found speech breathing for spontaneous speech to be far less systematic than for reading (also noted by Bless et al.) as the former was characterized by significantly fewer inspiratory pauses at major grammatical boundaries and significantly more inspiratory pauses at nongrammatical boundaries. It would be useful to study potential differences in speech breathing for reading and spontaneous speech with more sophisticated instrumental techniques (Baken, 1977; Hixon et al., 1973; Sackner, 1979) than employed by Goldman Eisler (1968).

An unresolved issue concerns the relationship between lung volume change and the length of major grammatical constituents. Horii and Cooke (1978) obtained nearly zero-order correlations between volume of inspired air and the length of following "breath groups," but Bless et al. (unpublished manuscript) and Wilder (1983) found greater volumes of expired air to be associated with greater phrase length. Actually, the former and latter findings are not necessarily inconsistent, because greater *expiratory* volumes could be used for longer phrases even if preutterance *inspiratory* volumes are independent of phrase length. Experimental work incorporating careful operational definition and manipulation of breath group length is needed to clarify the interrelations between preutterance inspiratory volumes and utterance length.

The dependence of certain features of speech breathing on linguistic structure suggests that respiratory function for speech is unique, and not simply a biological process serving an "overlaid" demand. Conrad and Schonle (1979) provided support for this view by demonstrating that the pattern of short inspirations–long expirations typically observed for speech production is approximated in *subvocal* tasks that demand no volume exchange but presumably involve speech–motor planning and covert articulatory processes. "Thus it can be concluded that resting respiration cannot be maintained during subvocal tasks and that the articulatory act alone changes the respiratory pattern automatically in the direction of speech respiration" (Conrad and Schonle, 1979, p. 260). The shortening of inspiratory refill time with increases in speaking rate reported by Grosjean and Collins (1979) is also consistent with this view, indicating an integration of breathing pause time with articulatory rate control. Finally, Hixon and associates (1976) have proposed that the constant muscular activity of the abdominal wall during speech should be regarded as a "speech-specific posturing" (p. 350) of the chest wall, because of the associated contribution to efficient speech breathing. The special status of speech breathing processes has been emphasized by von Euler (1982), who warns against trying to understand the neural processes associated with speech breathing by studying neural processes associated with "automatic" respiration (e.g., vegetative breathing).

The consistency of a speech-specific posturing of the respiratory system was replicated by Baken, Cavallo, and Weissman (1979) and Baken and Cavallo (1981) in a reaction-time type of experiment. As in the work by Hixon and co-author (1973), the chest wall adjustment prior to phonation was characterized by a larger rib cage size (volume) and smaller abdomen size (volume), relative to the size of these structures when the chest wall is relaxed at corresponding lung volumes. This prephonatory posturing of the chest wall was shown by Baken and his colleagues to be independent of the respiratory phase and volume within tidal breathing epochs, and to involve minimal overall changes in lung volume.

Studies of Disordered Speakers

Respiratory function for speech production by the hearing impaired has been studied recently by Forner and Hixon (1977), Itoh, Horii, Daniloff, and Binnie (1982), and Feudo, Zubick, and Strome (1982). Although the former two studies employed profoundly hearing-impaired young adults (with one exception of "severe" impairment in the Forner and Hixon [1977] study), subjects studied by Itoh and colleagues (1982) were orally trained, while those used by Forner and Hixon (1977) used manual communication exclusively or partially. In addition, Forner and Hixon's subjects were selected on the basis of a *perceived* "moderate-to-severe" speech breathing problem. Feudo and co-workers (1982) used subjects with bilateral sensorineural losses of at least 75 dB HTL, with primary orientation to oral communication. These differences in subject population notwithstanding, the results of these studies indicated for the most part that profoundly hearing impaired persons breathe for speech in much the same way as persons with normal hearing. Itoh and co-authors (1982), using standard aerodynamic techniques for measuring flow at the mouth, showed that for trains of repeated syllables the hearing impaired used approximately the same overall volumes as normal hearers, but expended more *volume per syllable* than normal hearers. This result suggests a laryngeal or supralaryngeal valving problem, or both, among the hearing impaired subjects (see also Whitehead and Metz, 1982). The kinematics analysis (Hixon et al., 1973) reported by Forner and Hixon (1977) suggested a normal "posturing" of the chest wall (see earlier discussion) and relative contribution of rib cage and abdomen during the speech of hearing impaired subjects. The one speech breathing abnormality observed among hearing impaired subjects was in the use of lung volume. Hearing impaired speakers initiated speech at *lower* lung volumes than normal hearers; many utterances were initiated within the tidal volume range, and three subjects often initiated speech below REL. Moreover, Forner and Hixon's (1977) subjects terminated most utterances below REL, a clear departure from the "normal" pattern. A similar finding has been reported by Feudo and co-workers (1982), especially for speakers who are judged as relatively unintelligible.

Initiation of utterance slightly above or below REL would seem to be grossly inefficient, as discussed above, but Hixon (1982) has suggested a reason profoundly hearing impaired persons may *choose* this range of lung volumes for speech production. Human sensitivity to *changes* in lung volume appears to be greater near and below REL, as compared to the midrange of lung volumes (Salamon, von Euler, and Franzen, 1975 [cited in Hixon, 1982]), so by speaking at lower lung volumes the profoundly hearing impaired person may enrich the impoverished feedback associated with his or her speech. Perhaps the heightened awareness of respiratory status allows the hearing impaired speaker to monitor vocal intensity more effectively than if speech was produced throughout the midrange of lung volumes. Experiments using subjects with normal hearing and temporary disruption of auditory feedback are needed to evaluate Hixon's (1982) hypothesis. For example, it might be predicted that in a graded vocal intensity task the lung volume range used for successive intensity increments will depend on the status of the auditory feedback channel.

Speech breathing characteristics associated with various dysarthrias have been described by Putnam, Hixon, and Stern (1981), Hunker, Bless, and Weismer (1981), and Hixon (1982). Putnam and associates (1981) performed kinematics analysis on a group of patients with amyotrophic lateral sclerosis, a degenerative disease of upper and lower motor neurons that often has a profound effect on speech production (see Darley, Aronson, and Brown, 1975, pp. 230–235). Although the 12 subjects in this study all had involvement of spinal motor neurons, only two demonstrated any abnormality for speech breathing. These two subjects used very limited lung volume ranges for speech, which may have been associated with their greatly reduced vital capacities.

Hunker and colleagues (1981) and Hixon (1982) used the kinematics technique in case studies of ataxic subjects. The subject studied by Hunker and associates (1981), a 69 year old woman, used highly variable initiation volumes for speech and frequently continued utterance into functional residual capacity. She also had abrupt shifts in the relative volume displacement of her rib cage and abdomen, a characteristic never observed in normal speakers and only rarely noted in disordered speakers (e.g., see Forner and Hixon, 1977, pp. 391–392). Hixon's (1982) ataxic subject was a 17 year old woman having moderate to severe paresis of the rib cage and diaphragm, and paralyzed abdominal muscles. When the patient spoke, her chest wall configuration was such that her rib cage was smaller, and her abdomen larger, than the size of these chest wall parts when relaxed at corresponding lung volumes. This is opposite to the speech-specific posturing of the chest wall described above, and provides an excellent real-life demonstration of the efficiency loss consequent to speaking with a relaxed abdomen. The patient's paralyzed abdominal wall could not resist the downward force applied to the diaphragm by the positive rib cage drive, and so it was displaced outward to sizes exceeding the relaxed size. This outward movement of the abdominal wall compromises the expiratory effort of the rib cage, which must be driven to smaller sizes to achieve the desired lung volume displacement.

A small amount of data concerning the speech breathing characteristics of persons with Parkinson's disease is also available. Both Kim (1968) and Hunker and co-workers (1981) reported that parkinsonian dysarthric patients may have "inflexible" respiratory patterns for speech. This inflexibility may be manifested by a reduction in lung volume excursions for utterance (Kim, 1968) or a restricted use of chest wall part combinations to achieve lung volume displacements (Hunker et al., 1981). These observations appear to be consistent with the generalized muscular rigidity that is characteristic of Parkinson's disease.

SUMMARY

It seems obvious that persons with speech disorders are quite heterogeneous with respect to the way they use the respiratory system for speech production. Some persons with disordered speech have essentially normal speech breathing characteristics, whereas others evidence abnormalities in lung volume range, chest wall configuration, or the coordination of chest wall parts for achieving lung volume displacements. Specific speech breathing abnormalities do not appear to be associated with specific disorders, and many patients who would seem to be likely candidates for chest wall control problems (e.g., those of Putnam et al., 1981) have normal speech breathing patterns. In those areas where only a small number of subjects has been studied, such as Parkinson's disease and cerebellar ataxia, more data are needed to describe the range of speech breathing behaviors that characterize the disorders. Clinical experience suggests that stuttering (see Hunker et al., 1981) and voice disorders are sometimes associated with speech breathing problems, so instrumental analysis might be fruitful in these areas. In a recent study by Baken, McManus, and Cavallo (1983) the prephonatory configuration of the chest wall of stutterers and normal speakers was shown to be essentially identical; however, more in depth analysis of chest wall behavior *during* speech is required before ruling out disturbances of speech breathing in stutterers.

FUTURE DIRECTIONS

In this author's opinion, research on speech breathing appears to be at a sort of plateau. The modern methods of respiratory physiology have been applied successfully to speech production behavior (Baken et al., 1979; Hixon et al., 1973, 1976), and many of the general questions about respiratory function for speech have been answered. There are several areas, however, in which knowledge is limited and more is needed for a complete account of speech breathing. For example, the function of specific respiratory muscles during speech production is not well understood, even though results from a fair amount of EMG work have been published (e.g., Adams and Munro, 1973; Draper et al., 1959; Eblen, 1963; Hoshiko, 1960; Munro and Adams, 1971). Because the pattern of rib cage intercostal activity is lung volume–dependent (Sears, 1971), investigators interested in intercostal activity during speech should sample EMG activity in multiple rib interspaces simultaneously. Single interspace sampling for external and internal intercostals, such as used by Draper and associates (1959) and Munro and Adams (1971), cannot provide representative views of overall intercostal contribution to compression or expansion of the rib cage. Similarly, EMG investigations of abdominal muscle activity during speech must sample the heretofore unstudied transverse abdominis muscle, which may be a high-risk structure for electrode insertion (because of its proximity to abdominal contents) but probably can provide the most effective displacement of the abdominal contents and thus of the diaphragm (see Strohl, Mead, Banzett, Loring, and Kosch, 1981). EMG studies that would attend to these methodological issues and be accompanied by movement data, via the kinematics technique, could provide a much more fine-grained understanding of speech breathing than is currently available.

To put the issue of neuromuscular control of speech breathing in a somewhat larger perspective, it would be useful to have a line of inquiry which might be directed at developing and clarifying a model of respiratory motor control for speech. One of the prerequisites for such a model—a firm understanding of the neuroanatomical structures directly and indirectly involved in the regulation of respiratory work—appears to be available, as recently reviewed by Kalia (1981). In a recent theoretical effort, Abbs and Cole (1982) offer speculation on the nature of articulatory motor control that may also be relevant for speech breathing motor control. They discuss the possible role of very fast afferent contributions, via suprabulbar pathways, in coordination of articulatory gestures. Although it is known that intercostal activity may be modulated by spinal level reflex arcs (via muscle spindle output [Sears, 1973]), Abbs and Cole (1982) are more interested in afferent influences on *voluntary,* or consciously prepared movement. Such influences might be useful in the respiratory system for coordinating the relative contribution of rib cage and abdomen–diaphragm to lung volume displacement, so as to maintain the speech-specific posturing of the chest wall throughout changes in lung volume. In this regard, it is noteworthy that Lansing and Meyerink (1981) obtained intended EMG reaction times (RTs) from abdominal muscles as brief as 40 to 60 ms and attributed these to central mechanisms. These intended RTs are sufficiently fast to suggest that afferent information could be used effectively to coordinate chest wall parts for speech breathing. The poor control of the relative contribution of rib cage and abdomen to lung volume displacement observed by Hunker and co-workers (1981) for an ataxic subject seems to make sense here, because the cerebellum is thought to be involved in intended reactions (see references in Abbs and Cole, 1982). Speech breathing characteristics of additional cerebellar ataxics should be studied in conjunction with independent measures of intended RTs (i.e., in the limbs or abdomen) to see if chest wall incoordination is correlated with increased "voluntary" RTs.

One study having the explicit purpose of exploring the nature of central control for speech breathing was reported by Hunker and Abbs (1982). This study demonstrated that chest wall configuration for utterance onset at a predetermined lung volume was *typically* variable, an observation readily inferred from inspection of graphs published by Hixon et al. (1973, pp. 94, 96, 99, 100, 102). Moveover, the concept of *motor equivalence* (Lashley, 1930), wherein the same goal may be accomplished by a variety of combinations of neuromuscular events, was invoked to explain the observation of different chest wall configurations associated with post hoc selected utterances having the same initial subglottal pressure. Motor equivalence would, in fact, seem to offer a reasonable conceptual framework for understanding the variability associated with chest wall configuration for repeated utterances by the same speaker.[4] Hixon and colleagues (1973), in considering this kind of variability in their data, noted that "there are a number of ways to achieve acceptable motions for utterances...whether the motion be in the chest wall or vocal tract" (pp. 107–108). Hunker and Abbs's (1982) data do not bear directly on this issue, however, because subglottal pressure—the "goal" they assume for speech breathing—is *not* the net output of chest wall configuration. Stated otherwise, the variable chest wall configurations observed by Hunker and Abbs (1982) can be related to volume *displacement,* but are not interpretable in terms of volume *compressions.* This is because a given chest wall configuration may be associated with a variety of subglottal pressures, depending on airway resistances at the glottal and supraglottal levels of the speech mechanism. The motor equivalence analysis makes sense only when a given configuration, or position of two or more structures (such as the upper and lower lip, and jaw, in Hughes and Abbs, 1976) yields *one possible output* (such as the amount of mouth opening described in Hughes and Abbs, 1976).

Perhaps one way to gain insight into motor control for speech breathing is to observe the respiratory system's response when normal function is altered either for an entire utterance or at unexpected times during utterance. There is a precedent for this kind of work in the articulatory system, either by the use of bite blocks to fix jaw position (e.g., Gay et al., 1981) or by unexpected perturbations of ongoing movement (Folkins & Abbs, 1975). In respiratory physiology, there is currently a fair amount of work concerning the effects of restricted rib cage or abdominal movements on vegetative aspects of respiratory functions (see Daubenspeck, 1981; DiMarco, Kelsen, Cherniack, Hough, and Gothe, 1981; Scheidt, Hyatt, Rehder, 1981; and various reports in Pengelly, Rebuck, and Campbell, 1974). The methods of these studies could be easily adapted to speech research, and could help answer some interesting questions about speech breathing. For example, if the central nervous system has as a control principle the initiation of utterance at lung volumes at which the alveolar relaxation pressure and subglottal pressure demand are roughly equivalent (Hixon et al., 1976), it might be expected that adjustments of the relaxation pressure function that result from rib cage or abdominal restriction (Scheidt et al,. 1981) would be associated with systematic changes in lung volume initiation levels for utterance. Also, when appropriate output parameters are chosen (i.e., pressure or volume displacement, depending on the type of load applied to the system), it would be interesting to observe neuromuscular and movement responses to unexpected loads, and the relationship of those responses to the variability of the output parameter. The results of DiMarco and associates (1981) would seem to predict that chest wall configuration for speech might be more readily perturbed by the application of rib cage, as compared to abdominal, loads. This result may relate to the fact that abdominal wall displacement must be about four times greater than rib cage displacement to achieve equivalent changes in lung volume.

Another need is for data concerning the development of adult-like speech breathing patterns. This information, which is virtually nonexistent at present, would be of great value not only to our general understanding of developing speech production skills, but also as a basic framework against which developmental speech disorders can be assessed. Although the use of techniques involving deep electrodes or pressure-sensing balloons (Hixon et al., 1976) is contraindicated in child subjects, the kinematics approach is essentially hazard-free and noninvasive. Wilder and Baken (1974) have applied this technique to the study of chest wall configurations associated with infant cry. Finally, there are very few data concerning respiratory–laryngeal interactions during speech production. Studies that would obtain data on various laryngeal functions under varying respiratory conditions (e.g., different starting lung volumes) might prove valuable in understanding how dysfunction of one subsystem can affect the function of another subsystem.[5]

[1]Some details of the "diaphragmatic tuning" explanation of abdominal activity during speech may require modification to be consistent with data reported recently by Braun, Arora, and Rochester (1982). Measurements of roentgenograms of diaphragmatic length and radius of curvature (the latter performed by J. Mead and S. H. Loring) showed a clear shortening of diaphragmatic fibers with increasing lung volume, but little corresponding change in radius of curvature. According to Braun and colleagues (1982), the relative doming of the diaphragm is fairly independent of diaphragmatic contraction; rather, the length of the muscle fibers determines how much contractile force the muscle can develop. The force–length data of Braun and co-workers, (1982) do seem to suggest a force peak at physiological rest length of diaphragmatic fibers, so the issue is whether or not "diaphragmatic tuning" would make sense in terms of fiber length alone, as opposed to relative doming of the diaphragm. Because any distortion of diaphragm fiber length from rest length should decrease the force-generating capabilities of the muscle, a postive Ppl applied to the diaphragm could reduce contractile efficiency by distorting diaphragmatic fibers regardless of the relative doming of the muscle. Thus, diaphragmatic tuning by abdominal muscle activity still seems to be a reasonable concept, but the effect on the diaphragm may not be to maintain the dome shape, but to prevent distortion of muscle fiber lengths.

[2]This pattern of muscular activity is not characteristic of conversational speech, in which the typical starting lung volume is such that the available relaxation pressure usually does not exceed the subglottal pressure demand (Hixon et al., 1976). The present discussion is more concerned with speaking tasks which, for example, start at very high lung volumes (e.g. sustaining a vowel) and continue to relatively low lung volumes. There are apparently some cases during conversational speech in which the speaker will take a deeper-than-normal inspiration and begin speaking at a lung volume where the relaxation pressure slightly exceeds the alveolar pressure demand (Hixon et al., 1976, p. 334).

[3]Unpublished manuscript, "Influence of mechanical and linguistic factors on volume changes during speech," made available to the author by Dr. D. M. Bless. See also Bless and Miller (1972).

[4]Another example of motor equivalence in speech breathing is the case of speakers with severely disordered breathing mechanisms who nevertheless manage to produce "normal-sounding" speech. Hixon, Putnam, and Sharp (1983) have recently described the physiological adjustments for speech breathing made by a 48 year old man with paralyzed rib cage muscles, abdominal muscles, and diaphragm. This patient generated and maintained adequate levels of P_s for speech by employing a combination of muscular mechanisms. To raise lung volume above REL, and so take advantage of the positive recoil pressures generated by the lung–thorax unit, the patient used so-called "accessory" inspiratory muscles to apply small lifting forces to the rib cage, and laryngeal and supralaryngeal muscles to pump air into the lungs ("frog breathing"). Once positive P_s had been generated by these actions, the natural recoil to REL was slowed by increased flow resistance at laryngeal and supralaryngeal valves. Hixon and colleagues (1983) suggest that such adjustments may not have to be learned following loss of function, but may be effected more or less automatically. This is reminiscent of bite-block studies (Gay, Lindblom and Lubker, 1981) in which subjects make automatic lingual compensations to adjust for a fixed jaw and produce an acceptable formant pattern for a vowel.

[5]The writing of this chapter was supported in part by NINCDS Award NS13274. I am deeply indebted to Susan Ellis Weismer, and especially to Diane M. Bless, for their valuable comments on earlier versions of the chapter. Ann Fennell also provided helpful comments on a later draft of the manuscript. My intellectual debt to Thomas J. Hixon should be obvious throughout the chapter, but any deficiencies or errors are my own responsibility.

REFERENCES

Abbs, J. H., and Cole, K. J. (1982). Consideration of bulbar and suprabulbar afferent influences upon speech motor coordination. In S. Grillner, A. Persson, B. Lindblom, and J. Lubker (Eds.), *Speech motor control.* New York: Pergamon Press.

Adams, C., and Munro, R. R. (1973). The relationship between internal intercostal muscle activity and pause placement in the connected utterance of native and non-native speakers of English. *Phonetica, 28,* 227–250.

Agostoni, E. (1970a). Statics. In E. J. M. Campbell, E. Agostoni, and J. Newsom Davis (Eds.), *The respiratory muscles: Mechanics and neural control.* Philadelphia: W. B. Saunders.

Agostoni, E. (1970b). Dynamics. In E. J. M. Campbell, E. Agostoni, and J. Newsom Davis (Eds.), *The respiratory muscles: Mechanics and neural control.* Philadelphia: W. B. Saunders.

Baken, R. J. (1977). Estimation of lung volume change from torso hemicircumferences. *Journal of Speech and Hearing Research, 20,* 808–812.

Baken, R. J., and Cavallo, S. A. (1981). Prephonatory chest wall posturing. *Folia Phoniatrica, 33,* 193–203.

Baken, R. J., Cavallo, S. A., and Weissman, K. L. (1979). Chest wall movements prior to phonation. *Journal of Speech and Hearing Research, 22,* 862–872.

Bishop, B. Abdominal muscle activity during respiration. (1974). In B. Wyke (Ed.), *Ventilatory and phonatory control systems.* London: Oxford University Press.

Bless, D. M., and Miller, J. F. (1972). *Mechanical and linguistic factors influencing lung volumes in speech.* Paper presented at the Annual Convention of the American Speech and Hearing Association, San Francisco.

Borden, G. J., and Harris, K. S. (1980). *Speech science primer: Physiology, acoustics, and perception of speech*. Baltimore: Williams & Wilkins.

Braun, N. M. T., Arora, N. S., and Rochester, D. F. (1982). Force-length relationship of the normal human diaphragm. *Journal of Applied Physiology: Respiratory, Environmental and Exercise Physiology, 53*, 405–412.

Campbell, E. J. M., and Newsom Davis, J. (1970). The intercostal muscles and other muscles of the rib cage. In E. J. M. Campbell, E. Agostoni, and J. Newson Davis (Eds.), *The respiratory muscles: Mechanics and neural control*. Philadelphia: W. B. Saunders.

Conrad, B. and Schonle, P. (1979). Speech and respiration. *Archiv fur Psychiatrie und Nervenkrankheiten, 226*, 251–268.

Daniloff, R. G., Schuckers, G. H., and Feth, L. (1980). *The science of speech and hearing*. Englewood Cliffs, NJ: Prentice-Hall.

Darley, F. L., Aronson, A. E., and Brown, J. R. (1975). *Motor speech disorders*. Philadelphia: W. B. Saunders.

Daubenspeck, J. A. (1981). Influence of small mechanical loads on variability of breathing pattern. *Journal of Applied Physiology: Respiratory, Environmental, and Exercise Physiology, 50*, 299–306.

Dickson, D. R., and Maue-Dickson, W. (1982). *Anatomical and physiological bases of speech*. Boston: Little, Brown and Company.

DiMarco, A. F., Kelsen, S. G., Cherniack, N. S., Hough, W. H., and Gothe, B. (1981). Effects on breathing of selective restriction of movement of the rib cage and abdomen. *Journal of Applied Physiology: Respiratory, Environmental, and Exercise Physiology, 50*, 412–420.

Draper, M. H., Ladefoged, P., and Whitteridge, D. (1959). Respiratory muscles in speech. *Journal of Speech and Hearing Research, 2*, 16–27.

Draper, M. H., Ladefoged, P., and Whitteridge, D. (1960). Expiratory muscles and airflow during speech. *British Medical Journal, 18*, 1837–1843.

Eblen, R. E., Jr. (1963). Limitations on use of surface electromyography in studies of speech breathing. *Journal of Speech and Hearing Research, 6*, 3–18.

Euler, C. von (1982). Some aspects of speech breathing physiology. In S. Grillner, B. Lindblom, J. Lubker, and A. Persson (Eds.), *Speech motor control*. New York: Pergamon Press.

Feudo, P., Jr., Zubick, H. H., and Strome, M. (1982). Air volumes during connected speech of normal-hearing and hearing-impaired adults. *Journal of Communication Disorders, 15*, 309–318.

Folkins, J. W., and Abbs, J. H. (1975). Lip and jaw motor control during speech. *Journal of Speech and Hearing Research, 19*, 207–220.

Forner, L. L., and Hixon, T. J. (1977). Respiratory kinematics in profoundly hearing-impaired speakers. *Journal of Speech and Hearing Research, 20*, 373–408.

Gay, T., Lindblom, B., and Lubker, J. (1981). Production of bite-block vowels: Acoustic equivalence by selective compensation. *Journal of the Acoustical Society of America, 69*, 802–810.

Goldman Eisler, F. (1968). *Psycholinguistics experiments in spontaneous speech*. London: Academic Press.

Grosjean, F., and Collins, M. (1979). Breathing, pausing and reading. *Phonetica, 36*, 98–114.

Hardcastle, W. J. (1976). *Physiology of speech production*. London: Academic Press.

Hixon, T. J. (1973). Respiratory function in speech. In F. D. Minifie, T. J. Hixon, and F. Williams (Eds.), *Normal aspects of speech, hearing, and language*. Englewood Cliffs, NJ: Prentice-Hall.

Hixon, T. J. (1982). Speech breathing kinematics and mechanism inferences therefrom. In S. Grillner, A. Persson, B. Lindblom, and J. Lubker (Eds.), *Speech motor control*. New York: Pergamon Press.

Hixon, T. J., Goldman, M., and Mead, J. (1973). Kinematics of the chest wall during speech production: Volume displacements of the rib cage, abdomen, and lung. *Journal of Speech and Hearing Research, 16,* 78–115.

Hixon, T. J., Mead, J., and Goldman, M. D. (1976). Dynamics of the chest wall during speech production: Function of the thorax, rib cage, diaphragm, and abdomen. *Journal of Speech and Hearing Research, 19,* 297–356.

Hixon, T., Weismer, G., and Putnam, A. H. B. (1979). *A tutorial requiem for the Edinburgh studies of speech breathing physiology.* Paper presented at the Annual Convention of the American Speech-Language-Hearing Association, Atlanta, Georgia.

Hofmann, W. W., Alston, W., and Rowe, G. (1966). A study of individual neuromuscular junctions in myotonia. *Electroencephalography and Clinical Neurophysiology, 21,* 521–537.

Horii, Y., and Cooke, P. A. (1978). Some airflow, volume, and duration characteristics of oral reading. *Journal of Speech and Hearing Research, 21,* 470–481.

Hoshiko, M. S. (1960). Sequence of action of breathing muscles during speech. *Journal of Speech and Hearing Research, 3,* 291–297.

Hoshiko, M. (1965). Lung volume for initiation of phonation. *Journal of Applied Physiology, 20,* 480–482.

Hunker, C. J., and Abbs, J. H. (1982). Respiratory movement control during speech: Evidence for motor equivalence. *Society for Neuroscience, 8,* 946. (Abstract)

Hunker, C. J., Bless, D. M., and Weismer, G. (1981). *Respiratory inductive plethysmography: A clinical technique for assessing respiratory function for speech.* Paper presented at the Annual Convention of the American Speech-Language-Hearing Association, Los Angeles.

Itoh, M., Horii, Y., Daniloff, R. G., and Binnie, C. A. (1982). Selected aerodynamic characteristics of deaf individuals during various speech and nonspeech tasks. *Folia Phoniatrica, 34,* 191–209.

Kalia, M. P. (1981). Anatomical organization of central respiratory neurons. *Annual Reviews of Physiology, 43,* 105–120.

Kim, R. (1968). The chronic residual respiratory disorder in post-encephalitic parkinsonism. *Journal of Neurology, Neurosurgery, and Psychiatry, 31,* 393–398.

Kunze, L. H. (1964). Evaluation of methods of estimating sub-glottal air pressure. *Journal of Speech and Hearing Research, 7,* 151–164.

Ladefoged, P. (1960). The regulation of subglottal pressure. *Folia Phoniatrica, 12,* 169–175.

Ladefoged, P. (1962). Sub-glottal activity during speech. In A. Sovijarvi and P. Aalto (Eds.), *Proceedings of the Ninth International Congress of Phonetic Sciences.* The Hague, Netherlands: Mouton & Co.

Ladefoged, P. (1964). Comment on "Evaluation of methods of estimating sub-glottal air pressure." *Journal of Speech and Hearing Research, 7,* 291.

Ladefoged, P. (1967). *Three areas of experimental phonetics.* London: Oxford University Press.

Ladefoged, P. (1974). Respiration, laryngeal activity and linguistics. In B. Wyke (Ed.), *Ventilatory and phonatory control systems.* London: Oxford University Press.

Ladefoged, P., Draper, M. H., and Whitteridge, D. (1958). Syllables and stress. *Miscellanea Phonetica, 3,* 1–14.

Lansing, R. W., and Meyerink, L. (1981). Load compensating responses of human abdominal muscles. *Journal of Physiology, 320,* 253–268.

Lashley, K. S. (1930). Basic neural mechanisms in behavior. *Psychological Review, 37,* 1–24.

Lieberman, P. (1967). *Intonation, perception, and language.* Cambridge, MA: MIT Press.

Lieberman, P. (1977). *Speech physiology and acoustic phonetics.* New York: Macmillan.

Loring, S. H., and Mead, J. (1982). Abdominal muscle use during quiet breathing and hyperpnea in uninformed subjects. *Journal of Applied Physiology: Respiratory, Environmental, and Exercise Physiology, 52,* 700–704.

MacNeilage, P. F. (1972). Speech physiology. In J. H. Gilbert (Ed.), *Speech and cortical functioning*. New York: Academic Press.

Munro, R. R., and Adams, C. (1971). Electromyography of the intercostal muscles in connected speech. *Electromyography, 3–4*, 365–378.

Newsom Davis, J. (1970). Introduction. In E. J. M. Campbell, E. Agostoni, and J. Newsom Davis (Eds.), *The respiratory muscles: Mechanics and neural control*. Philadelphia: W. B. Saunders.

Pengelly, L. D., Rebuck, A. S., and Campbell, E. J. M. (Eds.) (1974). *Loading breathing*. Edinburgh: Churchill Livingstone.

Putnam, A. H. B., Hixon, T. J., and Stern, L. Z. (1981). *Chest wall behavior in speakers with motor neuron disease*. Paper presented at the Annual Convention of the American Speech-Language-Hearing Association, Los Angeles.

Roussos, C., and Macklem, P. T. (1982). The respiratory muscles. *New England Journal of Medicine, 307*, 786–797.

Sackner, M. A. (1979). *Monitoring of ventilation without physical connection to the airway: A review*. Paper presented at the Third International Symposium on Ambulatory Monitoring, Clinical Research Center, Middlesex, United Kingdom.

Scheidt, M., Hyatt, R. E., and Rehder, K. (1981). Effects of rib cage or abdominal restriction on lung mechanics. *Journal of Applied Physiology: Respiratory, Environmental, and Exercise Physiology, 51*, 1115–1121.

Sears, T. A. (1971). Breathing: A sensorimotor act. *Scientific Basis of Medicine, Annual Reviews*, 129–147.

Sears, T. A. (1973). Servo-control of the intercostal muscles. In J. E. Desmedt (Ed.), *New developments in electromyography and clinical neurophysiology*. Basel: S. Karger.

Strohl, K. P., Mead, J., Banzett, R. B., Loring, S. H., and Kosch, P. C. (1981). Regional differences in abdominal muscle activity during various maneuvers in humans. *Journal of Applied Physiology: Respiratory, Environmental, and Exercise Physiology, 51*, 1471–1476.

Warren, D. W. (1976). Aerodynamics of speech production. In N. J. Lass (Ed.), *Contemporary issues in experimental phonetics*. New York: Academic Press.

Whitehead, R. L., and Metz, D. E. (1982). *The mechanics of abnormal laryngeal devoicing gestures exhibited by deaf persons*. Paper presented at the 103rd Meeting of the Acoustical Society of America, Chicago.

Wilder, C. N. (1983). Chest wall preparation for phonation in female speakers. In D. M. Bless and J. H. Abbs (Eds.), *Vocal fold physiology*. San Diego: College-Hill Press.

Wilder, C. N., and Baken, R. J. (1974). Respiratory patterns in infant cry. *Human Communication, 3*, 18–34.

Zemlin, W. R. (1968). *Speech and hearing science: Anatomy and physiology*. Englewood Cliffs, NJ: Prentice-Hall.

CHAPTER 3

A Phenomenological Model for Vowel Production in the Vocal Tract

Herbert M. Teager
Shushan M. Teager

There are perhaps three primary justifications for formulating alternative physical models to supplant "established" ones: utility, purity, and interest. Of these, utility might be the most objective and important. If a theory fits available experimental evidence and accurately predicts outcome, the normal tendency is to accept it. These criteria can, however, become very subjective if the accepted bounds of accuracy are too loose or the range of critical experimental tests too narrow to reveal the possibility of circular reasoning. Purity, on the other hand, is more concerned with natural laws. A physical model, even if it can be made to yield useful predictions, is suspect if the underlying physics is either demonstrably wrong or too inelegant. Indeed, some theories, because of their seeming elegance, are defended tenaciously even though they cannot predict accurately. Interest is the most subjective and treacherous of the three. Several areas of classical physics, believed to have been thoroughly codified and explored by eminent scientists of the past, are incomplete, but since technology has bypassed the need for particular devices, the fields have become moot or are left as interesting intellectual problems. This is the case for large areas of fluid dynamics and acoustic hydrodynamics in particular.

Physiological models, in general, have additional obvious and subtle difficulties. For example, complete and accurate fluid measurements cannot readily be made inside the tortuous internal geometries of a living system, nor can parameters be conveniently varied or even held constant. Moreover, such models might be intertwined with other models even less susceptible to experiment. This is especially true of speech, which is interlinked with hearing, because it requires feedback from the latter. Thus, speech models tacitly depend on the validity of models for hearing.

The established models for speech and hearing are strongly coupled in linear filter theory. In the current view, the voice produces pure-tone frequency components, and the ear, an imperfect Fourier analyzer, is believed to extract the magnitude of these objective components. Even Helmholtz (1954/1885), the founding father of this field, was aware of the fact that an animate ear had to include additional efficient means of locating and classifying transient noises in a natural, nontonal world. Further, if significant nonlinear effects exist in either the voice or hearing, they cannot be readily predicted, tested, or verified by linear theory.

Scientists are seldom so rash as to declare, or even imply, that a theory is perfect or complete in all respects. Scientific leadership, however, may differ greatly in its willingness to acknowledge anomalous findings. Past revolutions in "pure" science have begun over seemingly infinitessimal experimental discrepancies with theory. Indeed, much of the zest in modern physics seems to be derived from searching for such small anomalies. In the case of speech, it is believed by some that the source filter theory explains more than 90% of the observed effects. However, neither the remaining 10% nor the total range of effects ever seem to be specified. This being the case, we suggest our own list of anomalies, including some that the purist might consider "anecdotal" in the absence of footnotes, but which we nevertheless believe to be demonstrably true and readily confirmable.

1. Only highly limited and constrained speech recognition and speech generation devices have been developed over the past 50 years; compared to human abilities, they could be held as comparative failures. The current rationale allows that such failures are tolerable and not due to any inadequacies of the speech and hearing models, but rather hinge on our imperfect understanding of the human brain. If this is the case, how can we explain the abilities of a myna bird, a natural mimic who not only can repeat an astonishing repertoire of noises, but also can produce long passages of speech in a voice indistinguishable from that of its trainer? Yet the bird has a cochlea that is anatomically far too short for place frequency selection, lacks a standard vocal tract, and obviously has a limited cerebral cortex.

2. As von Kempelen (1791) pointed out nearly 200 years ago and a recent do-it-yourself book expounds (Newman, 1980), humans using their vocal tract apparatus are capable of generating a large number of clicks, whistles, snores, barnyard sounds, and other noises that do not fit a conventional source filter model because their sources are not glottal.

3. Theoretically, the formant values of speech depend solely upon the cross-sectional areas along the center line of the supraglottal vocal tract and are directly proportional to the velocity of sound in whatever gas fills the tract. How then can we explain the frequency changes in formants which occur in air at high or low pressure (Licklider and Kryter, 1958)? Similarly,

how do we explain the unexpectedly low formant shifts in pure helium and other gas mixtures at atmospheric pressure (Teager and Teager 1981; Wathen-Dunn and Michaels, 1968). Why are we unable to produce speech when our mouths and throats are parched, or after eating a dry cracker? Finally, how do voices change with illness and changes in the teeth that affect neither the glottis nor the tract area substantially?

4. Several anomalous observations can easily be made if a standard Fourier analysis is performed on a sustained vowel produced without changing the tract configuration. (a) During start up, the formant values take time to build up in amplitude and migrate to their final values, but they quench far more rapidly at their end. What is changing within the system? (b) During the "constant" portion of a sustained vowel with no variation in pitch, considerable variations in the pitch period–to–pitch period values (and occasionally location) of the formant spectral components have been found where theoretically none should exist. (c) Similarly, during this same constant portion, spectral zeros (a complete absence or cancellation) also appear, migrate, and disappear. The vocal tract ladder network "filter" cannot produce zeros. While the glottal "source" might be postulated to do so, such a zero would have to be of the absorption type.

5. It is generally believed that the time domain analysis of voice signals can offer no additional insights compared to vector harmonic frequency analysis. Although this may be trivially true in a mathematical world, it is not true in any finite, bounded, "efficient" processing system. Moreover, it is completely false if the generating system is nonlinear. In either case, if the theory is correct, time and frequency domain observations should not conflict.

Let us consider several cases in which they clearly do conflict. As a general rule, vowel time waveforms are singularly asymmetrical with respect to plus and minus wave shapes and swings, implying a harmonic bias. Further, for many sustained vowels, the first formant is found to build up quite rapidly over a single pitch period and then decay at a slower rate, going virtually to zero before the next pitch period begins. Similarly, the frequency of the formant, as determined from zero crossings, for example, can vary considerably over a single pitch period. Furthermore, the waveform shape remains essentially invariant as pitch is varied, although it might be truncated or expanded. An even stronger observation can be made in the case of some second formants. They not only rise and decay far more rapidly than the first formant, but also may do so one or more times during a single pitch period. Their timing and phase are generally random. Indeed, such second formants can, and often do, elicit a frequency domain zero by cancellation and not by a total absence. Obviously, neither phenomenon is consistent with a passive source filter model. The theoretical glottal source produces all harmonics of the basic pitch period, and unless we allow ourselves exceptional ad hoc harmonic control of the source wave shape, particularly as pitch is varied, adjacent higher harmonics of the glottal spectra are of similar magnitude. Yet, as pitch is varied, wave shape stays constant, a condition that requires a shift in harmonic balance. For a passive linear system to resonate at a formant frequency with an amplitude 5 or 10 times greater than that of the adjacent harmonics, a high Q system is required. The theoretical amplitude of the formant thus not only will be slowly varying over many pitch periods, but also will have the same rise and decay times. A multiply excited second formant, quite clearly, is not allowed by theory (Guillemin, 1949).

6. By neglecting flow effects, the accepted theory has not adequately addressed the mechanical energy balance in the vocal tract. If, as has been claimed (Flanagan, 1965), only a fraction of a percentage point of the energy from the lungs is propagated as an acoustic wave beyond the mouth, where then has the substantial balance of kinetic and potential energy gone? The Bernoulli equation, which holds along any actual path, or streamline, taken by air flow in the absence of loss, equates a pressure drop with velocity squared. The acoustic model insists that pressure and flow are in phase and in proportion to the acoustic impedance. Obviously, both equations cannot be correct simultaneously.

Although the above-mentioned anomalies have been known for relatively long periods of time, they have not, to our knowledge, been addressed directly, even though their solution requires no particularly unique experimental technique or instrumentation. We have, as has been pointed out in previous papers, been making air velocity and vibration measurements in the vocal tract for the past decade, and can append to these last six items an additional list of physical anomalies from our own work and other published papers concerned with flow (Teager, 1980; Teager and Teager, 1981).

7. During phonation, air flow in the mouth, and most probably in the rest of the vocal tract, is separated, not isotropic. That is to say, the flow, instead of being stable and uniform across any cross section during a single pitch period, is time varying, concentrated near surfaces, and can switch many times between those surfaces.

8. Formants are present in the interior flows that do not exist in the output sound, and vice versa. Formants also vary between flows measured in differing mouth locations.

9. Mouth flows and pressures are not related by the acoustic impedance of air. Our published work for the sustained front vowels, at normal volume, showed pulsatile first formant flows in the mouth going from approximately

3 cm/s to a peak of 300 cm/s in one pitch period. Flow in the mouth was measured at the back, where, because of the measuring array's size the minimum cross-sectional area was 5 cm². A maximum area of about 20 cm² was attained toward the front of the mouth. From the characteristic acoustic impedance of air in free space, this pulsating velocity of 300 cm/s could be equated to a corresponding pressure of 12,000 dynes/cm² or, an absurdly high value of 150 dB. The actual measured peak mouth pressure was close to 110 dB; in other words, there was a hundredfold discrepancy between the measurements and theoretical predictions. It might be postulated that an area function correction could reduce this by a factor of 4 or 5, but this still leaves a large amount of kinetic energy unaccounted for.

METHODS AND AEROACOUSTIC MEASUREMENTS

Our previously published work concentrated on the axial flow measurements taken across an internal cross section during phonation (Teager, 1980). Several years ago, in order to further explore the physical mechanisms of speech, we ran an additional series of sustained vowel measurements with probe trajectories along the geometric flow center line of the oral area, as shown in Figure 3–1, and externally across the front of the lips. In addition to the usual equilateral array of hot wire anemometers, as shown in Figure 3–2 (1 cm centers, top two horizontal, plane of sensor vertical) a wide-band miniature microphone (phase and amplitude checked against the external microphone located about 3 inches from the mouth) was placed in the array plane (Appendix 3–I). Since in the previous runs we had found only minor left–right flow differences in the middle of the mouth, the left axial hot wire sensor was replaced by one sensitive only to sidewise, or radial flows, in the plane of the cross section. These trajectories provided more insight into different vowel patterns and mechanisms. Only one vowel, however, is discussed here.

Figure 3–3 is a condensed, pitch-synchronous, multichannel set of tracings for an approximately center-line trajectory, starting from the back and out through the front of the mouth, during the sustained vowel "oo" in "book" (ʊ). Each trace is an average of four successive pitch periods starting with pitch period 4 and ending with pitch period 656. The probe was moved at a constant velocity during the experiment, whereas pitch period was held constant at about 5 ms. The columns of traces from left to right are as follows: external pressure microphone (sound), internal

Figure 3–1. Probe trajectory. Adapted from an actual x-ray transparency taken during the phonation of "oo" (book) (ʊ) without a probe.

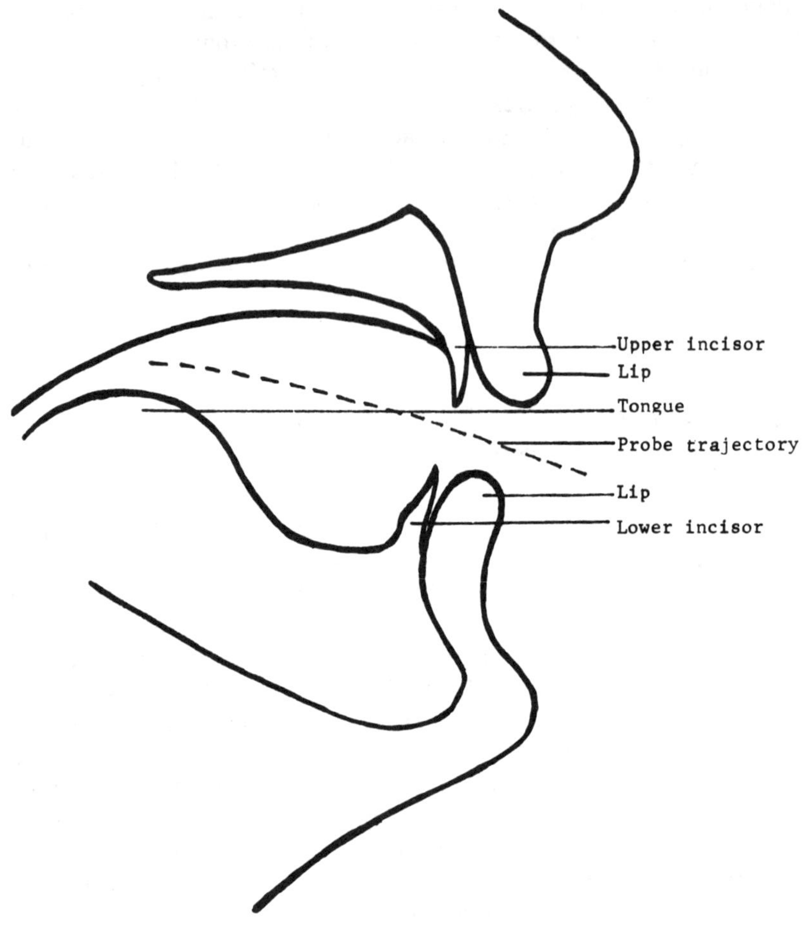

pressure microphone (mouth), top axial flow, top radial flow, and bottom axial flow. These are referred to as columns 1, 2, 3, 4, and 5, respectively. Pressures within the mouth were always positive, with peak amplitudes at 115 dB. Flow peaks were on the order of 5 ft/s (150 cm/s), while minima were on the order of 0.1 ft/s (3cm/s) with no evidence of flow reversals.

Figure 3–4 presents the corresponding data for a trajectory across the front of the lips, left to right, for the same vowel. The same convention detailed for Figure 3–3 is used. Since the trajectory outside the mouth is shorter, there are fewer pitch periods. For comparison with measured

Figure 3–2. Instruments used in aeroacoustic measurements. *A*, Detail of hot wire, supports, and protective wire (shroud). *B*, Normal (*1*) and axial (*2*) probe cartridges. Scale: 0.2 inch. *C*, Triple probe assembly without cartridges (*1*), surface accelerometer (*2*), and preamplifier (*3*). *D*, Oblique view of probe end, showing sockets, central light, angle spreader microphone, and finger switch.

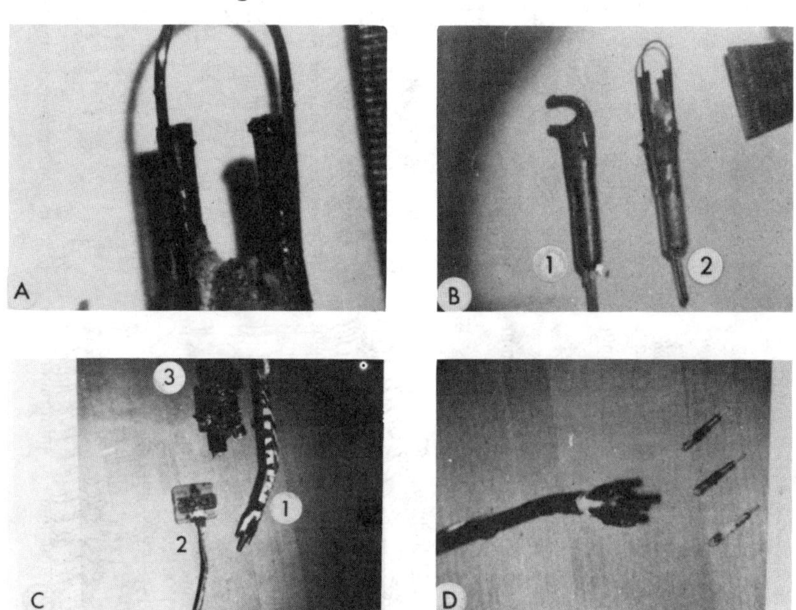

variables, synchronous "theoretical flow" curves, computed from the external sound integral, are shown under each column for both sets of trajectories.

Much of the formant frequency structure can be seen in these tracings before any Fourier analyses are performed. The pitch frequency is about 200 Hz; the first formant can be seen as an oscillation in the pressures occurring two to three times per period, that is, at about 600 Hz; the 2500 Hz second formant is visible as an additional low amplitude fluctuation superimposed on the traces. These are most clearly seen in Figure 3–3, columns 3 and 5.

Two versions of Figure 3–3 (*a* and *b*) have been included. The first (*a*) is marked and annotated, whereas the second (*b*) is left unmarked for clarity. From the wealth of qualitative data in the trajectories for this vowel, we point out only the most salient features and anomalies.

10. Flow not only is separated, as shown by the differences between the top and bottom axial traces (Figure 3–3, columns 3 and 5), but it also

Figure 3–3a. Annotated version of multichannel tracings for sustained "oo" vowel (book). Probe trajectory: from back of mouth to front of mouth.

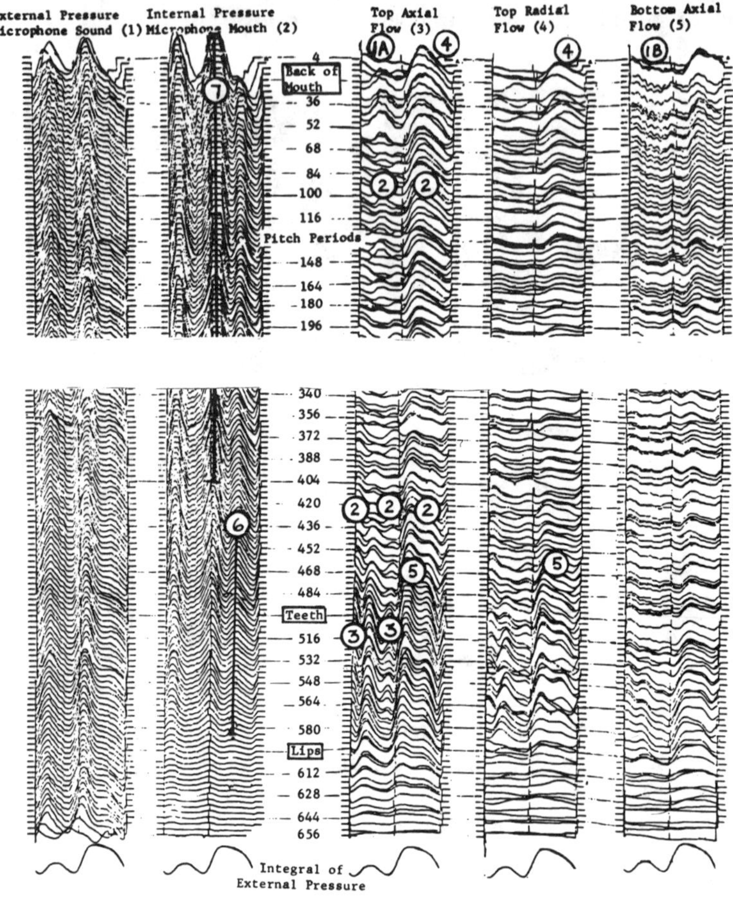

(1), 2500 Hz flow fluctuation is restricted to the back of the mouth. Fluctuations are out of phase, indicating a whistle source with the upper pharynx forming a cavity. (2), Distinct flow pulses. (3), Evidence of collisions at front of the mouth corresponding to pressure rises. (4, 5,) Evidence of swirl. (6), Rapid pressure loss behind lips. (7), Artifactual pressure clipping on positive peaks.

Figure 3–3*b*. Unmarked version of multichannel tracings for sustained "oo" vowel (book). Probe trajectory: from back of mouth to front of mouth.

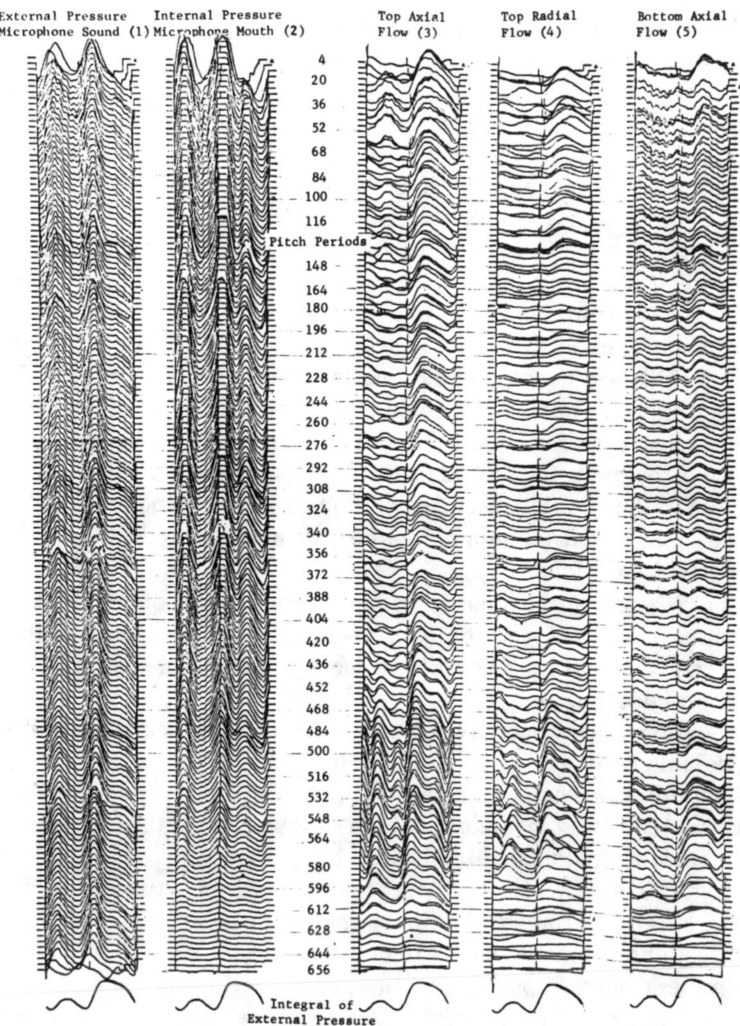

appears to travel as discrete *pulses* in time and space both within and beyond the mouth (Figure 3–3, column 3 [2]). These pulses show only minor delays consistent with near-sonic velocity. Pulse features occur at very nearly the same position within the pitch period over a long distance, indicating that the flow wave is not traveling at the speed of flow, but at a much faster, near-sonic, velocity.

11. The axial flow pulses at the back of the mouth and near the teeth in columns 3 and 5 are comparable to the simultaneous radial flows in column 4. These data indicate a sidewise swirl, and thus the presence of a vortex, whose axis is aligned along the probe trajectory. The axial vortex is inconsistent with a one-dimensional flow model.

12. There is evidence for high-frequency second formant (2500 Hz) flow oscillations at the back of the mouth seen as low-amplitude wiggles in each trace (Figure 3–3, columns 3 and 5 [1]). These are multiply excited during a pitch period, as shall be seen later. A close comparison of columns 3 and 5 will show that the upper and lower axial second formant flows are out of phase. The lack of a radial component (column 4) to this second formant flow indicates a deflection of the separated flow in the vertical plane. Furthermore, the second formant is less evident in the flows toward the front of the mouth; however, the second formant in the pressure waves remains unchanged (columns 1 and 2), demonstrating little amplitude change with position.

13. Whereas approximately 20 pitch periods are required before the sound reaches a steady state (Figure 3–3, column 1), it quenches in less than eight pitch periods, 648 to 656, without perceptible change in the vocal tract configuration.

14. Although the decrease in mouth pressure from back to front (Figure 3–3, column 2 [6] and [7]) might have the appearance of a standing wave in a quarter-wavelength chamber, this picture is not borne out by flow, which has its greatest magnitude at both ends with a pronounced minimum in the middle, analogous to half-wave behavior.

Figure 3–4 shows similar evidence of separation between axial flows for the left–right front of the lip trajectory for the same vowel, as well as indications of marked left-to-right asymmetry in the exit of individual flow pulses from the lips. Swirling flow, or an axial vortex, is more evident at the left and right corners than in the middle, where the radial flows are smaller in comparison to axial flows.

Additional, more qualitative conclusions can be drawn by examining the relevant Fourier analyses, shown in Figure 3–5, of the sound and flow data in Figure 3–3. The frequency response for both the flow sensors and the external microphones was flat over the range shown. The subminiature mouth microphone had a loss in its response below 1 kHz. The additive

Figure 3–4. Multichannel tracings for sustained "oo" vowel (book). Probe trajectory: Left to right in front of mouth (outside). Five pulse positions, labeled 1 to 5, are shown. Pulses 1 and 3 disappear at the right side of the mouth. Pulses 2 and 5 are not present at the left side of the mouth. Pulse 4 is uniform on both sides of the mouth.

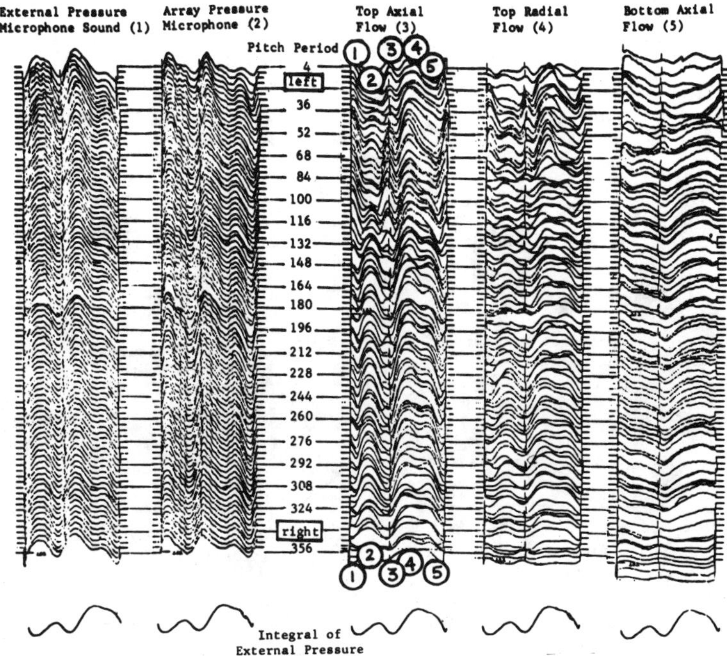

correction for calibration is shown on the mouth pressure response curves ([*3*] in both series). Fourier analyses of normalized data are shown for four pitch periods of data taken at the back of the mouth (pitch periods 20 to 23, series 1) and near, but behind, the teeth (pitch periods 500 to 503, series 2). These components are plotted on the familiar logarithmic amplitude scale (10 dB/division) and on a linear scale for frequency (1000 Hz/division). It should be noted that a decibel scale can obscure rather large variations, so that an error of ±30% in an expected value, which might horrify an experimentalist, only amounts to 3 dB. Plots for the relative phase information between pressures and flows have not been provided because they showed little or no consistency.

15. High-frequency spectral amplitudes of pressures and flows show very large pitch period-to-pitch period variability, as seen by the scattered

Figure 3–5. Fourier analysis of simultaneous pressures and flows for "oo" vowel (book). *1,2,* **the formant at 2500 Hz (1) is multiply excited per pitch period, with a time varying phase shift between mouth pressure and output sound pressure, leading to false zeros (2).** *3,* **Additive calibration correction.** *4,* **Solid line is plotted through average of spectral values for four sequential pitch periods.**

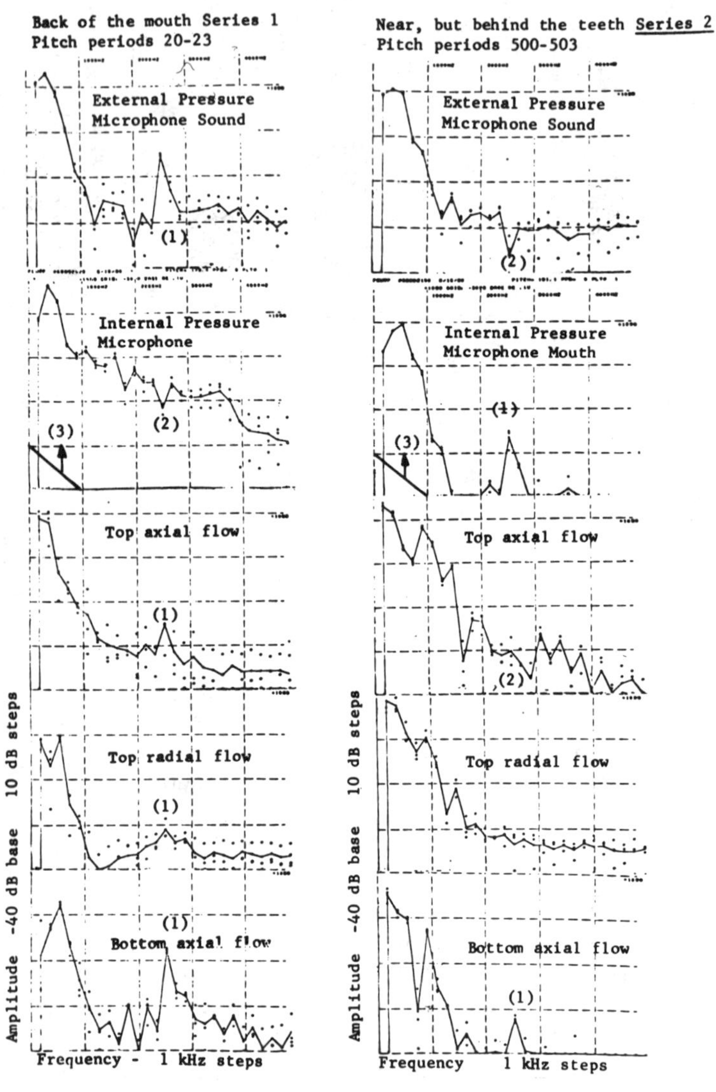

points around the averaged response lines (Figure 3–5, *4*). This variability in high-frequency spectra for sound and mouth pressures is, in part, due to the turbulent air flow generating high-frequency, random, shot-type noise at the lips.

16. The relative sizes of the first five low-frequency harmonics in both series are inconsistent in pressures and flows, as evidenced by the wide variability in spectral shapes. There is too little second harmonic, for example, to account for the second harmonic pressures compared to those of the first harmonic.

17. The 2500 Hz formant plays an all-or-nothing role, appearing as either a zero or a pole in various flows and pressures (Figure 3–5 [*1*] and [*2*] in both series).

18. Whereas peak mouth pressures are far higher and flows somewhat lower than was the case for the front vowels (anomaly 9), the ratio of flow to pressure is an order of magnitude greater than that predicted by acoustic impedance.

MODEL PHYSICS

Physiological model building must rest on a reasonably solid base of known physics if it is to succeed. For the source filter theory, that base is the branch of mathematical physics known as acoustics. Passive linear filter theory modeling is possible because the equations of acoustics are linear and solvable (Morse, 1938; Rayleigh, 1894/1945). Although one might quibble about an occasionally distressing concert hall, acoustic models work fairly well in the design of such zero-average flow transducers as microphones and loudspeakers. In the case of wind instruments, including the human voice, objections that the assumptions and acoustic equations were incorrect in a fundamental and important way were raised in the late 1920s, notably by Bouasse (1929a, b), but seldom heeded. Virtually all theoretical and experimental work with air flows stopped after the 1920s. Since then tests have been conducted with sinusoidal signals from loudspeakers, which produce no apparent average flows and are only monitored with pressure-sensitive microphones. Yet the flow kinetic energy present and available in air-driven sound systems can easily be orders of magnitude greater than the pure acoustic energy tied up in the rate of change of flow. This ignored energy need not quietly disappear in the vocal tract. The deeper we delve into fluid dynamic acoustic interactions, the more we are struck by the paucity of solid physical theory to guide our understanding. While purists might argue that a numerical solution to vocal tract physics can be obtained from the complete nonlinear Navier-Stokes equations, aerodynamicists have always been much more cautious about their validity and verification, particularly in the nonsteady state. Thus, we must proceed cautiously, even if a numerical model might be easier to construct than a physical one.

Flow kinetic energy can produce active, self-excited oscillations and other nonlinear effects forbidden to a passive system. An acoustic filter, on the other hand, is limited to the total acoustic energy in the *exact* frequency bands delivered to it by the source. The energy emerging from the filter in each of the frequencies must always be *less* than the energy of the input.

For an example of active nonlinearity, consider the interaction of a jet and cavity described in a previous paper (Teager and Teager, 1981). A steady jet of air, disregarding the small amount of turbulent noise generated at its edges, produces no acoustic energy since there is no rate of change of flow. However, because of its velocity, the jet obviously contains a prodigious amount of kinetic energy, which is proportional to the source pressure. When the jet excites a cavity, intense sound is produced. From the experimental evidence of the jet's deflection into and out of the cavity described in that paper, we know that the sound energy came from the conversion of a fraction of the jet's kinetic flow energy. The same experiment also determined that a vortex existed within the cavity and that the output sound wave contained strong phase-locked harmonics. The frequency of the system could be altered ±50% by varying the source pressure. The sound amplitude also changed with flow rate and went to zero at high and low limits. It was not mentioned in the paper cited above that the sound was significantly amplitude modulated at the precession rate of the cavity vortex. A linear system could have no such variability.

Another example, known since antiquity, is that an obstacle in the path of a laminar air stream generates a pure "aeolian" tone, and such outstanding scientists as Prandtl (1952) and von Karman and Rubach (1911/1965) studied the problem empirically. They were interested in the effect since it caused substantial drag in wire-braced aircraft. Even von Karman and Rubach, however, chose to study the far simpler problem of downstream vortex stability and spacing in the flow regimens where such vortexes are shed rather than the dynamics of vortex motion. The mechanisms of sound generation *at velocities even below those wherein those vortexes are shed were left unexplored.* Despite all the experimental evidence for its existence, a vortex is incompatible with acoustic theory. Furthermore, although it is known that a vortex moving at constant velocity is silent, it can be detected by sonar, since it reflects sound in much the same fashion as a solid object does. Vortexes themselves are also internally unstable, and can oscillate in a variety of modes (Widnall, 1975).

Although there is a vast gulf in the detailed understanding of separated flows and the dynamics of their associated jets and vortexes, much can be inferred from basic physics and experimental observations, such as the following:

1. The basic conservation laws of mechanics hold true:
   a. Conservation of energy along a streamline—Bernoulli's law.
   b. Conservation of linear and angular momentum during collisions and deflections.
2. Jets, whether free or attached to a wall, always produce vorticity due to the conservation of angular momentum. This vorticity coalesces to produce circulating flows (eddies and vortexes) that grow, in both magnitude and size, with time.

It is generally assumed (Schlichting, 1968) that the pressure in a free or wall-bound jet is zero, all the energy being kinetic, leaving unanswered questions on how energy (pressure) is transmitted when jet flow velocity is changed, as, for example, in a pulse. It is also generally concluded from experimental evidence, and also confirmed by our measurements, that a change in flow speed propagates along a jet at near-sonic velocity, whereas the coupled second-order changes in the jet's spread angle propagate at speeds closer to stream velocity. But does the corresponding propagating pressure wave, predicted by acoustic theory, exist both within and without the jet? Fluid considerations would confine the pressure wave to an area within the jet. Our own experiments on pulsating wall flow seem to rule out energy traveling as an acoustic pulse of pressure and flow on the following grounds:

1. The velocity of the flow pulse, while much faster than stream velocity, seems to be comparable to the velocity of sound, perhaps slightly slower.

2. Pressure always appears to be highly uniform across cross sections, which may include areas of differing flows. The differential pressure along the flow axis is generally smaller, by orders of magnitude, than that which would be predicted by acoustic impedance between pressure and flow magnitudes.

We believe that these flow momentum waves must propagate as solitons (as in a tidal bore), without a corresponding pressure pulse. As solitons, they are nonlinear and nonsuperposable. If they collide with each other or a vortex, they do not pass through one another invisibly, as a sound wave would, but are observed to collide and rebound. When such collisions occur, time-varying pressures (and therefore sounds) which can be computed from the resulting changes in vector momentum, are generated. (see Appendix 3–II). Such collision events easily generate pressure harmonics absent in the original flow frequencies.

Before we proceed to our models for speech, which clearly depend on a very complex internal geometry, let us consider how even a simple cavity excited by a pulsating flow is capable of highly nonlinear behavior. If the cavity geometry is such that an inlet jet does not strike a wall before exiting, the cavity will have no effect whatsoever on the output flow, or sound, and might as well not exist except for second-order effects. If, however, the cavity is large, with an inlet designed to prevent separation and promote internal air mixing, and the system is driven by a unidirectional pulsatile flow source, then the cavity becomes *a resonator for all frequencies and a strong harmonic generator* for the following reason: Flow entering the cavity is integrated to produce a cavity pressure, whereas the exit flow velocity is proportional to the square root of the internal pressure, as dictated by the Bernoulli equation. Thus, if the internal pressure is a sinusoid with a positive minimum value, proportionately less air will leave during positive swings than during negative ones; consequently, the size of the swings and the average cavity pressure value will increase. Furthermore, the output flow will be nonsinusoidal and therefore the cavity will behave as a nonlinear filter.

The foregoing description of the physics is admittedly cursory. As has been indicated before, there is a dearth of applicable hydrodynamic theory that corresponds to readily observable physical effects. Nevertheless, enough is known about the dynamics of separated flows to postulate probable effects in the vocal tract. Further exploration of the hydrodynamic acoustic interactions involved seems worthwhile in order to arrive at a qualitative mathematical description rather than continued adherence to exact linear equations, which, however elegant, fail to predict observed phenomena.

SUGGESTED VOCAL MODELS

We do not propose an overall model that holds true in detail for all phonemic subgroups of vocalization. Instead, we pose a phenomenological explanation that can be applied separately to each phoneme, since we believe that each such sound is, in fact, primarily generated at a different location, taking full advantage of the local shapes and flow instabilities available along the tortuous course of the vocal tract. We do not claim to have completely "proved" our models, but we believe that we have significant verifications.

As suggested earlier, human experimentation is not always practicable, whereas physical model construction and testing have intricate requirements of their own, which cannot be met without deep and extensive experimentation. Let us consider separately how the suggested models apply to the subglottal, glottal (including the larynx), and supraglottal spaces.

Subglottal: Trachea, Bronchi, Lobes, Diaphragm, and Intercostal Muscles

The source filter theory assumes that the subglottal portions of the respirtory system serve as a constant pressure source of air and are driven by the diaphragm and chest muscles during vocalization. The normal argument advanced is that the trachea and bronchi are too short to resonate as a tube at the 100 to 300 Hz frequencies of vocal pitches. Moreover, since the piping cross section increases from trachea to alveoli, any acoustic wave should be completely absorbed at the far end. Experiments, however, seem to indicate otherwise. Measurements taken from probes connected to the trachea show a very large, pitch-synchronous, pressure swing (Koike and Hirano, 1973). Our own measurements, taken with sensitive, ultra-low-mass accelerometers mounted on the chest, demonstrate each lobe of the lungs to be vibrating with different coupled characteristics. The accelerometers are sensitive in the plane in which they are applied and only detect motions perpendicular, or normal, to that plane. These chest wall vibrations, overlying the four major lung lobes, do not show the same structures in either time or frequency domain analysis, and pitch harmonic phase differences can approach 180 degrees between lobes. The left lobes, for example, carry more of the high frequencies. Converted to sound, these vibrations have little in common with the exterior voice. Thus, they are most likely to be real, reflecting underlying lobe motions and air pressures, rather then being artifacts from body-transmitted glottal vibrations.

Let us, therefore, temporarily assume that the lungs are resonant, albeit with the high damping of a "thud" rather than the low-loss "bong" of a bell. Let us further seek a resonance, or rather a set of resonances, that can vary with the lung's physiological state. Since we accept the stricture that the "laws" of acoustics cannot allow a conventional resonance, we must take a deeper than usual look at the physiology of breathing for an explanation. The linear physiological model of the lungs assumes that, during breathing, air moves uniformly into and out of all available paths down to each and every air sac. A little reflection and self-experimentation, listening to our own breathing on a sleepless night, suggest otherwise. The vital parts of the lungs are the air sacs or alveoli, which actually exchange O_2 and CO_2 between blood and air. There is, however, a large volume of air retained in the bronchi and tubing that must be cleared before fresh air reaches the alveoli. During shallow breathing, the tidal volume of fresh air would never get past the inactive conduits if air flow were uniform and laminar. CO_2 and O_2 could then only move slowly by the mechanism of diffusion, and we would die of asphyxiation in our sleep. Luckily we do not breathe in that manner, using the entire lung capacity at all times; instead we use only a few lobes or portions thereof at a time, and thus we have a very efficient respiratory system with fresh mixed air reaching all the way to the alveoli because the flow is separated. Whereas direct air flow measurements within the lungs are generally not feasible, blood flow studies of the lungs show this identical principle in action. Lung lobes are far from equally perfused, and perfusion changes with the pattern of breathing. Consider how this design feature might be implemented.

The common analogy likening the lungs to a set of bellows is highly misleading. In ordinary bellows, the internal air currents take up a negligible amount of energy. The lungs, on the other hand, are excited by local displacements of the surrounding chest wall and diaphragm muscles. The effect is to sequentially squeeze and flatten the air sacs, layer by layer, expelling the air inside with a substantial velocity—and hence with momentum and energy—but with no corresponding pressure rise unless the air is blocked downstream. Thus, the usual physiological technique of estimating dynamic lung air pressures with an esophageal transducer is highly suspect. Such a momentum wave keeps its kinetic energy largely intact as it separates and proceeds along the bronchial surfaces. It will be joined by others similarly induced and travel downstream toward the glottis, without taking any sharp backward turns at convening Y bifurcations. Indeed, some of the air at these branches will be induced to join the downstream flow by aspiration. At a T junction, however, the momentum wave may well split and proceed both upstream to another lobe and downstream to the trachea. The momentum wave, traveling at sonic velocity, will set the flow lines by which bulk gas will move at stream velocity. During inspiration, because of separated flow and the ramified structure of the bronchi, the cycle will not be exactly reversed, but, as the surrounding muscles relax, the air sacs, in the reverse sequential order, can again regain a spherical shape and reinflate themselves from the connecting bronchial air. This part of the cycle sends a negative momentum wave back toward the trachea. The exhalation wave flow pattern differs from the inspirational one with the result that circulating flows, or vortexes, develop at the bifurcations (West, 1977). Such a system can be resonant since pressure energy can be stored both at the glottal end, in the usual acoustic fashion, and as elastic energy in the air sac wall at the alveoli involved.

Although this seems contrary to our usual notion that the walls of a balloon hold only a small fraction of the compression energy released when it is punctured, the ratio of shared energy in elastic walls to volume is 1/radius and alveoli are exceedingly small, with a total surface area equal to that of a football field!

The vortexes and separated flows in the bronchi not only provide nonlinear coupling between the glottis and air sacs, but also allow for the existence of multiple modes of oscillation which can be influenced by the state of lung inflation and by the tension of the intercostal muscles and diaphragm. A simple analogy might be the motion observed in two waterbeds, of different volume, connected by large hoses.

Resonance effects, such as those just described, would not normally be expected in ordinary breathing, but can and do show up with chest percussion and auscultation. The top end of the trachea, however, can be occluded, as it is during phonation, and can reflect momentum waves, in which case we would have a nonlinear coupled system of glottis and lungs that would be phase locked with the lung resonances indicated. We will not explore the implications of this model of the subglottal system further except to note that there should be substantial changes with impaired or abnormal lung function, and that lung resonance effects cannot be ignored.

Glottis (Including the Larynx)

It cannot be claimed that the glottis is a neglected part of the vocal tract. Judging by the number of papers and conferences, it has been the "hottest" and most openly controversial area in vocal model literature over the last few decades. Yet despite static physical model evidence recently presented by several groups showing "separated" air flow at the glottis (Gauffin, Nguyen, Ananthapadmanabha, and Fant, 1981; Titze, Baer, Cooper, and Scherer, 1981), the nonlinear implications upon glottal function do not seem, thus far, to have been considered. The major efforts seem related to a search for mechanisms of motion which can produce both the glottal area–time functions inferred from inverse filtering of speech, and the three-dimensional surface motions observed during phonation. If a fixed passive filter exists, it is clear that only the source is left with which to explain any bothersome anomalies.

There seem to be three basic areas that any glottal model must address:
1. What is the timing mechanism?
2. Where does its exciting energy come from?
3. What are the usual characteristics of exit air flow at the glottis?

1. With respect to timing, most distributed and lumped glottal models assume some variation on coupled masses and springs, which result in a period of oscillation primarily dependent upon the mechanical properties of glottal tissue. This being the case, helium speech poses immediate

difficulties because not only do formants go to higher frequencies, albeit far less than theory predicts, but in addition voice pitch itself goes up by about the same factor as the formants. *The pitch should not change with gas if system timing were determined solely by tissue stiffness and mass.*

2. When we consider the energetics of a self-excited glottis, the current explanations are inconsistent with fluid dynamics. The major difficulty lies in the misapplication of the Bernoulli equations for aerodynamic glottal forces. In the Bernoulli equation, which is a statement of energy conservation, the sum of kinetic (velocity squared) plus potential (pressure) energy is constant and holds *only along the stream path.* If a flow issues from a slit in the form of a slowly spreading jet, downstream velocities—and thus pressure—depend upon the actual jet area and not the available cross-sectional area of the chamber into which it flows. Further, Bernoulli's forces are conservative and are identical for the same glottal edge positions regardless of whether the cords are opening or closing. *Thus, no net energy can be extracted when such forces are integrated over a complete cycle unless there is a dynamic asymmetry in pressure upstream and downstream to pump net energy into the vibrating system.* If the subglottal pressure remains constant, the system cannot oscillate unless separated flow effects intervene.

3. Other workers have shown separated jet flow issuing from static, two-dimensional models of the glottal cross section (Gauffin et al., 1981; Titze et al., 1981). There is a limit to how far analytical glottal models that neglect the effect of separated flow can be carried before they lead to serious errors. Realistic physical models are essential, however, and a great deal can be learned from quite simple ones, particularly about the range and conditions under which such models will not oscillate and the form of the resulting air flow. This is particularly true if the model is adequately instrumented with hot wire anemometers and miniature microphones to study pressure and flow while wall motions are observed stroboscopically.

We constructed such a glottal device several years ago, utilizing a cylindrical plastic form (a syringe case with beveled edges) and thin rubber sheeting with a beaded edge, as shown in Figure 3–6A. The device produced a high-pitched sound for a very narrow range of pressures only. At high or low pressure it would blow open and remain so. If driven directly from a large constant pressure tank, it would not oscillate at all, but it required an upstream impediment to flow to allow its "subglottal" pressure to swing. Attempts to lower the pitch by reducing tension or by adding mass in the form of silicone along the "cord" edges failed to produce oscillations, as did all configurations that left a gap between the "cords."

In our experiments to find dynamic air flow patterns over a cycle of oscillation, we observed that the jet flow varied in all three space dimensions

Figure 3-6.

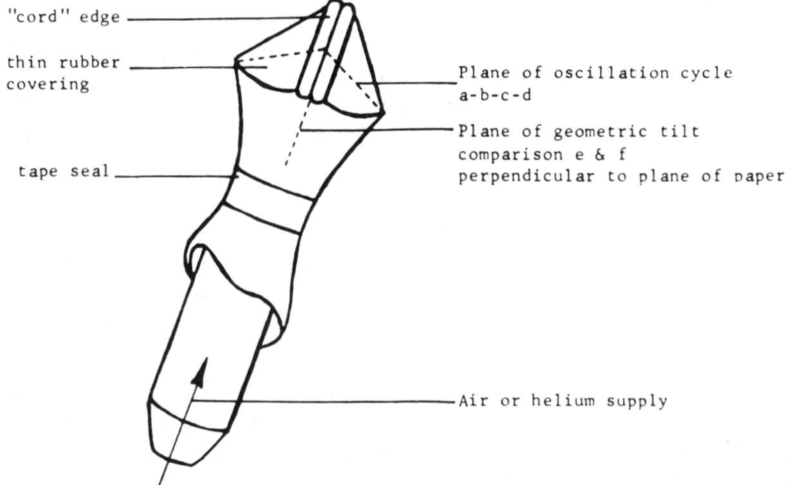

A, Glottal device, to scale, made from a 3½ inch syringe case.

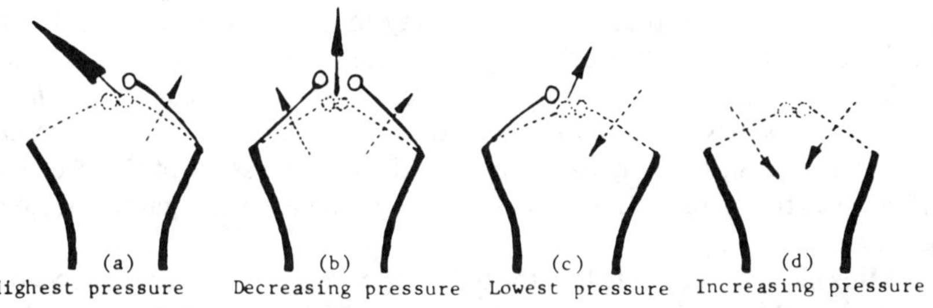

B, Sequence of events over a single cycle of oscillation. *a–d*, Dashed lines represent rest position of rubber covering. Solid arrows represent exit flow magnitude and direction. Dashed arrows indicate wall motions.

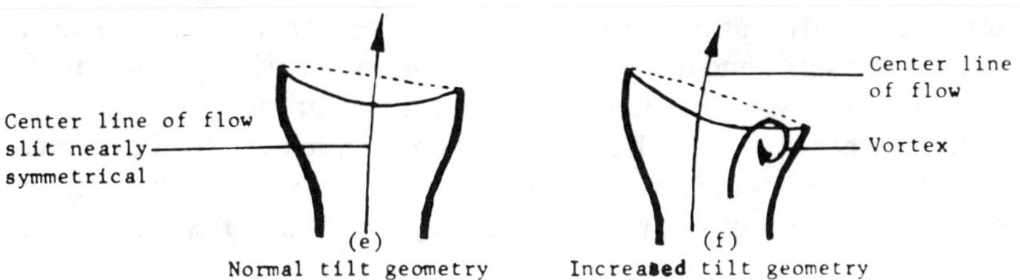

C, Tilt geometry comparison (*e, f*).

as well as in time. Figure 3–6*B, a–d* shows the sequence of events over a single cycle of oscillation through a cross section perpendicular to "cord" motion. At time *a* the right lip moves outward and upward and a narrow, very high-velocity jet of air issues to the far left. From *a* to *b* the jet widens, deflects to the middle, and loses velocity. From *b* to *c,* the jet continues to deflect to the right, starts to narrow, and picks up velocity as the slit closes. Because of lower subslit pressure, its velocity is then much less than it was at the same area while the slit was widening. The time spent in the opening phase is shorter than that spent in closing, and although it can increase with upstream constrictions, the "cords" remain closed at *d* for a very small fraction of the cycle. Neither particle velocity nor volume velocity was proportional to slit area. Only a small part of this discrepancy can be accounted for by the cyclic variation of pressure immediately below the "cords."

When driven by helium, the device produced a 60% higher pitch. When exhausting into an open room, the device is almost completely defined by its "subglottal" pressure. When its "cords" are closed, pressures increase to their highest; the "cords" are then literally blown open, accompanied by a corresponding fall in the "subglottal" pressure. Wall motion is parallel to its plane and not perpendicular to the flow axis, as would be the case for Bernoulli-driven effects. At its widest opening, position *b,* chamber pressure is on its way to a minimum, but does not begin to rise until the "cords" are perhaps half closed, at which time the cycle is repeated. *Thus, the force–distance curve of the "cords" exhibits a positive hysteresis and net energy gain per cycle.* There is no apparent rebound, and although elastic energy undoubtedly assists in the process of closure, the system rapidly dissipates any kinetic energy gained during the cycle.

It is interesting to note that the behavior of this physical device depends greatly on the relative wall geometry above and below the "cords." An increased tilt in the geometry, as in Figure 3–6*c, f,* drastically changes the air flow pattern along the slit, so that both motions and air flows are concentrated at the acute angle, and there is evidence for a vortex beneath the obtuse angle, which can influence the pulsatile flow. If a chamber is formed by hands cupped above our glottal device, its pitch lowers, its sound becomes less shrill, and the system will oscillate over a wider pressure range.

As stated earlier, we have made no claim that our glottal device is anything other than a rough analogue of one possible mode of dynamics. Its major value lies in its simplicity, allowing the physics of its operation to be verified. Our primary interest in the glottis is the effect of complex wall geometry of the larynx, including false folds and epiglottis above the folds per se, on its separated, time-varying vector air flow. Because of difficulties in visually tracking the relative position of intralaryngeal hot wires during phonation, particularly during those vowels for which the epiglottis obstructs a clear view, these experiments have not yet been duplicated in vivo, nor have the expected effects been confirmed with a more realistic mechanical model. However, based upon our general experiences with the effects of walls and cavities on separated flows, we can speak of the likelihood of certain consequences being present. *One conclusion is that is is the detailed three-dimensional shape of the walls, because of their effect upon separated and rotating flows, rather than the enclosed cross-sectional areas, which is most important in determining whether a possible qualitative mode of oscillation can occur.* From our glottal device data, it is reasonable to expect that the flow from in vivo folds is in the form of a similar deflecting and time-varying, fan-shaped jet, whose plane is in the lateral glottal axis, and whose deflection is side to side with an anterior–posterior tilt. In the course of its deflection, the jet can strike both the side walls and roof (epiglottis) of the larynx. A free jet is highly influenced by surrounding walls, even though the jet itself occupies only a small portion of the available volume. Secondary flows in the form of vortexes will build up and cause the jet to adhere to and switch between opposite walls during a single cycle.

Internal larynx geometry is variable, and very much a function of what is being voiced. The walls are not shaped simply, but include two lateral cavities, the sinus of Morgagni, which are particularly well developed in adult males. The effects of such cavities on the flow issuing from the larynx can range from profound to minor, depending upon the coupling of the jets and cavities. At a minimum such cavities can be expected to promote and hold growing vortexes whose flow pattern will influence a passing jet. If the jet actually deflects a part of its energy into these cavities, an active, self-excited oscillation, or a least a damped oscillation, will be set up, as demonstrated in our analysis of the jet cavity whistle (Teager and Teager, 1981). Finally, depending on the relative incidence angle of the epiglottis to the jet cavity, the jet may, upon leaving the larynx, have its long axis rotated 90 degrees to the horizontal plane.

To elucidate exactly what is happening within the larynx during the different phonemes, experiments on realistic models are quite obviously required. Whether a realistic numerical model experiment, based on Navier–Stokes equations, is either feasible or potentially accurate in such a clearly nonisotropic, nonsteady state situation, remains to be seen.

Supraglottal Spaces: Throat, Mouth, and Beyond the Mouth

Our direct experimental knowledge of flow and pressure patterns at the lips, mouth, and pharynx area diminishes with our ability to both access the area and simultaneously ascertain sensor position and orientation relative to interior surfaces. Although it is possible to collect data with sensors in fixed positions at or beyond a constriction, obtaining data along a known trajectory becomes more difficult. In the case of varying vocalizations, such as diphthong, change of pitch, or a change of volume, spacial variations become inseparable from temporal ones. Because of the great range of space and time variation in flow, data along a fixed trajectory, with no "wall" motions or sound variation, are vital. However, a sufficient variety of unique, vowel-specific, flow-dynamic patterns for sustained vowels have been recorded by sensor trajectories to draw reasonable inferences for other sounds and areas.

Throat. We have been able to observe the separated flow patterns for the open vowels "uh" (ʌ) and "ah" (ɑ) in the upper pharynx, where those vowels are primarily shaped. For "uh" (ʌ), flow appears primarily separated in the lateral plane with flows entering alternatively from the left and the right sides of the throat over the course of a pitch period. "Ah" (ɑ), on the other hand, has a smaller left–right time variation but a large separated flow in the frontal plane, switching between the back and front walls of the throat at the first formant frequency. It is our deduction that the nasopharynx and sinuses are providing the cavity with which the wall-bound jets actively interact, with the positive feedback of a cavity whistle mechanism, to generate the "ah" (ɑ) formant.

Throat vortexes with axes aligned perpendicular to flow are present for "ah" (ɑ) and "uh" (ʌ). We believe such throat vortexes are also responsible for the observed flow separation and first formant switching between tongue and mouth roof, previously observed and reported for the front vowels. For the lax vowels, there is also the possibility of an axial, swirling vortex in the throat, which can act as an additional active source of sound energy, using the vortex whistle mechanism (Chanaud, 1965; Vonnegut, 1954). *Thus, the throat is primarily implicated in first formant generation.*

Mouth. Our experimental understanding of flow acoustic effects has concentrated on flow and pressure in the mouth. Based on our observations and deductions from separated and circulating flow, we have sought coupled, dynamic, regenerative mechanisms for active sound generation and modulation throughout the vocal tract. We are not unhappy with acoustic models in essentially still air, but when flow energies that are orders of magnitude greater than those predicted by acoustic impedance from measured pressures are present inside and along side walls of a closed chamber such as the mouth cavity, they cannot be ignored. Flows in the pharynx can diverge along a number of pathways, but these flows must converge in the mouth, where they might collide, be trapped, or dissipated because of their directions and angular momenta. At the mouth exit, both angular and linear momenta accrued from wall flows must be conserved, and these manifest themselves as greater or lesser amounts of pressure depending upon the extent to which collisions are elastic. As mentioned earlier in this chapter, our data suggest that soliton flow waves, which we have called flow momentum waves, do not behave in the accepted linear fashion of acoustic waves. A separated flow momentum wave may be reflected or absorbed, but it must produce pressure when it collides, elastically or inelastically, with a separated or circulating flow moving in a different direction.

In the lower portion of the vocal tract, we considered vortexes as essentially passive barriers to air flow, whose motions and effects can influence the observed wall flow switching in the first formant range. In the mouth, however, they appear to interact with separated flow in a more active way to produce second formant pressures in the output sound, which may have no direct counterpart in the mouth flows. Vortexes can also pump energy into the mouth from the outside.

Swirling axial vortexes, from typhoons to water drains, or a submicroscopic "bojum," have almost no lower limit on physical scale, but even the smallest can amass significant amounts of energy when losses are low. Even a static vortex, such as a smoke ring, is also resonant (Widnall, 1975) and, with the appropriate geometric constraints, can exchange energy regeneratively with its flow and pressure surroundings to produce sustained oscillations, as in a "vortex whistle" (Vonnegut, 1954).

To make a regenerative oscillator out of a passive cavity like the mouth, a means of adding energy synchronously with the pressure swings within has to be found. Thus, either a net flow has to be pushed in when cavity pressure is high, or a net flow has to be pulled out when cavity pressure is low. For an integrating cavity, energy will be added if there is a nonlinear obstruction at the exit, which opens more fully when the pressure is at its lowest and is least open when pressure is at its peak. An axial, pulsating, swirling vortex at the exit can have this effect. As pressure in the cavity rises, the vortex is pushed into a convergent space at the front, but since angular momentum is conserved, the vortex velocity increases, and the resulting collisions deflect a larger fraction of the flow away from the mouth exit. Conversely, as pressure decreases, the vortex velocity decreases and deflects a smaller fraction of the flow away from the mouth exit. *Thus, the axial vortex at the exit can act as a nonlinear plug.*

A nonlinear modulator is one that can transform energy from one frequency into another and thus can produce output energies at frequencies not present in inputs. In a cavity, such important modulation effects can be expected from nonlinear collisions between jets and vortex blockages. Momentum must be conserved even if the collision of two air streams is inelastic, and the resulting pressure generated will correspond to the squares and cross products of stream velocities. In other words, *a pulsating flow that intersects a second flow can be expected to generate self- and cross-harmonics of all the frequencies in the two flows.* Another nonlinear vortex–flow pressure interaction, which may be important for the second formants of some vowels, can take place with a vortex whose axis is perpendicular to mouth flows, and whose ends can communicate with the mouth exterior, at the corners for example. If such a vortex cylinder is deformed or squashed into an ellipsoid at one frequency, the flow emerging along the axis will be at approximately twice the excitation, since the volume has two minima per cycle.

Beyond the mouth. Finally, we consider the situation at the exits of the vocal tract, primarily the lips. It should be clear from the experimental data shown that flow from the mouth is still separated, and the output jets appear at different places and directions along the lips over a pitch period, as in Figure 3–4. The resulting air motions are certainly not coherent enough to be replaced by a "vibrating piston" (Flanagan, 1965; Morse, 1938). Moreover, the conversion of excess kinetic energy into sound pressure seems to occur over a distance of several inches beyond the lips. The conversion of an oscillating motion into a radiating pressure wave is more complex than is stated in textbooks.

We have described models for an essentially static model of the vocal tract, based on our work with sustained vowels—models in which boundaries and walls are more or less fixed, and only flow instabilities are important. Speech is obviously a dynamic process in which walls and boundaries such as the larynx, tongue, and lips are required to move as the tract assumes a different configuration. *Such wall motions not only change the shape of the cavities but also create new air flows and influence existing jets and vortexes as a byproduct of their motions.* These "motional" flows may be comparable to glottal flows in magnitude and can easily give rise to additional transient instabilities and sounds that we have not yet considered, but which may be important in phoneme production.

There are four common threads among the interactions described in the various sections of the vocal tract:

1. Separated wall flows.

2. Axial and radial swirling air flows in cavities formed by local flows and walls.
3. Nonlinear coupling of pressures and flows resulting in active and regenerative feedback between the jets and vortexes in the different sections of the tract.
4. Nonlinear modulation and the generation of harmonics from momentum wave interaction.

It is our observation that the patterns of flow, including jets and vortexes resulting from definite three-dimensional tract shapes, have specific instabilities unique to each phonemic sound. Lungs, larynx, pharynx, nose, mouth, teeth, and lips form a coupled system in which all parts interact. Each part is at least resonant, but each can also be oscillatory, as we have tried to show in our discussion.

CONCLUSIONS

There is much that we have left implicit in our models of the vocal tract. We have not explicitly delineated how and where these models explain each item in our list of anomalies. Nonetheless, we believe that the salient features of the system, *vowel-specific active regeneration and flow pattern nonlinearity in space and time throughout the tract, have been demonstrated and their effects indicated.* However, passive acoustic effects also influence and enhance output sound. Formant resonance locations, as derived from area function data, are not incompatible with our measurements and deductions.

We have specifically shunned unvoiced and time-varying phonemes and have not elaborated on how the differing flow patterns and formants for each vowel sound are related in a cause-and-effect way. We have covered neither the reason for differing speech in a population of speakers nor for that of the same speaker at different times. These involve matters of perception beyond our present scope and subtleties in the generation mechanisms we have discussed. We do not claim to be fluid dynamicists or physicists, and thus we look forward to alternative and better explanations of our findings as well as experimentation with realistic, air-driven vocal tract models. A reconstruction and study of von Kempelen's 1775 speaking machine might be a welcome new starting point. The prevailing attitude that the only physical effects that can occur are those for which we have elegant linear equations handed down a century ago is hampering scientific progress.

REFERENCES

Blackwelder, R. F. (1981). Hot-wire and hot-film anemometers. In L. Marton and C. Marton (Eds. in Chief), *Methods of experimental physics, Vol. 18-A, Fluid dynamics* (pp. 259–314). New York: Academic Press.

Bouasse, H. P. M. (1929a). *Instruments a vent* [Wind instruments]. Paris: Librairie Delagrave.

Bouasse, H. P. M. (1929b). *Tuyeaux et resonateurs* [Pipes and resonators]. Paris: Librairie Delagrave.

Chanaud, R. C. (1965). Observations of oscillatory motion in certain swirling flows. *Journal of Fluid Mechanics, 21*, (1) 111–127.

Flanagan, J. L. (1965). *Speech analysis synthesis and perception.* New York: Springer-Verlag, Academic Press.

Gauffin, J., Nguyen, B., Ananthapadmanabha, T. V., and Fant, G. (1981). Glottal geometry and volume velocity waveform. In D. M. Bless and J. H. Abbs (Eds.), *Vocal fold physiology, contemporary research and clinical issues* (pp. 194–201). San Diego, CA: College-Hill Press.

Guillemin, E. A. (1949). *The mathematics of circuit analysis.* New York: Wiley.

Helmholtz, H. (1954). *On the sensations of tone* (A. J. Ellis, Trans.). New York: Dover Publications. (Original work published in 1885.)

Karman, von Th. V., and Rubach, H. L. (1965). In S. Goldstein (Ed.), *Modern Developments in Fluid Dynamics,* Vol. II. New York: Dover Publications. (Original work published in 1911 *Göttinger-Nachrichten* [pp. 509–517] and 1912 [pp. 547–556] and in *Physik. Zeitschr, 13* [1912], pp. 49–59.)

Kempelen, W. von (1791). *Le méchanisme de la parole, suivi de la description d'une machine parlante.* (The mechanism of speech, followed by the description of a speaking machine). Vienna: J. V. Degen. (English translation in press. Belmont, MA: Venerable Press)

Koike, Y., and Hirano, M. (1973). Glottal-area time function and subglottal-pressure variation. *Journal of the Acoustical Society of America, 54*, (6), 1618–1627.

Licklider, J. R. C., and Kryter, K. D. (1958). Articulation tests of standard and modified interphones conducted during flight at 5000 and 35,000 feet. OSRD Report 1976, Psycho-Acoustic Laboratory, Harvard University, 1 July, 1944 (PB 5505). In Stevens, S. S. (Ed.), *Handbook of experimental psychology* (2nd ed.). New York: Wiley.

Melnik, W. L., and Weske, R. F. (Eds.). (1967). Advances i hot wire anemometry. In *Proceedings of the International Symposium on Hot Wire Anemometry.* University of Maryland Department of Aerospace Engineering, March 20–21.

Morse, P. M. (1938). *Vibrations and sound.* New York: McGraw-Hill.

Newman, F. R. (1980). *Mouth sounds.* New York: Workman Publishing.

Prandtl, L. (1952). *The essentials of fluid dynamics.* London: Blackie.

Rayleigh, J. W. S., Lord. (1945). *The theory of sound (Vol. I & II).* New York: Dover Publications. (Original work published by MacMillan Co., London, in 1894 and 1896).

Schlichting, H. (1968). *Boundary layer theory.* New York: McGraw-Hill.

Teager, H. M. (1980). Some observations on oral air flow during phonation. *IEEE Transactions on Acoustics, Speech, and Signal Processing, ASSP Vol. 28* (5), 599–601.

Teager, H. M., and Teager, S. M. (1981). The effects of separated flow on vocalization. In D. M. Bless and J. H. Abbs (Eds.), *Vocal fold physiology, contemporary research and clinical issues* (pp. 124–143). San Diego, CA: College-Hill Press.

Titze, I. R., Baer, T., Cooper, D., and Scherer, R. (1981). Automated extraction of glottal graphic waveform parameters and regression to acoustic and physiologic variables. In D. M. Bless and J. H. Abbs (Eds.), *Vocal fold physiology, contemporary research and clinical issues* (pp. 146–154). San Diego, CA: College-Hill Press.

Vonnegut, B. (1954). A vortex whistle. *Journal of the Acoustical Society of America, 26,*(1), 18–20.

Wathen-Dunn, W., and Michaels, S. B. (1968). Some effects of gas density on speech production. *Annals of the New York Academy of Science, 155,* 368–378.

West, J. B. (Ed.) (1977). *Bioengineering aspects of the lung* (Vol. 3). New York: Dekker.

Widnall, S. E. (1975). The structure and dynamics of vortex filaments. *Annual Review of Fluid Mechanics, 7,* (8070), 141–165.

APPENDIX 3-I

HOT WIRE ANEMOMETRY

Hot wire anemometry is based upon temperature-induced resistance changes in a short thin wire due to integrated differences between electrical power input and the convective heat transfer of a moving stream. This technique has a long history in acoustics, but its modern "constant temperature" form owes its development to the growth of precise aerodynamic measurements during the 1930s. It would be digressive to detail the vast literature on this technique here (Blackwelder, 1981; Melnik and Weske, 1967); suffice it to say that in wind tunnel work, flow measurements of 0.1% accuracy in flow magnitude and flow direction out to frequencies of 100,000 Hz are commonplace. For our initial purposes, 5% accuracies and 8000 Hz bandwidth were quite adequate. Only the most important sources of potential error with the method will be considered here. These are the directionality of the sensor, the nonlinearity of the sensor and its associated electronics, the bandwidth limitations on the system as a function of wire temperature, and the in vivo experimental hazards to the wire.

The heat transfer rate of a hot wire depends on the component of flow *perpendicular* to the wire. Thus, to resolve flow magnitude and direction, more than one orthogonally oriented wire or spacial shrouding technique should be used. Typically, any upstream barrier will shield the flow, by separation, for a downstream distance comparable to the barrier width.

A block diagram of the bridge circuit for a constant temperature hot wire apparatus is shown in the Figure 3-7 inset, page 104. The bridge apex is driven by a difference amplifier with input voltages from the arm midpoints. For the resistance values shown, the bridge is in balance for no flow when the hot wire has the same resistance as the control resistor. As flow increases, the power loss at the hot wire is made up by driving the bridge, which remains balanced, with a higher voltage. The output voltage change follows very nearly a square-root relationship with flow rate because of the nonlinearity of heat transfer. It is obviously monotone, as can be seen in the static calibration curves of Figure 3-7.

If the overheat ratio is set too low, the system will lose high-frequency bandwidth. If it is too high, the wire will burn out. The low- and high-pass filters between V_{bridge} and V_{out} can also introduce phase shifts and information loss if carelessly set. More sophisticated "modern" constant temperature systems may include an electronic linearizer, which, if incorrectly set, can completely distort the output.

Surprisingly, hot wires have never proved dangerous to a subject since their miniscule energy is easily absorbed by the moisture of tissue, and the amount of energy is too small to inflict burns. Hot wires, typically of 5 μm diameter platinum-plated tungsten, are subject to easy breakage and surface contamination due to polymerization of plaque if they are allowed to touch tissue. If polymerized, the wire's bandwidth and sensitivity can be drastically reduced. The hot wire cartridges, shown in Figure 3-2*A* and *B*, were evolved to minimize such difficulties.

Hot wire anemometry is not a trivial technique that can be easily mastered during one afternoon. Available alternatives, on the other hand, have their own deficiencies: tracer technique such as laser Doppler anemometry, for example, offers poorer spacial and timing accuracy, even if an illuminated source of particles could be provided in the vocal tract during phonation. Accurate pulsatile measurements with hot wires can be assured if appropriate calibration techniques are developed for the physiological velocities of interest, as these are learned with experience.

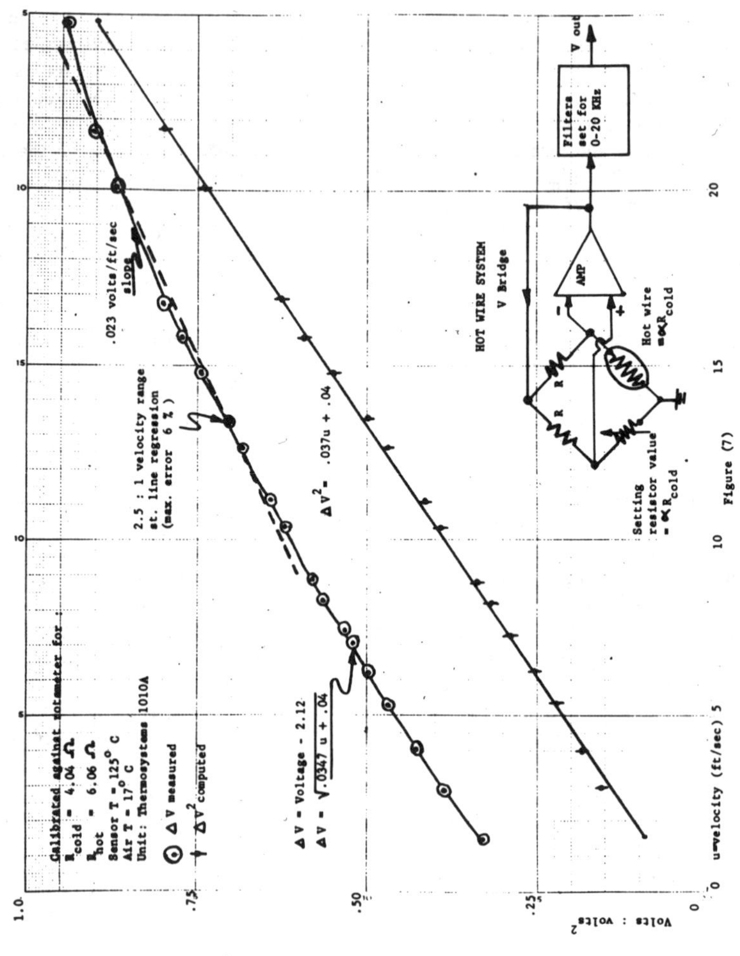

Figure 3–7. Static calibration curve for temperature hot wire anemometer. Inset: Block diagram for bridge circuit.

Figure 3-8. Calibration devices. *A*, Vitalometer. *B*, Specific parts of calibration device: *1*, rotameter; *2*, turbine; *3*, regulator; *4*, siren wheel; *5*, gauge. *C*, Siren calibrator. *D*, Reciprocating calibrator: *1*, drive motor and belt; *2*, pump; *3*, end bell and screen; *4*, mirror for video; *5*, pump pulley with position sensor.

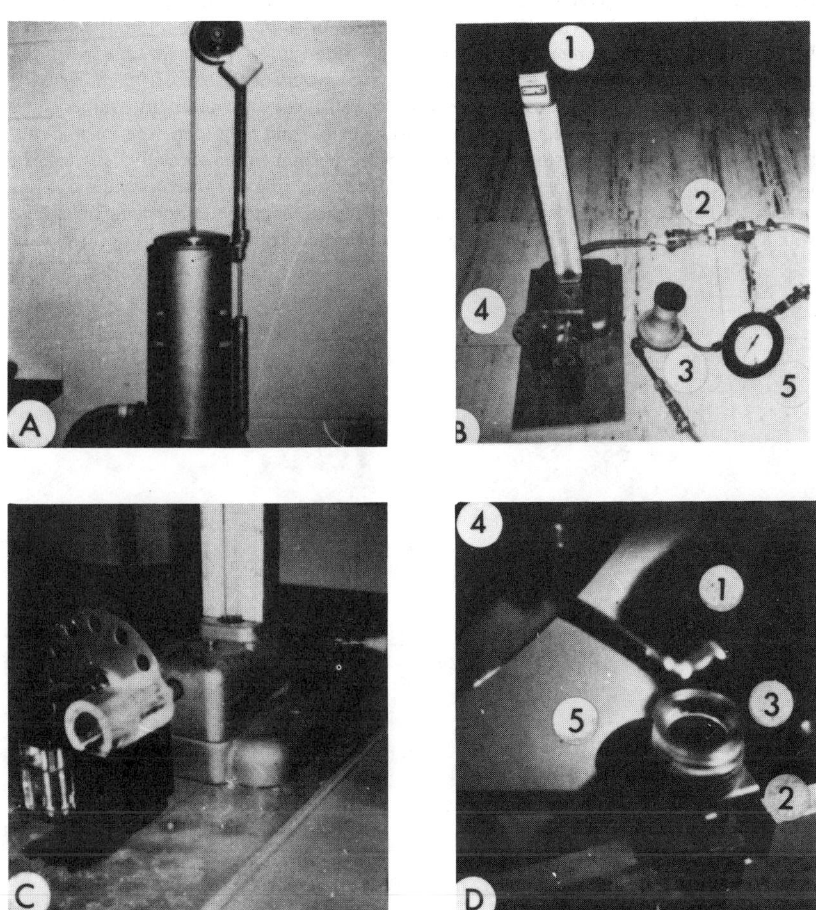

The most necessary calibration device for hot wire anemometry is a fixed graduated volume, such as a water-filled beaker, bellows, or a Vitalometer, as shown in Figure 3–8*A,* in which constant air flow rate can be integrated over a low-gauge pressure. The next need is for a regulated source of quiet air at low pressure that can be connected to a good, low-bandwidth, low-pressure drop, flow *rate* device such as a rotameter or digital turbine, as in Figure 3–8*B,* which can then be connected to the Vitalometer and calibrated against it. A test section with a converging throat, to avoid separation and provide a uniform velocity, can then be substituted for the Vitalometer and used for *static* velocity calibrations of the hot wire system. To make pulsatile calibrations of a *single* hot wire, the variable speed disc siren system in Figure 3–8*C* was used, but an expansion system downstream of the siren failed to provide a uniform, large area flow because of wall flows and vortex instabilities.

To calibrate an anemometer array dynamically before and after each experimental run, a variable speed, constant displacement, reciprocating pump with a specially designed exit bell throat (to eliminate the persistent and unstable vortex ring due to exit separation) was developed (Figure 3–8*D*). This device provided a 1/2-inch diameter, uniform air flow field, with a frequency, and thus velocity, that could be measured against the anemometer signals.

APPENDIX 3-II

FLUID MECHANICS

Acoustic models, such as those used in the source filter theory, neglect the effects of both steady flow and separation. These effects, however, are far from negligible, as we shall see. In the following discussion we assume that the flow rate is low enough to avoid turbulence.

The general equations of flow, neglecting viscosity, apply to both the usual "potential," or uniform flow, and separated flow.

The general dynamic equations of motion for compressible flow along a streamline, assuming elastic collisions, are Euler's equations:

$$-\frac{1}{\varrho 2}\frac{\delta p}{\delta s} = v\frac{\delta v}{\delta s} + \frac{\delta v_s}{\delta t} \quad \text{(along a streamline)} \quad (1)$$

$$\frac{1}{\varrho}\frac{\delta \varrho}{\delta n} = \frac{v^2}{r} + \frac{\delta v_n}{\delta t} \quad \text{(perpendicular)} \quad (2)$$

where p = pressure, v = velocity, v_s = velocity along a streamline, v_n = velocity normal to the streamline, r = radius of curvature of flow, ϱ = density, n = normal direction, (δs) = an increment of length along a streamline, (δn) = an increment perpendicular to the streamline, and t = time.

In acoustics it is customary to neglect the first terms on the right-hand sides in order to linearize the equations, but this adjustment is less justifiable in the presence of an average flow than it is in a flow that is merely oscillating.

Equation 1 can be integrated along a streamline to yield an arbitrary time function $f(t)$:

$$\int_{s_1}^{s_2}\frac{\delta v}{\delta t}\,\delta s + \left[\frac{v^2}{2} + \int_{v_1}^{v_2}\right.\left.\int_{s_1}^{s_2}\frac{1}{\varrho}\frac{\delta p}{\delta s}\,\delta s\right] = f(t) \quad (3)$$

For a constant density, Equation 3 yields the unsteady-state Bernoulli equation:

$$\frac{1}{2}\left(v_2^2 - v_1^2\right) + \frac{p_2 - p_1}{\varrho} + \int_{s_1}^{s_2}\frac{\delta v}{\delta t}\,\delta s = 0 \quad (4)$$

An obvious consequence of this equation (which is a statement of conservation of energy) is that steady flow through a hole is proportional to the *square root* of the pressure difference, or equivalently, a pressure difference is proportional to a velocity *squared* difference.

For an example of a usual application of Bernoulli's equation, consider a section of cylindrical pipe of cross section A_1 that is between two smaller pipes of area A_2. The inlet, outlet, and central pressures depend on the behavior of the streamlines. If we assume a uniform potential flow, the inlet and outlet pressures are equal, and the pressure *rise* within the chamber is proportional to

$$\Delta p = \frac{\varrho}{2} \, v_1^2 \left[1 - \left(\frac{A_1}{A_2} \right)^2 \right] \tag{5}$$

However, if the flow is separated, as is usually the case, not only will there be a pressure loss across the chamber, but in addition the internal pressure rise will be much less than that indicated in Equation 5. Moreover, the streamlines may be unstable, and if the flow is swirling, the effective output flow area may be considerably reduced because of the centrifugal forces of Equation 2.

MOMENTUM RELATIONS

When flows are separated, equations based on the conservation of energy no longer apply, but momentum equations remain valid. In fluids, as in solid mechanics, momentum is conserved while energy may be lost due to inelastic collisions.

Momentum relations in fluids equate vector force applied to a fluid with the rate of change of momentum in the direction of the force. Linear momentum is equal to mass times velocity, and since mass is equal to the product of velocity, area, density, and time, a rate of change of momentum is proportional to the velocity squared times area times density, thus:

$$\overrightarrow{\text{Momentum pressure}} = \vec{v_1} \cdot v_1 \cdot \varrho_{in} - \vec{v_2} \cdot v_2 \cdot \varrho_{out}$$

Thus:

$$\overrightarrow{\text{Pressure in a direction } x} = 2 \times \overrightarrow{[\text{energy carried in—energy carried out}]}$$

where pressure is in the direction of the energy difference. Although the momentum theorem is usually applied to the forces that have to be applied to bent pipes carrying fluids, it can also be applied to the interface between colliding fluid streams. We can thus understand the pressure-generating effects of colliding flows by considering the effects of inelastic collisions of masses, where the velocities in the following equations are *vectors* having both magnitude and direction.

Initial energy: $\frac{1}{2} m_1 v_1^2 + \frac{1}{2} m_2 v_2^2$

Initial and final momentum: $m_1 v_1 + m_2 v_2$

Final velocity: $\dfrac{m_1 v_1 + m_2 v_2}{m_1 + m_2}$

Final energy: $\dfrac{1}{2} \dfrac{(m_1 v_1 + m_2 v_2)^2}{m_1 + m_2}$

$$= \frac{1}{2} \left(\frac{m_1}{m_1 + m_2}\right) m_1 v_1^2 + \frac{1}{2} \left(\frac{m_2}{m_1 + m_2}\right) m_1 v_2^2 + \left(\frac{m_1 m_2}{m_1 + m_2}\right) v_1 v_2$$

$$\text{Energy loss} = \frac{1}{2} \left[\left(\frac{m_2}{m_1 + m_2}\right) m_1 v_1^2 + \left(\frac{m_1}{m_1 + m_2}\right) m_2 v_2^2 - \left(\frac{m_1 m_2}{m_1 + m_2}\right) (v_1 v_2)\right]$$

$$= \frac{1}{2} \left(\frac{m_1 m_2}{m_1 + m_2}\right) (v_1 - v_2)^2$$

substituting $m_1 = \varrho A v_1; \ m_2 = \varrho A v_2$

$$\text{Therefore the pressure} = \frac{1}{2} \varrho \left(\frac{v_1 v_2}{v_1 + v_2}\right) (v_1 - v_2) \tag{6}$$

The exact direction in which the interfacial pressure is expected, and the effects it will produce, will of course depend upon the direction and magnitude of the colliding streams as well as the internal geometry of the containing vessel near the collision.

Clearly, the pressure generated will be at a maximum when flows collide head on, and at a minimum when the flows "rear end." In these cases the pressures will act to either speed up or slow down the flow in the direction in which it is already moving. "Sidewise" collisions, on the other hand, can generate pressures in perpendicular directions.

From the form of Equation 6, it is clear that collisions lead directly to a variety of cross modulations, depending upon the frequency, magnitude, and direction of time-varying flows. Thus, flows of frequencies f_1 and f_2, when colliding, can easily produce $2f_1$, $2f_2$, $f_1 - f_2$, $f_1 + f_2$, as well as higher order harmonics.

CHAPTER 4

Identification of Speech and Speechlike Signals by Hearing Impaired Listeners

M. F. Dorman
Maureen T. Hannley

Individuals with hearing impairment due to cochlear pathology frequently experience a deficit in speech understanding. The mechanisms that underlie the deficit are not well understood. There is, to be sure, a rich psychoacoustic literature describing aberrations in frequency resolution, temporal resolution, and loudness growth in individuals with hearing impairment. A survey of this literature leaves little doubt that cochlear pathology can alter peripheral processing in each of the physical domains of the speech signal—time, frequency, and intensity.

There is, however, a gap between our understanding of how cochlear pathology disrupts the processing of simple signals such as pure tones and our understanding of how cochlear pathology disrupts the processing of complex signals such as speech. In this chapter both the recent psychoacoustic literature and the recent literature on phonetic identification to gain a better understanding of the mechanisms that might underlie poor phonetic identification are reviewed.

One mechanism which clearly results in impaired phonetic identification is an elevation in auditory threshold. The effects of threshold elevation, or, alternatively, signal attenuation, have been well described and will not be dealt with here. Instead we concentrate on two phenomena that co-vary with elevated auditory thresholds—poor temporal resolution and poor frequency resolution. Our chapter, thus, is divided into three sections: the first is a brief history of the materials and methods used to study phonetic identification in the hearing impaired; the second is a brief review of psychoacoustic studies of temporal resolution and a longer review of studies of phonetic identification when stimulus duration is varied; and the third is a brief review of psychophysical studies of frequency resolution and a longer review of studies of phonetic identification when changes in formant frequency underlie identification.

MATERIALS AND METHODS FOR STUDYING SPEECH INTELLIGIBILITY

A variety of speech materials have been used to investigate the disordered speech perception associated with sensorineural hearing impairment. These materials range in complexity from nonsense syllables (Dubno, Dirks, and Langhoffer, 1982) through single words (Egan, 1948; Hirsh, Davis, Silverman, Reynolds, Eldert, and Benson, 1952; Owens and Schubert, 1977; Tillman and Carhart, 1966) to third-order sentential approximations delivered with competing speech (Jerger, Speaks, and Trammell, 1968). Such a range of materials, of course, presents a range of acoustic, phonetic, linguistic, and lexical variables that may influence performance.

We can identify at least four different approaches to analyzing subject responses to these materials. In each, the analysis addresses a different aspect of speech processing and thus yields data which make cross-study comparisons difficult.

The traditional *audiometric approach,* for example, uses (mainly) single-syllable words selected for familiarity and for phonemic balance within lists. Here, the usual procedure is to score using a binary criterion; a response is either correct or incorrect. This criterion is applied whether there has been a substitution, omission, or addition of a phoneme to a word, whether a response involves an error in only one phoneme or all phonemes in a word, or whether the distortion is so great as to render the stimulus altogether unintelligible to the listener and leave him or her in bewildered silence. Although this approach can easily quantify the listener's error rate across lists, it has the implied, and probably incorrect, assumption that all errors are of equal importance. Moreover, little insight into mechanisms contributing to disordered speech perception is afforded by this approach.

A second approach to response analysis is the construction of a *phonetic confusion matrix.* This technique might be likened to a physiological input–output function in the sense that the listener's response is compared, phoneme for phoneme, with the stimulus. Using this approach, patterns of phoneme confusions typical of sensorineural hearing loss have emerged, but the mechanisms underlying those patterns remain obscure.

A corollary approach, *linguistic feature analysis,* has been used by some to study speech perception in the hearing impaired. This approach has proven to be no more satisfactory than the previous two, for it is the case that linguistic features do not map directly onto the acoustic characteristics of a phone. That is, a single linguistic feature, such as voicing, may have multiple acoustic cues. If the voicing feature, for example, is misperceived, then, the acoustic underpinnings of that error are still unknown.

Two decades of research using these three methods led to the following broad conclusions about phonetic perception in hearing-impaired listeners:

1. Vowel identity is well perceived.
2. Consonant recognition is better in syllable-initial position than in syllable-final position.
3. Voicing and manner of articulation are the linguistic features most likely to be correctly identified.
4. The feature of place of articulation is not as well identified as other linguistic features.
5. Both the audiogram configuration and the severity of the hearing impairment affect phonetic identification.

In the 1970s a number of researchers turned to a fourth approach, *speech synthesis,* as a tool to probe the mechanisms that underlie poor speech understanding. Speech synthesis is attractive as a tool for several reasons. One reason is that signals can be created in which the spectral, temporal, and intensity characteristics vary independently. This, in principle, allows investigators to separate the relative contribution of the various signal parameters to overall speech intelligibility. A second attraction of synthetic signals is their malleability to a continuum—a set of signals which differ along a single physical dimension or small set of physical dimensions. The use of a stimulus continuum offers a significant refinement in the evaluation of disorders of phonetic identification and discrimination. Consider that when listeners are presented a minimal contrast between a naturally produced voiced and voiceless stop consonant (e.g., /ba/ and /pa/), the voice onset time (VOT) of the voiced member of the pair might be 2 ms whereas that of the voiceless member of the pair might be 70 ms. If hearing impaired listeners are able to differentially identify or to discriminate between these signals, we know only that his or her auditory system is not so damaged as to prevent the resolution of this rather large acoustic difference. This outcome does not allow the investigator to infer that hearing impaired listeners are as sensitive as normal listeners to small differences in VOT. Such a conclusion *could* be reached, however, if it were shown that the hearing impaired listeners identified or discriminated among members of an entire stimulus continuum in the manner of normal listeners.

The use of speech synthesis as a tool is a major addition to the armamentarium of those who wish to understand the mechanisms underlying poor speech understanding. In the following review of research conducted in the past 5 years, we concentrate on studies which have used synthetic speech to probe the processing of spectral and temporal information by hearing impaired listeners.

TEMPORAL RESOLUTION

Psychophysical Studies

The cochlear damage that results in a loss of auditory sensitivity also results in a loss of temporal resolution. In the past several years temporal resolution for nonspeech signals has been assessed by a host of measures and procedures: gap detection (Fitzgibbons and Wightman, 1982; Irwin, Hinchcliffe, and Kemp, 1981; Stoker, 1978; Trinder, 1979; Tyler, Summerfield, Wood, and Fernandes, 1982); gap difference limens (Tyler et al., 1982); temporal difference limens (Tyler et al., 1982); detection of stimulus onset asynchrony (Bosatra and Russolo, 1976); forward masking (Festen and Plomp, 1983; Nelson and Turner, 1980); backward masking (Festen and Plomp, 1983); and temporal windows (Festen and Plomp, 1983; Zwicker and Schorn, 1982).

The several studies of gap detection have consistently found elevated thresholds for hearing impaired listeners. For example, Tyler and colleagues (1982) reported that when narrow band noise signals were presented to normal and hearing impaired listeners at equal sound pressure level (SPL), the gap detection threshold for the normal listeners was 13.3 ms for a 500 Hz signal and 7.4 ms for a 4000 Hz signal. In contrast, the hearing-impaired means were 22.9 ms and 11.6 ms, respectively. Although the group means differed significantly, a great deal of intersubject variability was evident in the hearing impaired sample independent of hearing sensitivity levels. In the 500 Hz condition, 37.5% of the hearing impaired listeners achieved gap detection thresholds within one standard deviation of normal; in the 4000 Hz condition 50% of the listeners fell within one standard deviation of normal. If the three subjects who were over 70 years of age are excluded from the analysis (the normal listener's mean age was 23 years), the thresholds of 46% of the listeners fell within one standard deviation of normal at 500 Hz and 61% at 4000 Hz. Given the substantial individual differences in threshold for gap detection, it is not surprising that the correlation between auditory sensitivity and gap detection thresholds (for the younger hearing impaired listeners) is modest at best.

Another estimate of the relationship between the magnitude of sensitivity loss and gap detection threshold has been derived from a study of chinchillas with temporary threshold elevation due to noise exposure.

Girandi-Perry, Salvi, and Henderson (1982) reported that with 15 dB elevation in threshold, no increase in gap detection threshold was found. With a 30 dB elevation in sensitivity threshold, the gap detection thresholds were elevated when measured at equal SPL, but not when measured at equal sensation level (SL). With greater than 40 db elevation in sensitivity, thresholds for gap detection were elevated in both equal SPL and equal SL comparisons. These animal data are somewhat more orderly than those reported for humans with hearing loss of heterogeneous causes. One listener in the study of Tyler and colleagues (1982) evidenced an 80 dB loss at 4000 Hz but showed a gap detection threshold within normal limits. It appears that the cause of impairment must be seriously considered as a factor underlying the variable performance of human listeners.

Despite substantial differences in gap detection threshold among hearing impaired listeners, as a group the impaired listeners perform less well than normal listeners. A similar conclusion obtains from two other measures of temporal resolution used in the studies of Tyler and associates (1982). Gap difference limens (DLs) for signals with 30 and 100 ms standards at 500 and 4000 Hz were found to be elevated for the hearing impaired group by 20 to 25 ms at both frequencies and durations. Again, a number of hearing impaired listeners showed gap DLs within the normal range; and again, with elderly listeners omitted from the data pool, 34% reached normal performance in the 30 ms standard condition and 65% in the 100 ms condition.

Temporal difference limens, that is, the DL for a filled interval rather than a silent interval, were also elevated in the hearing impaired. The mean DL for normals was 18.8 ms for the 500 Hz signal and 17.9 ms for the 4000 Hz signal. The corresponding values for the hearing impaired listeners were 48 ms and 41.8 ms. In this stimulus condition, in striking contrast to the other conditions, *all* hearing impaired listeners showed poorer than normal thresholds for at least one frequency. Thus, the nature of the task, in this case the detection of a filled versus unfilled interval, makes a difference in the number of listeners who show poorer than normal detection thresholds and suggests that the mechanisms underlying performance in the two tasks are not identical.

In summary, the data from a variety of tasks indicate that hearing impaired listeners as a group generally show poorer than normal temporal resolution. The magnitude of the disability is related in only a moderate degree to the magnitude of the loss in sensitivity and may vary with age and cause of the impairment (see Bosatra and Russolo, 1976, for comments on listeners with Meniere's disease, and Zwicker and Schorn, 1982, for differences among listeners with noise-induced hearing loss, presbycusic loss, and sudden, idiopathic hearing loss).

Word Intelligibility in Noise

Impaired temporal resolution is correlated significantly with poor identification of speech in noise. Tyler and colleagues (1982) report correlations ranging from − .62 to − .74 for the measures of gap detection and temporal difference limen and the measure of percent correct word identification in noise. When statistical maneuvers are performed to remove the effects of pure tone thresholds, the correlations remain significant but drop to − .36 and − .48. The fact that the correlations remain significant indicates that losses in auditory sensitivity and losses in temporal resolution ability exert independent effects on word intelligibility in noise (see also Festen and Plomp, 1983). However, the magnitude of the correlation indicates that differences in temporal resolution ability account for only a very small portion of the variance on the task.

Phonetic Identification Studies

A number of acoustic cues to phonetic identity are based on temporal aspects of the signal. It is of interest, therefore, to determine whether impaired temporal resolution for nonspeech signals is reflected in the resolution of temporal aspects of speech. In this section are reviewed experiments in which phonetic identification is cued by differences in stimulus duration in order to determine whether poor temporal resolution affects phonetic perception.

The differences in temporal resolution ability between normal and hearing impaired listeners are relatively small in terms of the absolute shift in threshold. For example, at one extreme Tyler and associates (1982) found a mean difference of only 4.2 ms in gap detection threshold at 4000 Hz. At the other extreme, a 31.2 ms difference was found in temporal DL at 500 Hz. Are these differences sufficient to affect phonetic identification or discrimination deterimentally?

To answer this question, let us look first to the magnitude of the durational differences which separate minimally contrastive phones in English (ignoring, for a moment, the fact that minimally contrastive phones do not differ in duration alone).

- The VOT of voiced and voiceless stop consonants in English may differ by as much as 100 ms (Lisker and Abramson, 1964).
- The formant transitions which distinguish stop consonant and semivowel manner at the same place of articulation differ in duration by at least 50 ms (Liberman, Delattre, Cooper, and Gerstman, 1956; Schwab, Sawusch, and Nusbaum, 1981).

- The presence of a stop consonant in a fricative stop vowel sequence, for example, "stay," is signaled by a silent interval of greater than 60 ms, while the absence of the stop in "say" is signaled by an interval of less than 20 ms.
- When vowel duration varies before voiced and voiceless stop consonants in word final position, the durational differences range from 1.25:1 to 2.3:1 (Raphael, 1971).

From this partial listing it would seem that the differences between phones, when stimulus duration is at issue, may be so large that small decrements in temporal resolution ability may go unnoticed. Here, then, the use of natural or synthetic speech continua can be of assistance—by creating such continua the identification or discrimination of small differences in stimulus duration can be readily assessed.

Identification Based on VOT

In syllable–initial position voicing, contrasts among stop consonants are realized by changes in the time of voicing onset relative to the time of the release of articulatory occlusion. Voiced stops are typically produced with a short delay in voicing onset (mean of /b d g/ = 9 ms), whereas voicless stops are produced with longer delay (mean of /p t k/ = 69 ms) (Lisker and Abramson, 1964). These differences in timing of laryngeal versus articulatory events creates a lengthy inventory of acoustic differences between voiced and voiceless stops. Voiced stops are characterized by a short interval between burst release and F_1 onset, an extensive rise in F_1 (at least for open vowels) from a low onset to the steady state of the following vowel and a rising pitch contour over the initial portion of the utterance. The voiceless stops are characterized by a relatively long interval between burst and F_1 onset, aspiration in the upper formants during F_1 delay, a high starting point of F_1, a small rise or no rise to the F_1 of the following vowel, and a falling pitch contour over the onset of the utterance (see Darwin and Pearson, 1982, and Summerfield, 1982, for recent comments and experiments on the acoustic cues to voicing). It is critical to remember that although voicing contrasts can be quantified by measuring only one temporal variable (the time between burst release and voicing onset), there are multiple acoustic events, spread over time, that are the consequences of the differences in articulatory gestures.

The data on the identification of voicing in natural speech signals in quiet and in noise indicate that hearing impaired listeners perceive voicing well. Erber's (1972) experiments indicate that even congenitally hearing impaired children with severe impairment can identify stop consonant

Figure 4–1. Identification and discrimination of stimuli from a /da/ to /ta/ continuum. Note the ability of patients identified as severe –10 and profound –2 to discriminate between stimuli they could not differentially identify.

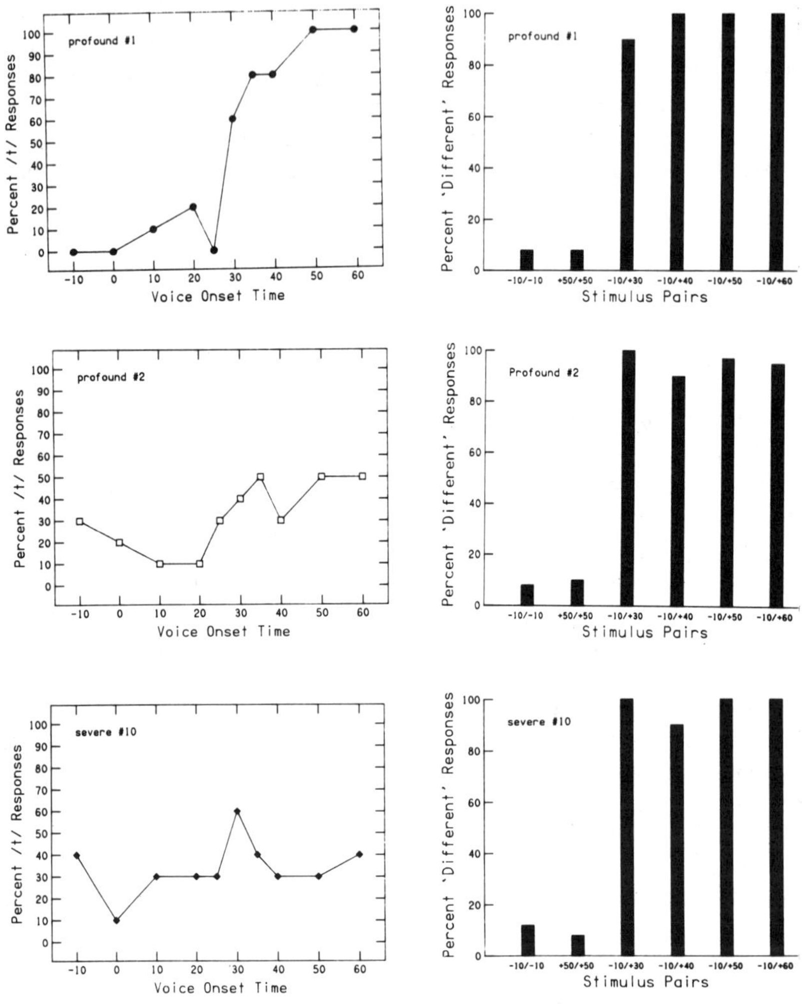

voicing with 85% accuracy. Adult listeners with adventitious losses evidence 94% accuracy on the voicing feature when the signals are embedded in noise at a +6 dB signal-to-noise ratio (Tyler et al., 1982). As noted earlier, although these experiments establish that the voicing feature is well identified in stop consonants, they do not establish that hearing impaired listeners are as sensitive as normal listeners to the acoustic cues to VOT. It is this question that must be answered if we are to learn the consequences of cochlear pathology on the resolution of small differences in the duration of cues to voicing. Four experiments—two using children as subjects and two using adults—have addressed this issue.

Parady, Dorman, Whaley, and Raphael (1981) synthesized stimuli to form a /da/ to /ta/ continuum for presentation to children with moderate, severe, and profound hearing impairment. All of the listeners with moderate to moderately severe impairments showed normal phonetic boundaries. Of the ten children with severe impairment, five showed normal boundaries. Three showed a longer boundary and a shallow slope and low asymptote to the labeling function. An additional two could not label the stimuli differentially. The latter two subjects began hearing aid use at a much later age (5 and 10 years) than the other severely impaired children (mean age of amplification was 2.5 years). Of the listeners with profound hearing loss, one with relatively late onset of impairment (3 years) generated a normal labeling function in terms of both absolute boundary and slope of the function. Two other profoundly hearing impaired listeners were unable to identify the stimuli.

To determine whether the listeners who could not differentially identify the stimuli could nonetheless discriminate between the stimuli, the listeners were presented VOT stimuli in an A to X discrimination task in which the reference stimulus was a −10 ms VOT /da/ and the comparison stimuli varied in VOT from +30 to +60 ms. As shown in Figure 4-1, two listeners, one severely and one profoundly hearing impaired, were able to discriminate a 40 ms difference in VOT without being able to differentially identify the two signals (see Blumstein, Cooper, Zurif, and Caramazza, 1977, for a similar outcome with aphasic patients). This outcome suggests that the peripheral auditory system was able to transduce the difference in VOT of the signals, but the information was not usable for phonetic identification.

The data of Parady and colleagues (1981) suggest that (1) the cochlear damage that underlies moderate, severe, and even profound hearing losses does not *necessarily* impair the resolution of VOT; (2) age of onset of sensitivity loss may play a role in labeling performance; (3) age at which amplification is initiated may play a role in labeling performance; and (4) identification and discrimination tasks can tap different levels of auditory processing of signals.

Results similar to those found by Parady and associates for children and adolescents with early onset of hearing loss have been reported by Tyler and co-workers (1982) for adults with adventitious hearing impairment (see also Ivory and Brandt, 1982). The individuals with mild to moderately

Figure 4–2. A profoundly hearing impaired listener's identification of stimuli from VOT continua. *A;* When tested with stimuli from one place of articulation at a time, the listener's phonetic boundary falls at normal values. *B;* When tested with stimuli from all three places of articulation in one test order, the phonetic boundaries shift to extreme values of VOT.

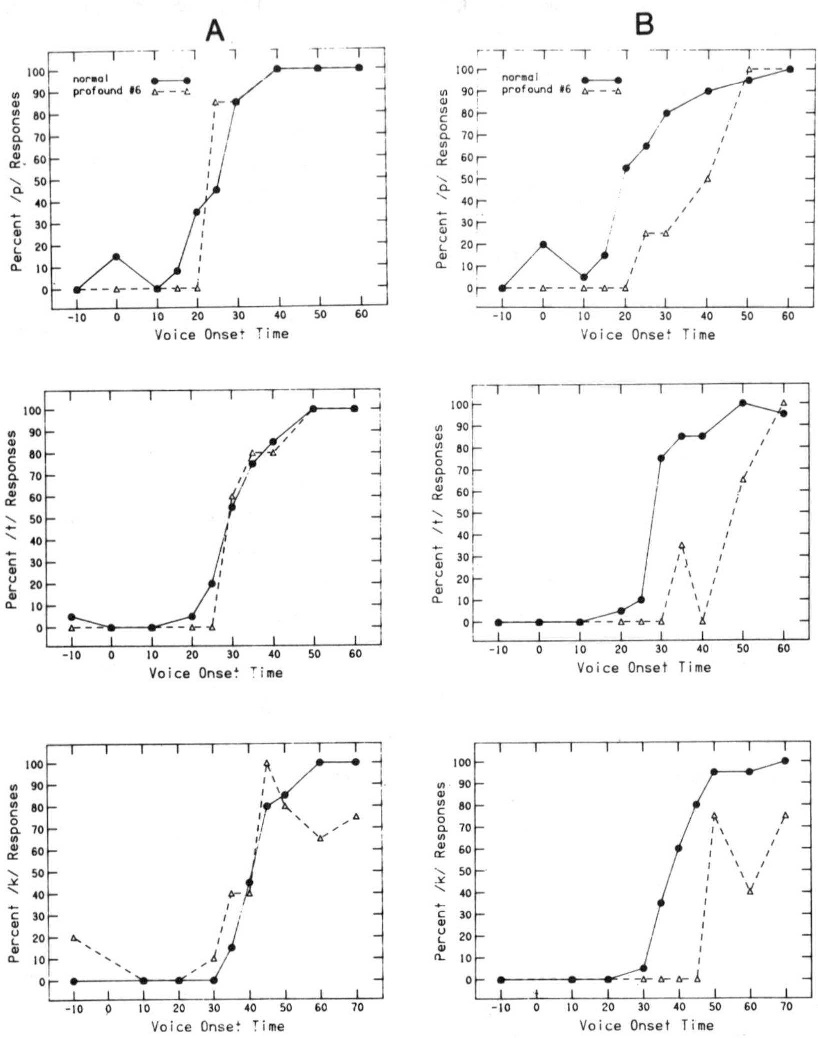

severe hearing impairment in this experiment showed normal phonetic boundaries and normal slopes to the labeling function for a /b/ to /p/ contrast in /a/ and /i/ environments. Both the normal and hearing impaired listeners shifted boundary locations from one vowel context to the other. In doing so, the impaired listeners showed normal sensitivity to the spectral changes which alter the VOT boundary in the two contexts.

The results of the Parady and colleagues and the Tyler and colleagues identification experiments must, however, be interpreted with some caution. Since a stimulus continuum at only one place of articulation was employed, the binary choice of /d/ or /t/, or /b/ or /p/ could overestimate the listener's ability to identify voicing in the natural context of three places of articulation. To investigate this possibility, Johnson, Whaley, and Dorman (1984) presented children and adolescents with mild, moderate, severe, and profound hearing impairment with stimuli from along /ba/ to /pa/, /da/ to /ta/ and /ga/ to /ka/ continua. The tests were divided into three two-choice tests, one four-choice test (/b p d t/), and one six-choice test (/b p d t g k/). The listeners in the mildly and moderately hearing impaired groups showed normal identification performance. The listeners in the severely impaired group deviated from normal in two ways. First, although their VOT boundaries were within the normal range for each place of articulation, further analysis revealed that the VOT boundaries did not vary systematically with place of articulation, as was the case in normal listeners. That is, the boundary for the labial place should be shorter than the boundary for alveolar place, which in turn should be shorter than that for velar place. In the six-response condition, none of the severely hearing impaired listeners showed the normal progression in boundaries. Second, in the six-response condition, response variability was much greater than normal. That is to say, at extreme values of VOT, where identification performance should be very stable, performance was, instead, variable.

Three of six listeners with profound hearing loss could establish phonetic boundaries in the two alternative conditions. In most instances the boundaries were within the outer limits of normal. One listener, who was able to identify the stimuli in a normal manner on the two-response conditions, was able to differentially identify the stimuli in the four- and six-response conditions, but needed abnormally long VOTs to reach asymptotic labeling for the voiceless category. This prodigious performance is worthy of note and is illustrated in Figure 4–2.

Correlation Between Nonspeech and Speech Measures of Temporal Processing

Tyler and colleagues (1982) have addressed the question, central to this section, of whether individuals who show poor temporal resolution on psychophysical tests also demonstrate poor identification of speech when phonetic identity is based on a difference in temporal structure. Since the hearing impaired and normal listeners in their study did not differ in identification of VOT, but did differ in temporal resolution ability, the correlation between the several measures of temporal resolution and phonetic identification was nonsignificant. Thus, listeners who have demonstrably poor temporal resolution can identify stimuli that differ in VOT in a normal manner.

If a discrimination task instead of an identification task is used, and the standard and target stimuli differ acoustically but not phonetically, then performance on nonspeech and speech tasks *is* found to be significantly correlated. Tyler and co-workers created two discrimination tasks for their listeners. In one the standard was a 15 ms /ba/; in the other the standard was a 30 ms /pa/. In the former task, when VOT was incremented, the task could be solved phonetically (since the phonetic boundary was at +23 ms). The latter task could be solved only acoustically. Only in this condition was performance on the psychophysical tasks correlated significantly with performance on the VOT tasks. We can phrase this outcome another way: When the listener's response was based on a phonetic decision, then neither the identification nor discrimination test results were correlated with performance on the psychophysical tests.

Comment on VOT Studies

First, we should reiterate that, although acoustic differences among voiced and voiceless stop consonants can be referenced to a single temporal variable, voiced and voiceless stop consonants vary acoustically in a great number of ways. It is by no means clear which of the many cues to voicing a listener uses when all are available in the signal. Indeed, it is reasonable to assume that a perceiving system uses all the information available to it. From this point of view we must be careful when we use stimuli that differ in VOT as tests of "temporal processing." We must also be careful in inferring "normal processing" of VOT from studies that use a stimulus continuum at only one place of articulation.

With these caveats in mind, the results of the studies reviewed here indicate that the cochlear damage that produces mild, moderate, and moderately severe hearing impairment does not alter the resolution of VOT to the extent that phonetic identification is altered. However, the cochlear damage underlying severe hearing impairment does alter the fine-grained processing of VOT. This deficit is exposed only when listeners are forced to process the cues for place of articulation as well as for voicing. These results can be summarized with the observation that the information that specifies VOT is sufficiently robust to withstand degradation from high sound pressure levels and major loss of sensory receptors in the cochlea.

Identification Based on Friction Duration

Several phonetic contrasts in English can be created by varying the duration of friction noise. None of the contrasts in their natural form rely solely on friction duration, but all can be created artificially by holding another, normally co-varying, parameter constant. In this way, the ability of hearing impaired listeners to base phonetic judgments solely on difference in stimulus duration can be assessed. Three recent experiments have used such a procedure.

Dorman and Marton (1981) created a "shop" to "chop" continuum from a recording of the word "shop" by (1) reducing the rise time of the friction envelope to 50 ms; (2) making "center cuts" in the friction so that the onset and offset times of the friction noise would be unchanged; and (3) creating friction noises with durations of 60 ms through 140 ms in 10 ms steps. The stimuli were presented to listeners with hearing loss due to presbycusis and to young and elderly listeners with normal hearing. The three groups did not differ in location of the phonetic boundary. Thus, neither age nor hearing impairment plus age affected identification performance.

Ginzel, Pederson, Spliid, and Anderson (1982) have also assessed phonetic identification in presbycusic listeners using stimuli that differed in friction duration. The results of the identification tests showed that the presbycusic listeners needed slightly longer friction duration (10 ms) to reach asymptotic performance in each of the categories. Unfortunately, neither audiometric data nor statistical tests of the differences between groups were provided by the authors. Moreover, an equal age control group was not provided for the presbycusic listeners so that age per se cannot be ruled out as a factor contributing to the differences in performance between normal and presbycusic listeners.

In a third experiment in this tradition, a "toe" to "sew" continuum was created by synthesizing friction plus vowel syllables in which the friction noises varied in duration from 20 ms to 100 ms (Williams, Whaley, and Dorman, 1981). Age-matched children with normal sensitivity and those with mild, moderate, and moderately severe hearing losses identified the stimuli in similar manner. However, 3 of the 12 hearing impaired listeners who were tested could not identify the signals differentially. The listeners with severe impairment fared even less well: only two of six could identify the stimuli differentially and those two placed the phonetic boundary at greatly abnormal values. For these subjects, the sensitivity loss may have rendered the aperiodic noises so close to detection threshold that identification was impossible.

Identification Based on the Duration of a Periodic Signal

Several groups of investigators have created continua in which the duration of a voiced signal cues phonetic identity. Godfrey and Millay (1978) synthesized a /be/ to /we/ continuum by varying the duration of the formant transitions in two-formant stimuli. Across the continuum, the rise time of the amplitude envelope of the signals was fixed. When the stimuli were presented at equal sensation level (SL) to the normal and hearing impaired listeners, 9 of 15 moderately hearing impaired adults established phonetic boundaries in a normal manner. The six listeners who did not classify these stimuli in a normal manner did not differ from those who did in terms of audiogram contour or degree of loss. Given that the stimuli were synthesized with a minimum number of formants and a fixed amplitude rise time, the difficulty in identification shown by the six listeners could have been due to the stimuli not fitting the listeners' internal "template" of what a /b/ or /w/ should sound like. If so, the poor performance of the six listeners does not necessarily imply poor temporal resolution for moving formants. This interpretation receives support from a second study by Godfrey and Millay (1980), who found that each of 15 hearing impaired listeners was able to label the stimuli from a /ba/ to /wa/ continuum synthesized with five formants. For these stimuli the rise time of the amplitude envelope *did* vary with formant duration. Eleven of the 15 listeners were able to identify the stimuli from a /da/ to /ja/ continuum in a normal manner. Since both continua were synthesized with five formants an account of the poor performance of the five listeners in the /da/ to /ja/ continuum cannot be attributed to minimal synthesis. Rather, the relative difficulty may be due to the presence of falling F_2 and F_3 in the /da/ to /ja/ series, as opposed to the rising F_2 and F_3 in the /ba/ to /wa/ series. Hannley and Dorman (1983) have reported that hearing impaired listeners have more difficulty identifying place of articulation for stop consonants when the cue is a falling second formant transition than when the cue is a rising second formant transition. Thus, falling formant transitions may pose slightly more of a problem in resolution than a rising transition.

Results consistent with Godfrey and Millay (1980) have been obtained by Dorman and Marton (1981). In this experiment the phonetic boundary along a two-formant /ba/ to /wa/ continuum, in which the amplitude envelope co-varied with formant duration, did not differ among presbycusic listeners with mild and moderate hearing impairment, elderly normal hearing, and young normal hearing listeners.

Identification of periodic signals which do not change in frequency over time has also been examined in hearing impaired listeners. Ginzel and co-workers (1982) synthesized a continuum in which steady state vowel duration was varied over the range of 100 to 200 ms to create a contrast between Danish "laese" (short vowel duration) and "lasse" (long vowel duration). The results of the identification test indicated that presbycusic listeners showed a phonetic boundary within 10 ms of that established by younger, normal hearing listeners.

Another indication of sensitivity to differences in vowel duration can be extracted from an experiment by Revoile, Pickett, Holden, and Talkin (1982). Normal listeners and listeners with mild to severe hearing impairment were presented stimuli in which the several cues for the voicing characteristics of syllable-final consonants were altered. In the baseline condition, the vowel duration preceding the voiceless stop consonant was shorter than the vowel duration preceding the voiced stop consonant. When the duration of the vowel was neutralized between conditions, that is, the shorter vowel made longer by about three pitch periods, normal and hearing impaired listeners showed equivalent reductions in accuracy in identifying the stimulus as voiceless. In the case when the vowel preceding the voiced stop was made shorter, the hearing impaired listeners showed a greater than normal sensitivity to the change. Thus, it appears that hearing impaired listeners are at least as sensitive as normal listeners to relatively small changes in vowel duration when vowel duration is one of the cues to final consonant voicing.

Identification Based on the Duration of a Silent Interval

The relative duration of a silent interval can signal several phonetic contrasts in English, for example, the distinction between fricative and affricate in syllable-final position, the presence or absence of a stop consonant in a consonant cluster, the voicing of a stop consonant in word-medial position, and the distinction between single and double stop consonants.

The ability of hearing impaired listeners to identify stimuli in which silent gap duration has been varied has been studied by two groups of investigators. Dorman and Marton (1981) created a "slit" to "split" continuum by varying the duration of a silent interval between /s/ and "lit." The results of the identification test showed that young normal listeners established a phonetic boundary at 77 ms; elderly normal listeners established a boundary at 72 ms; and presbycusic listeners with mild to moderate losses established a boundary at 65 ms. The performance of the presbycusic group differed from that of the young normal group but not the elderly normal group. This outcome suggests that age per se plays a role in the boundary shift shown by the presbycusic individuals. The performance of the presbycusic listeners differed from normal in terms of the distribution of phonetic boundaries. The young normal listeners showed a nearly uniform distribution of phonetic boundaries within the range of 65 ms to 95 ms. However, for both the elderly normal and the presbycusic group, a clump of scores fell at 51 ms, whereas other scores spanned the region 65 ms to 95 ms. The subjects with a short boundary and those with a longer boundary did not differ in any obvious manner, specifically, in auditory thresholds or frequency resolution. An outcome similar to this one has been reported using a "say" to "stay" continuum (Ivory and Brandt, 1982). Ivory and Brandt reported that of seven mildly to moderately hearing impaired listeners, five showed labeling functions similar to those of normals. One listener had difficulty identifying the stimuli and one showed a very short boundary.

We note parenthetically that, although the "slit" to "split" and "say" to "stay" continua seem well suited to measuring gap detection in a phonetic mode of perception, they suffer, in fact, from an overabundance of cues to stop manner. Not only is the duration of a silent interval a manner cue; so also is the rate at which the friction noise offsets and the duration and rise time of the initial portion of F_1 in the vocalic portion of the signal. Thus, if hearing impaired listeners process the friction noise abnormally, or respond to the onset of the "lit" or "ay" abnormally, then a non-normal labeling function may be attributed incorrectly to abnormalities in processing silent gap duration. Another problem is that the friction and vocalic portions of the signal fall in frequency regions of generally very different sensitivity—that is, acuity is poorer in the /s/ region than in the F_1/F_2 region of the vowel. This may lead to differences in loudness growth for the two portions of the signal. In summary, although a good deal is known about the acoustics of "slit" versus "split" and "say" versus "stay" the contrasts may be too complex acoustically to be useful as a test of temporal processing ability. They may, however, be useful in experiments on cue salience or dominance for normal and hearing impaired listeners.

Further evidence that mildly and moderately hearing impaired listeners detect the duration of silent gaps well enough for normal phonetic identification can be gleaned from Revoile and colleagues (1982). In this experiment, referred to previously, changes were made in the acoustic structure of CVCs to assess the cue value of the several acoustic features which co-vary with final consonant voicing. In one condition the duration of the stop closure and closure murmur, which ordinarily varies between voiced and voiceless stops, was neutralized; in other words, the murmur was deleted and the silent interval made longer than normal for voiceless stops and shorter than normal for the voiced stops. The results showed that identification accuracy for stop voicing decreased slightly, about as much for the normal hearing listeners. Thus, the hearing impaired listeners as a group showed a sensitivity to the small change in closure duration, just as they had done for a small change in vowel duration.

Summary

We have reviewed the results of experiments carried out in the tradition of creating a series of stimuli that vary along a single acoustic dimension, or at least a small set of acoustic dimensions, for presentation to listeners in identification or discrimination tasks. A common finding has been that mildly and moderately hearing impaired listeners as a group show normal ability in using stimulus duration to cue phonetic identification. This outcome has been obtained for both periodic and nonperiodic signals and for signals that varied in formant onset asynchrony (or VOT), stimulus ontime, and stimulus offtime.

Listeners with severe hearing impairments have been tested extensively only with stimuli that differ in VOT. In these experiments a rather subtle deficit was found, which arose from the interaction of processing the cues for voicing and the cues for place of articulation. A similar interaction for mild to moderately hearing impaired listeners may be inferred from the data of Godfrey and Millay (1980).

FREQUENCY RESOLUTION

Psychophysical Studies

Frequency resolution, the ability to detect one signal in the presence of another, is poorer in hearing impaired listeners than in normal hearing listeners. This is the common conclusion of experiments measuring frequency resolution by psychophysical tuning curves (Pick, Evans, and Wilson, 1977; Thornton and Abbas, 1980; Wightman, McGee, and Kramer, 1977; Zwicker and Schorn, 1978), by masking patterns (Florentine, Buus, Scharf, and Zwicker, 1980; Jerger, Tillman, and Peterson, 1960; Martin and Pickett, 1970; Rittmanic, 1962), and by critical bands (deBoer and Bouwmeester, 1974). (For a critical review of this literature, see Humes, 1983.) These psychophysical results are in turn broadly consistent with data obtained in physiological investigations of neural tuning curves in animals with reversible and irreversible hearing impairment (Evans and Klinke, 1974; Kiang, Liberman, and Levine, 1976; Kiang, Moxon, and Levine, 1970).

Psychophysical tuning curves in hearing impaired listeners are characterized by a higher "tip," reflecting a loss of sensitivity for the probe tone and a reduced distance in decibels between the masking effectiveness of frequencies remote from the probe and those near the probe. The slope of the tuning curve depends in part on experimental conditions, such as whether a simultaneous or forward masking procedure is used (Wightman et al., 1977), whether the probe is presented at equal SL or SPL to the normal and hearing impaired listeners (Carney and Nelson, 1982), and the distance in hertz between the probe and the masker frequencies near the probe. The results of psychophysical tuning curve experiments with hearing impaired listeners have consistently led to the following conclusions: (1) Tuning curves can be flattened on the low-frequency side of the probe, implying upward spread of masking; (2) the curves can be flattened on the high-frequency side of the probe, implying downward spread of masking; (3) they can be flattened on both sides of the probe; or (4) they can assume a "w" shape. Such abnormalities are generally found when the sensitivity loss for the probe exceeds 30 to 40 dB.

The correlation between absolute sensitivity and frequency resolution tends to be greater than that between sensitivity and temporal resolution, depending on, of course, the measures used to assess these functions. Pick, Evans, and Wilson (1977) have reported correlations ranging from .41 to .61 between thresholds in quiet and thresholds in the presence of comb-filtered noise maskers. Others, using pure tone maskers, have reported correlations as high as .66 (Florentine et al., 1980) and .68 (Tyler, Summerfield, and Wood, 1982). When normal and elderly subjects are removed from the data pool, however, the correlation between sensitivity loss and frequency resolution is reduced.

Word Intelligibility in Noise

Both reduced auditory sensitivity and impaired frequency resolution are correlated significantly with poor speech understanding in noise. For example, Bonding (1979) reports correlations of $-.54$ between the mean threshold at 0.5, 1, and 2 kHz and word recognition in noise and of .69 between frequency resolution at 1 kHz and word recognition in noise. However, the correlation between frequency selectivity and word identification in noise is nonsignificant when auditory sensitivity is partialed out (Tyler et al., 1982). This does not mean that poor frequency resolution plays no role in word identification in noise. Rather, it indicates that either frequency selectivity and sensitivity are so highly correlated that it is difficult to assess their effects independently, or that both are related to a third variable, which is highly correlated with poor word intelligibility in noise.

Phonetic Identification Studies

There are two aspects of impaired frequency resolution which should produce detrimental effects on speech recognition *in quiet*. One is that a reduction in frequency resolution should blur formant peaks in the spectrum (see Bailey, 1983, p. 19). The other is that, given greater than normal upward spread of masking, information carried on the second and third formants may be masked by the more intense energy in the first formant. To facilitate our assessment of whether or how either of these related aspects of impaired frequency resolution affects phonetic identification, we have grouped recent studies into the categories of vowel and stop consonant recognition.

Vowel Recognition. If both frequency resolution and frequency discrimination are poorer in hearing impaired listeners than in normal hearing listeners (Turner and Nelson, 1982), it might be expected that the difference limen (Δf) for steady state formant frequencies would be larger for hearing impaired listeners than for normal listeners. Two recent studies have addressed this issue.

Millay and Godfrey (1980) synthesized two series of vowels, one in which the first formant varied in equal log frequency steps while F_2 and F_3 were fixed in frequency, and one in which F_1, F_3, and F_4 were fixed and F_2 varied in equal log steps. These series were presented to normal and hearing impaired listeners. The Δf necessary to detect a difference in the vowel set in which F_1 varied did not differ between the two groups.

This outcome is not surprising, since both groups had normal or near-normal sensitivity in the F_1 region. However, when the stimuli were varied in the region of the hearing impairment, that is, when F_2 varied, the four hearing impaired listeners showed difference limens four times larger than those of the normal listeners.

To assess the generality of this finding, Dorman and Marton (1981) synthesized stimuli in which F_1 was fixed at 335 Hz and F_2 varied in frequency over the range 924 to 1688 Hz. The F_2 of the "standard" stimulus in the A to X discrimination task was at 1230 Hz. For normal listeners, the point of 75% "different" responses fell at approximately 100 Hz. The listeners with mild and moderate sloping hearing impairment differed greatly in performance—some showed normal DLs in spite of their hearing loss, while others demonstrated DLs in excess of 456 Hz.

Interpretation of these two studies is made difficult by the fact that, as the comparison and standard stimuli move apart in frequency, a subtle phonetic as well as acoustic difference exists between the stimuli. It is possible that some hearing impaired listeners simply waited to hear a phonetic change between the standard and comparison stimuli before responding with "different" even though they were instructed to make such a response to *any* difference between the signals.

Another, more indirect method of estimating sensitivity to small changes in steady state formant frequency is to determine the slope of the phonetic identification function for stimuli that vary in steady state frequency. Godfrey and Millay (1980) reported normal slopes to the labeling functions of a group of 15 mildly to moderately hearing impaired listeners tested on /o/ to /a/ and /u/ to /o/ continua. Thus, there is little evidence that the large DLs showed by some hearing impaired listeners affect vowel recognition. Of course, it is possible that, by chance, the subjects in the phonetic identification experiment were those with normal DLs. On the other hand, it is possible that the relationship between vowel discrimination in a nonphonetic mode and vowel identification is similar to the case of VOT discrimination in a nonphonetic mode and VOT identification— abnormalities in discrimination are not sufficient to alter identification. Experiments in which the same listeners are tested on both discrimination and identification tasks would settle the issue.

Since hearing impaired listeners with mild to moderate hearing impairments identify vowels synthesized with only steady state formant cues in a normal manner, we would expect high identification accuracy for "natural" vowels. This is indeed the case. In a frequently cited article, Owens, Talbott, and Schubert (1968) reported 94% correct vowel identification (range, 84% to 99%) for hearing impaired listeners in a four-alternative forced-choice (4-AFC) task. The stimulus with the highest error

rate was /ɔI/ (24%). Not surprisingly, /ɔ/ was the most common substitute
for /ɔI/. The monothong with the highest error rate was /ɔ/ at 16% —
/ɔI/ and /ʌ/ were the most common substitutions. Unfortunately, the range
of hearing impairments over which this exemplary performance can be
reached is not clear. The listeners were described only as having
"sensorineural" losses, with scores on the relatively easy W-22 word list
ranging from 20% to 70% correct.

To assess whether the 4-AFC task artificially inflated vowel
identification by narrowing the range of responses to vowels in the front
or back environment, Dorman and Marton (1981) presented ten vowels in
b-vowel-t (/bVt/) format to presbycusic listeners with mild to moderate
impairments, normal listeners matched to the presbycusic subjects for age,
and young, normal hearing listeners. The results are shown in Figure 4–3.
The presbycusic listeners showed a mean score of 90% correct. Only one
vowel (/ɔ/) produced a concentration of errors. The error responses for
/ɔ/ were equally divided among /æ/ and /ʌ/—that is, vowels with similar
F_1 frequencies (585 Hz for /ʌ/, 605 Hz for /æ/, and 683 Hz for /ɔ/). Given
the similar vowel formants of these three vowels, we might expect that the
elderly listeners who showed poor identification (7 of 22) would have poorer
frequency resolution than those who achieved 100% correct. This was not
the case, at least in the lowest frequency region tested (1000 Hz). The
masking patterns of a 1000 Hz probe tone did not differ between the two
subgroups of listeners.

When interpreting the low error rates for vowels in natural context,
it should be remembered that natural vowels differ in several dimensions
in addition to F_1–F_2 space. For example, they differ in the relative
amplitude of the formants and in vowel length. Moreover, the presence
of formant transitions into and out of the vowel nucleus can aid greatly
in vowel identification (Verbrugge, Strange, Shankweiler, and Edman, 1976).
Thus, there are many cues to vowel identity in addition to those of F_1 and
F_2 steady state that a hearing impaired listener may exploit in a vowel
identification task. Here, then, is where Godfrey and Millay's (1980)
identification data with synthetic vowels are important: When only F_1
differed among the stimuli in the /u/ to /o/ continuum and when F_1 and
F_2 varied in small steps in the /o/ to /a/ continuum, the mildly and
moderately hearing impaired listeners showed normally sharp labeling
functions. It appears, therefore, that normal identification of vowels by
hearing impaired listeners need not be contingent on the presence of
multiple cues to vowel identity.

When cochlear damage is so great as to produce a severe loss of
sensitivity, vowel recognition, even with all of the natural cues in place,
is significantly impaired. As shown in Figure 4–4, Hack and Erber (1982)

Figure 4-3. Percent correct identification of vowels in /bVt/ format by young normal hearing listeners (top entry in each cell), elderly normal hearing listeners (middle entry), and presbycusic listeners (bottom entry).

<table>
<tr><td rowspan="2"></td><td colspan="10" align="center">Stimulus</td></tr>
<tr><td>i</td><td>I</td><td>e</td><td>ɛ</td><td>æ</td><td>ɔ</td><td>ʌ</td><td>o</td><td>u</td><td>ɝ</td></tr>
<tr><td rowspan="3" align="center">i</td><td>100</td><td>*</td><td>*</td><td></td><td></td><td></td><td></td><td></td><td>*</td><td></td></tr>
<tr><td>98</td><td>1</td><td>*</td><td></td><td></td><td></td><td></td><td></td><td>1</td><td></td></tr>
<tr><td>92</td><td>*</td><td>1</td><td></td><td></td><td></td><td></td><td></td><td>*</td><td></td></tr>
<tr><td rowspan="3" align="center">I</td><td>*</td><td>100</td><td></td><td></td><td></td><td></td><td></td><td></td><td></td><td></td></tr>
<tr><td>*</td><td>99</td><td></td><td></td><td></td><td></td><td></td><td></td><td></td><td></td></tr>
<tr><td>1</td><td>98</td><td></td><td></td><td></td><td></td><td></td><td></td><td></td><td></td></tr>
<tr><td rowspan="3" align="center">e</td><td>*</td><td>*</td><td>100</td><td></td><td></td><td></td><td></td><td>*</td><td>*</td><td></td></tr>
<tr><td>2</td><td>*</td><td>98</td><td></td><td></td><td></td><td></td><td>*</td><td>*</td><td></td></tr>
<tr><td>6</td><td>1</td><td>98</td><td></td><td></td><td></td><td></td><td>5</td><td>9</td><td></td></tr>
<tr><td rowspan="3" align="center">ɛ</td><td>*</td><td>*</td><td></td><td>100</td><td></td><td></td><td>*</td><td></td><td></td><td></td></tr>
<tr><td>*</td><td>*</td><td></td><td>87</td><td></td><td></td><td>*</td><td></td><td></td><td></td></tr>
<tr><td>1</td><td>1</td><td></td><td>86</td><td></td><td></td><td>6</td><td></td><td></td><td></td></tr>
<tr><td rowspan="3" align="center">æ</td><td></td><td></td><td>*</td><td>*</td><td>100</td><td>*</td><td>*</td><td></td><td>*</td><td></td></tr>
<tr><td></td><td></td><td>2</td><td>13</td><td>100</td><td>1</td><td>*</td><td></td><td>*</td><td></td></tr>
<tr><td></td><td></td><td>1</td><td>14</td><td>99</td><td>20</td><td>1</td><td></td><td>1</td><td></td></tr>
<tr><td rowspan="3" align="center">ɔ</td><td></td><td></td><td></td><td></td><td>-</td><td>98</td><td>*</td><td></td><td></td><td></td></tr>
<tr><td></td><td></td><td></td><td></td><td>-</td><td>88</td><td>*</td><td></td><td></td><td></td></tr>
<tr><td></td><td></td><td></td><td></td><td>1</td><td>63</td><td>1</td><td></td><td></td><td></td></tr>
<tr><td rowspan="3" align="center">ʌ</td><td></td><td></td><td></td><td></td><td></td><td>2</td><td>100</td><td></td><td></td><td></td></tr>
<tr><td></td><td></td><td></td><td></td><td></td><td>11</td><td>100</td><td></td><td></td><td></td></tr>
<tr><td></td><td></td><td></td><td></td><td></td><td>17</td><td>92</td><td></td><td></td><td></td></tr>
<tr><td rowspan="3" align="center">o</td><td></td><td></td><td></td><td></td><td></td><td></td><td></td><td>100</td><td>*</td><td>*</td></tr>
<tr><td></td><td></td><td></td><td></td><td></td><td></td><td></td><td>99</td><td>*</td><td>*</td></tr>
<tr><td></td><td></td><td></td><td></td><td></td><td></td><td></td><td>90</td><td>5</td><td>5</td></tr>
<tr><td rowspan="3" align="center">u</td><td></td><td></td><td></td><td></td><td></td><td></td><td></td><td>*</td><td>100</td><td></td></tr>
<tr><td></td><td></td><td></td><td></td><td></td><td></td><td></td><td>1</td><td>99</td><td></td></tr>
<tr><td></td><td></td><td></td><td></td><td></td><td></td><td></td><td>3</td><td>85</td><td></td></tr>
<tr><td rowspan="3" align="center">ɝ</td><td></td><td></td><td></td><td></td><td></td><td></td><td></td><td>*</td><td></td><td>100</td></tr>
<tr><td></td><td></td><td></td><td></td><td></td><td></td><td></td><td>*</td><td></td><td>100</td></tr>
<tr><td></td><td></td><td></td><td></td><td></td><td></td><td></td><td>2</td><td></td><td>95</td></tr>
</table>

Response

Figure 4-4. Percent correct identification of vowels in /bVb/ context by six children with severe to profound hearing impairment who obtained 80% to 100% correct recognition of spondees. From Hack, Z., and Erber, N. (1982). Auditory, visual, and auditory-visual perception of vowels by hearing-impaired children. *Journal of Speech and Hearing Research*, *25*, 100–107. Reprinted by permission.

	Stimulus									
Response	i	I	ɛ	æ	ɑ	ɔ	U	u	ʌ	ɝ
i	93						3	50		
I	7	67	3		3		13	13		
ɛ		27	23	7		7	17		10	7
æ			60	83	20				10	
ɑ				3	60	17	3		33	
ɔ				7	10	57			10	
U		3				7	23	3		3
u							17	33		7
ʌ			13		7	10	13		37	
ɝ		3				3	10			83

report vowel identification rates ranging from 93% for /i/ to 23% for /ɛ/ and /U/ in a sample of severely hearing impaired children with "good" word recognition abilities. Severely impaired children with "intermediate" word recognition skills showed poorer vowel identification—only /i/ and /I/ were identified with better than 50% accuracy.

Factors other than poor frequency resolution may contribute to poor vowel identification in this population. Since the onset of the hearing loss was prelingual, the children may not have all of the English vowels in their productive or perceptive repertoire. Thus, the poor identification of some vowels may reflect unfamiliarity with those phones as well as poor discrimination of the acoustic cues to vowel identity. The poor performance may also have been influenced by the nature of the task. The children were presented the stimuli in b-vowel-b (/bVb/) environments, but were given a set of "key words" with which to match the vowel in the /bVb/ stimulus. This is not an especially easy task even for the proverbial college sophomore and may have contributed in a small way to the error rate.

As we would expect from the spacing of vowel formants in F_1–F_2 space, Hack and Erber (1982) found fewer errors in front vowel environments and, as we would expect, incorrect error responses were generally vowels with similar formant frequencies. An interesting asymmetry in error responses was found for /I/ and /ɛ/: /ɛ/ was the dominant error response for /I/ and /æ/ was the dominant error response for /ɛ/. This pattern suggests a bias for vowels with either lower F_2 frequencies or high F_1 frequencies. A rather different pattern of errors occurred for /u/: 50% of the error responses were /i/. This outcome speaks to the importance of F_1 in determining error responses.

Poor identification of vowels is not a necessary consequence of a severe hearing impairment. We have recently tested an individual with postlingually acquired severe sensorineural hearing impairment on a bVt identification task. At 110 dB SPL presentation level, when the inherent variation in vowel duration was normalized and vocalic nucleus duration made brief (approximately 60 ms), this individual reached 90% identification accuracy. Confusions occurred only for /a/, which was heard as /ʌ/ 40% of the time, and for /i/, which was heard as /u/ 20% of the time. Although this is but a single case, it appears that vowel identification can remain accurate even in the face of severe hearing impairment.

In contrast, we have also tested a *prelingually* hearing-impaired listener with sensitivity 20 dB better than that of the patient described above. Vowel identification on the bVt series averaged only 81% correct, with errors distributed over /i,ɛ,ɔ,æ,ʌ, u/. Factors other than frequency resolution obviously play a role in determining errors in vowel identification.

Lesions to the central auditory system may cause more difficulty in vowel identification than peripheral lesions. We have reviewed the errors on a word identification test of a group of hearing impaired listeners with cochlear damage and a group of 12 listeners with confirmed acoustic neurinomas who were matched for degree and configuration of hearing loss. As expected, at moderate signal presentation levels, the retrocochlear group made more errors on both consonants and vowels than the peripherally impaired group. However, the ratio of vowel to consonant errors was similar between the groups. At high signal presentation levels, the ratio of vowel to consonant errors increased significantly for the retrocochlear group but not for the cochlear group. Thus, the "rollover phenomenon," poorer speech intelligibility at high than at moderate signal presentation levels (Jerger and Jerger, 1971), was due in significant measure to increased errors of vowel identification.

The interpretation of errors in open set word intelligibility testing is complicated by several factors. First, there may be no response to the stimulus; in this case, transmitted and perceived phones cannot be compared. Second, the listener's response is likely to be influenced by linguistic constraints in giving a meaningful word response, especially when there are multiple phoneme errors within the word. Third, the accuracy of the transcribed errors is attendant on the tester's perception in recording the response. Fourth, phoneme omissions and additions are often not recorded in a confusion matrix. Hence, the actual incidence of all phoneme confusions is not known. These problems of interpretation lead to the following question: Is the high error rate on vowels in retrocochlear eighth nerve disorder an artifact of open set testing? The vowel identification data from at least one patient suggest that it is not. We have tested with a closed set of 10 /bVt/ stimuli a patient with normal hearing sensitivity bilaterally (brought to our attention and made available to us for testing by J. Jerger) who had an astrocytoma in the cerebellopontine angle involving the eighth nerve. Overall vowel recognition was 56% correct with high identification accuracy only for the front vowels /i I e/. Thus, the high error rates for vowels in eighth nerve disorders does not seem, at first inspection, to be simply an artifact of open set testing. Rather, retrocochlear disruption of neural encoding may be far more detrimental to vowel recognition than is moderately severe loss of hair cells and aberrant peripheral encoding.

Summary and Comment. Vowel identification at adequate suprathreshold levels is robust in the face of poorer than normal frequency resolution and larger than normal difference limens for detection of differences in steady state formant frequency. When errors in vowel identification occur, they tend to be for the back vowels (mainly /ɔ/) with similar formant frequencies in F_1–F_2 space. A part of the stability of vowel identification in the face of a deterioration in frequency selectivity may be the several sources of vowel information in addition to steady state frequencies in the syllabic nucleus. Another contribution to the stability may be related to the generous spacing between English vowels in the F_1–F_2 domain. It could be the case in a language with a greater density of vowels (e.g., with both front and back rounded and unrounded vowels) that moderate hearing impairment would have a greater effect on vowel recognition.

Stop Consonant Recognition. To understand how poor frequency resolution and upward spread of masking (which poor frequency resolution usually entails) might affect the recognition of stop consonant place of articulation, the first thing to determine is acoustic cues for place of articulation. These include formant transitions caused by the movement of the articulators into the position of articulatory closure, the silent interval produced by vocal tract occlusion, a burst of energy produced at the moment of release of occlusion, friction as a consequence of turbulence in the still narrow opening between articulators, aspiration during the period before voicing onset, and finally, formant transitions produced by the movement of the articulators from the point of occlusion to the following vowel. Stop consonants which differ in place of articulation differ acoustically in terms of (1) the duration, amplitude, and spectrum of the burst, (2) the duration of the formant transitions, (3) formant onset frequency and direction of formant movement, and (4) voice onset time. When appropriate precautions are taken to neutralize other cues, each of these acoustic events can be shown to have value as a cue to place of articulation.

The strategy used by the listener to process this array of information is still a matter of considerable debate. Some researchers have argued that the processing system tracks the changing acoustic information given by the bursts and formant transitions to make decisions about place of articulation (Cooper, Delattre, Liberman, Borst, and Gerstman, 1952; Dorman, Studdert-Kennedy, and Raphael, 1977; Liberman, Delattre, Cooper, and Gerstman, 1954). Others argue that the speech processor looks to a static template of spectral tilt following the onset of acoustic energy (Blumstein and Stevens, 1980; Stevens and Blumstein, 1978; but see Blumstein, Isaacs, and Mertus, 1982, and Walley and Carrell, 1983, for evidence to the contrary). Still others believe that both static and dynamic templates are used by the processor (Kewley-Port, 1982, 1983). Whatever the theoretical position taken, there is little argument that the onset frequency of the formants, the energy distribution of the burst, and the trajectories of F_2 and F_3 can be used as information by the speech processor for stop consonant recognition.

Studies with Nonspeech Signals

Given the importance of the burst spectrum and F_2–F_3 onset frequencies as cues to place of articulation, researchers have asked whether hearing impaired listeners differ from normal in two important respects. First, do they experience greater than normal difficulty in discriminating between the onset frequencies of tone glides that mimic the behavior of isolated formant transitions? Second, do they experience greater than normal backward masking of brief noise bursts (which mimic the release bursts in speech)? These experiments represent an attempt to bridge the gap between psychoacoustic studies and studies of speech recognition by using nonspeech analogues which preserve certain dynamic properties of speech without its phonetic content. In this way, presumably, auditory perception can be assessed independently of phonetic contributions.

Tyler, Wood, and Fernandes (1983) presented 50 ms tone glides to mildly to moderately hearing impaired listeners in a 3-AFC task. In one condition the task was to detect the difference between the frequency of the constant frequency standard and the constant frequency target. In another task, the standard was held constant in frequency but the targets were frequency ramps rising to the frequency of the standard. In a third task, both the standard and the targets were rising in frequency. Across the three tasks for the 4000 Hz standard only three or four listeners performed worse than normal. Collins (in preparation) has extended this type of experiment to two situations in which a steady state frequency follows or precedes the tone glide (thus simulating a portion of both formant transition and steady state vowel in CV and VC syllables). The hearing impaired listeners exhibited larger DLs than normal, with the greatest deviation from normal occurring for VC analogues. Van Tassel (1980) has carried this type of experiment one step farther by presenting four mildly to moderately hearing-impaired listeners with isolated second formants in a discrimination task. When the standard was a formant with no initial transitions and the targets were synthesized with a transition rising to the steady state frequency of the standard, two of the listeners evidenced difference limens near the normal mean of 23 Hz while two others evidenced abnormally large difference limens (72–75 Hz). These results are quite similar to those reported by Tyler and colleagues (1983) in the sense that poor resolution of the starting frequency of a frequency-modulated signal such as a formant transition is not an inevitable consequence of a mild to moderate loss in auditory sensitivity.

The second question—whether hearing impaired listeners suffer greater than normal backward masking of brief noise bursts—has been addressed by Revoile, Pickett, and Wilson (1981). Severely hearing impaired listeners were presented 50 ms low- (500 to 1500 Hz), mid- (1500 to 4000 Hz), and high- (4000 to 6000 Hz) frequency noise bursts in quiet and followed after 10 ms with a 200-ms two-formant approximation to the vowels /a/ and /i/. The detection thresholds for the noise bursts in the masked condition did not differ from those in quiet. On the basis of these data, backward detection masking of release bursts by a following vowel does not seem a likely explanation for imperfect recognition of place of articulation. These data can be extrapolated to speech, however, only with caution. The bursts used by Revoile and colleagues were much longer in duration than those found in speech. Moreover, in natural speech, alveolar and velar bursts differ little in burst center frequency in front vowel environments (Dorman et al., 1977), but differ significantly in the distribution of energy, which is narrow for velars and spread for alveolars. Finally, Revoile and co-workers assessed detection, not recognition masking. This is an important distinction to make, for in speech, it is the perceived location and shape of the burst spectrum rather than its detectability, that we assume to be relevant for stop consonant recognition. We return to this issue again in discussing the results of experiments on the identification of stop consonants synthesized with and without a burst.

Studies with Natural and Synthetic Speech

Research with nonspeech signals can provide a strong inference about mechanisms underlying poor speech recognition. Experiments in which aspects of the speech signal are directly manipulated in order to make the signal more or less intelligible can provide more convincing evidence as to underlying mechanisms.

We begin our analysis of stop consonant recognition in speech with a review of recent experiments in which stops were presented to hearing impaired listeners at sound pressure levels that ensured that the information-bearing aspects of the signal were at suprathreshold levels. These experiments address a key question: When attenuation of information is not at issue and only the distortion engendered by cochlear pathology affects recognition, how well are stop consonants recognized? The answer, for voiced stops in initial position, is quite well. Van Tassel, Hagen, Koblas, and Penner (1982) report a mean score of 91% correct (range 73% to 99%) for natural speech /b d g p t k/ in the vocalic environments /i a u/. When the same listeners were presented stimuli synthesized with burst and five formants from a /ba/ to /da/ to /ga/ continuum, identification performance was again very good, yielding a correlation coefficient of .84 with performance on the natural speech task. Normal identification of signals from a /ba/ to /da/ to /ga/ continuum synthesized with burst and five formants has also been reported by Raz and Noffsinger (1979). Normal identification of these stimuli also extends to presbycusic listeners (Hannley and Dobbins, 1981). Indeed, even when the duration of "full cue" stimuli is reduced to two pulses, hearing impaired listeners perform about as well as normal listeners (Van Tassel et al., 1982).

Listening to speech at a level that ensures that the cues for stop consonant recognition are all suprathreshold may be an uncommon experience for many hearing impaired listeners with poor sensitivity in the 2 to 4 kHz region. The more common situation may be one in which the alveolar bursts, velar bursts in front vowel environments, and third formant transitions are near detection threshold. How is stop consonant recognition affected in situations such as this?

The ability of hearing impaired listeners to recognize stop consonants without burst cues has been studied extensively only in the /a/ environment—the environment in which burst removal makes little difference in recognition for normal listeners (Dorman et al., 1977). In this environment hearing impaired listeners as a group show a selective difficulty in stop consonant identification. For example, Turek, Dorman, Franks, and Summerfield (1980) synthesized a three-formant /ba/ to /da/ to /ga/ continuum for presentation to nine bilaterally hearing impaired listeners with moderate flat and sloping audiometric configurations. Performance on the task ranged from normal (two listeners) to extremely poor. Common abnormal response patterns included those with a /ba/ or /da/ category but no others; and those with /ba/ and /da/ category but no /ga/ category. A similar experiment and similar outcome has been reported by Raz and Noffsinger (1969). High error rates on stop consonants synthesized without a burst are not unique to the situation in which stimuli from along a continuum are presented to listeners. Hannley and Dobbins (1981) reported error rates of 14% for /ba/, 4% for /da/, and 46% for /ga/ when single tokens of three formants /ba/ to /da/ to /ga/ were presented to presbycusic listeners with mild and moderate losses. Across the three experiments reported here, identification of /ga/ tended to suffer most from the absence of a release burst.

In instances of poor phonetic identification the question should be asked whether listeners can discriminate between items that are identified as the same phone. Such an outcome was reported by Parady and co-workers (1981) for severely and profoundly hearing impaired listeners when the stimuli differed in a timing cue—voice onset time. A rather different outcome has been obtained when the stimuli differed in F_2 and F_3 onset frequencies. Stewart (1980) presented a three-formant /ba/ to /da/ to /ga/

continuum to 16 mildly to moderately hearing impaired listeners in both identification and discrimination tasks. In only 2 of 90 stimulus contrasts was discrimination markedly better than identification. Of course, performance on this type of experiment is critically dependent on the magnitude of the difference between the stimuli classified as belonging to the same category. It would not be surprising to find, if /ba/ and /ga/ were both labeled /da/, for example, that a listener could discriminate between these extreme tokens along a continuum. There is evidence, albeit scarce, that listeners with one broad category spanning /b d g/ can indeed hear some differences in the stimuli. Figure 4–5 (Turek et al., 1980) shows the labeling performance for a three-formant /b d g/ continuum of a moderately hearing impaired listener. Note that, although all stimuli are labeled /da/ for more than 60% of the time, inflection points in the identification function correspond to the location of phonetic boundaries for normal listeners.

Stimuli lacking a release burst are still relatively complex acoustically. To further simplify the formant patterns that specify place of articulation, investigators have used two-formant patterns in recognition experiments with hearing impaired listeners.

As a group, hearing impaired listeners experience great difficulty in identifying two-formant /b d g/. Marton and Dorman (1981) reported that mildly to moderately hearing impaired presbycusic listeners showed aberrant identification of the stimuli from all three phonetic categories. Of the three phones, /b/ was the best identified, and /g/ the poorest. Poor identification of two-formant /b d g/ is not limited to presbycusic listeners. As shown in Figure 4–6, young listeners with noise-induced hearing loss and listeners with Meniere's disease, as well as presbycusic listeners, show poor identification of /g/, better identification of /d/, and near-normal identification of /b/ (Hannley and Dorman, 1983; see Ivory and Brandt, 1982, for an experiment in which better performance on two-formant stimuli was elicited).

The difference in ability of hearing impaired listeners to identify full-cue and partial-cue stimuli when all cues are suprathreshold is striking. Whereas most mildly to moderately hearing impaired listeners perform normally with full-cue stimuli, when partial-cue stimuli are presented only a few of the same listeners perform in a resolutely normal manner.

The Upward Spread of Masking Hypothesis

There are two prevalent views of why stop consonant recognition is relatively poor in partial-cue contexts. One is that the poor recognition

Figure 4–5. Identification of stimuli from a /ba/to/da/to/ga/ continuum by normal listeners (A) and by a listener with moderate flat hearing impairment (B). Note that although this listener identifies all stimuli as /d/, inflection points in the function correspond to the locations of phonetic boundaries for normal listeners. (From Turek, S., v. deG., Dorman, M. F., Franks, J. R., and Summerfield, A.Q. (1980). Identification of synthetic /bdg/ by hearing impaired listeners under monotic and dichotic formant presentation. *Journal of the Acoustical Society of America, 67,* **1031–1040. Reprinted with permission.**

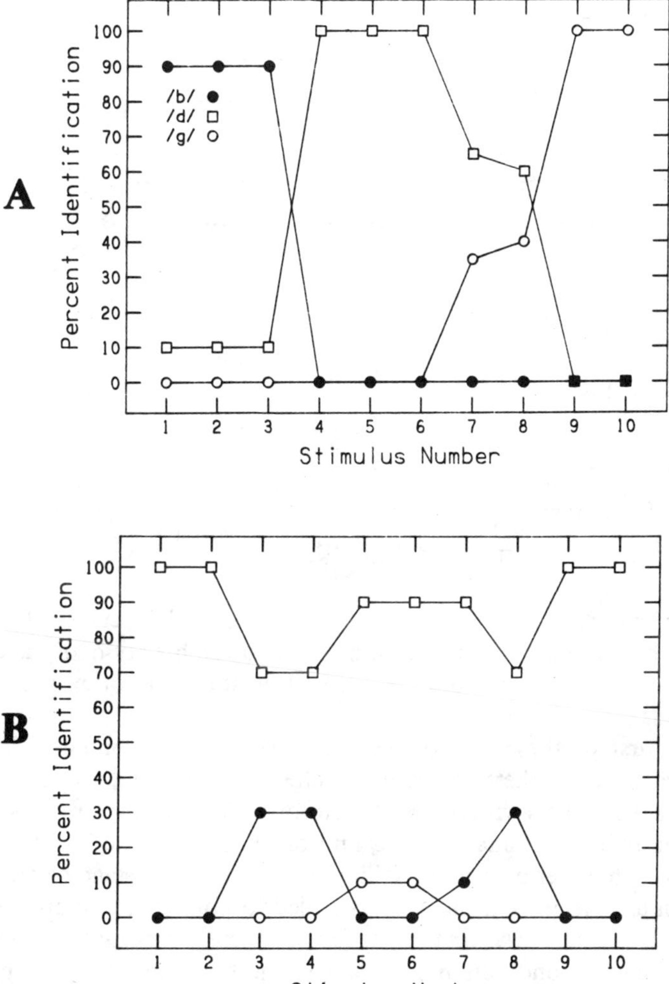

Figure 4–6. Identification of two-formant /ba/, /da/, and /ga/ by normal listeners and listeners with hearing impairment due to noise exposure, Meniere's disease, and aging (presbycusis). The order of the group data is the same for /d/ and /g/ as for /b/.

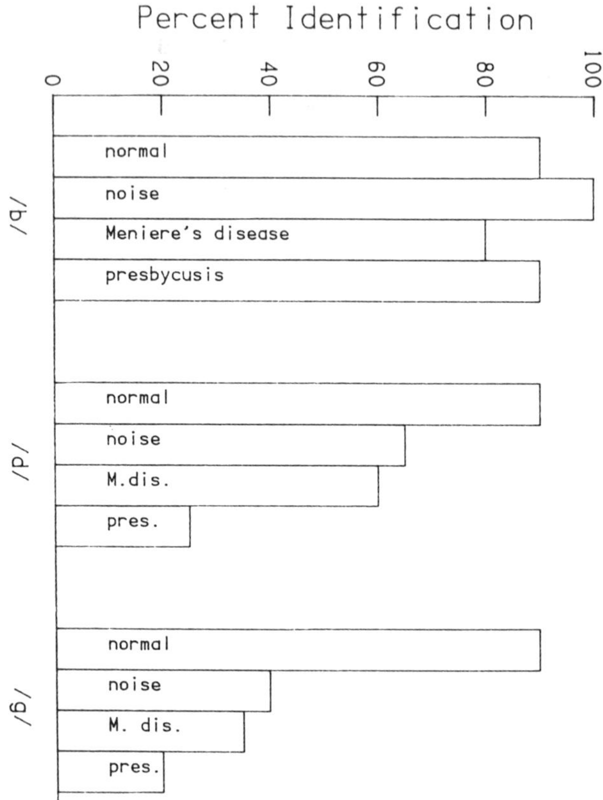

is due to upward spread of masking by F_1 on the place cues in F_2 and F_3. Another is that poor recognition is due to the brevity of F_2 and F_3 transitions (when contrasted to the longer transitions in, for example, the semivowels).

The first of these hypotheses is derived from a seminal series of experiments by Pickett, Martin-Danaher, and colleagues. In these experiments, listeners with severe and profound hearing impairments were presented, in a discrimination task, an isolated steady state formant as a standard with either a rising or falling transition to the steady state as a target. In another task a flat F_1 was added to both standard and target stimuli. The outcome was that the Δf for "different" responses was greater in the F_1 plus F_2 condition than in the F_2 alone condition. Upward spread of masking was entertained as a mechanism underlying the increased Δf

because it could be reduced by presenting F_1 to the opposite ear, by reducing the intensity of F_1, and by delaying the onset of F_1 (Pickett and Danaher, 1973).

In the years following the publication of these experiments it has become common to cite upward spread of masking as a probable mechanism underlying poor recognition of place of articulation. Less commonly cited are two other aspects of Pickett's and Danaher's experiments: (1) When tested at equal SPL, normal and hearing impaired subjects performed *equally.* This suggests that distortion due to high SPL, rather than distortion due only to cochlear pathology, was responsible for the large DLs reported. (2) The subject population was a special one—it was composed of severely and profoundly hearing impaired listeners, some of whom were congenitally hearing impaired. There is no guarantee that mildly or moderately impaired listeners with late onset of auditory dysfunction behave in the manner of those tested by Pickett and Martin-Danaher. Indeed, the results of a recent experiment suggest that at least some do not. Van Tassel (1980) reported extreme variability in performance on a task similar to that used by Pickett and Martin-Danaher. Depending on whether the steady state frequency of the isolated F_2 was at 1100 Hz or at the /b/to/d/ phoneme boundary, one of four listeners or three of four listeners did *not* show poorerΔfs in the F_1 plus F_2 condition than in the F_2 alone condition.

The small size of the subject sample and the large difference in performance of the listeners makes generalization from Van Tassel's study unwise. Further evidence of upward spread of masking in impaired phonetic identification should be sought in experiments with /ba/, /da/, and /ga/ in which F_1 has been reduced in amplitude or presented dichotically.

The results of an experiment that compared the identification of /ba/, /da/, and /ga/ in monaural and dichotic (i.e., F_1 to one ear and F_2-F_3 to the other ear) have been presented by Turek and colleagues (1980). Identification of the three-formant stimuli in the monaural conditions was poor. Identification in the dichotic conditions was consistently better for only one or two of the nine hearing impaired listeners. Similar results (little or no benefit of dichotic presentation) using filtered natural speech have been reported by Haas (1982), Foster, Glynn, Haggard, Trinder, and Fernandes (1980), and Kaplan and Pickett (1982).

A systematic exploration of the effect of a reduction in F_1 intensity has been reported by Hannley and Dorman (1983) for two-formant stimuli. In that experiment, four 10-step /ba/ to /da/ to /ga/ continua were synthesized and presented for identification to hearing impaired listeners. The continua differed in the level of F_1 relative to F_2; F_1 was synthesized at 0, -6, -12, and -18 dB relative to F_2. The results of the identification

Figure 4–7. Identification of two-formant /ba/, /da/, and /ga/ when F$_1$ amplitude is at 0, -6, -12, and -18 dB relative to F$_2$ for normal listeners (●) and listeners with hearing impairment due to noise exposure (0), Meniere's disease (□), and aging (Δ).

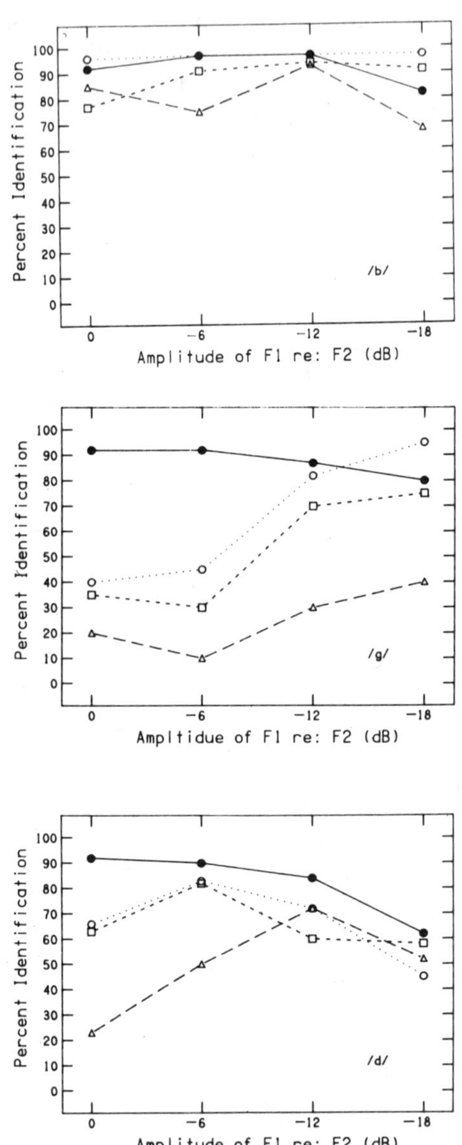

task are shown in Figure 4–7. In this figure the responses to stimuli 1, 2, 3; 5, 6, 7, and 9, 10 were combined to form /b/, /d/, and /g/ categories, respectively. Identification accuracy for /b/ was high among all groups. Identification accuracy for /d/ described an inverted U-shaped function for all groups. Of the hearing impaired listeners, those with presbycusic losses performed significantly more poorly than the others for all phoneme categories. In the -6 dB condition, both the Meniere's disease group and the noise-induced hearing loss group reached a normal level of performance. The largest effects, however, were seen in /g/ identification accuracy. At 0 and 6 dB attenuation, all hearing impaired groups showed very poor identification accuracy. With further reduction of F_1, both the noise-induced loss group and the Meniere's group reached normal levels of performance.

These results, especially for /g/ identification, provide compelling evidence that upward spread of masking can be of sufficient magnitude that phonetic identification is adversely affected. Why then is dichotic presentation of F_1, which should eliminate spread of masking by removing the putative masker from the same cochlea as the F_2-F_3 target, so ineffective in reducing errors in identification?

One possibility is that the cochlear damage that results in reduced sensitivity, reduced frequency resolution, and reduced temporal resolution also results in impaired dichotic fusion, the ability to combine signals presented simultaneously to the two ears. If this were so, the failure to find better intelligibility with dichotic presentation of F_1 and F_2-F_3 would not speak to the hypothesis of upward spread of masking. In the absence of converging evidence on the issue, this interpretation cannot be easily discarded. We suspect, however, that upward spread of masking affects phonetic identification only in cases of minimal stimulus information for place of articulation, that is, for two-formant stimuli. In this stimulus setting, in which there is simultaneous onset of F_1 and F_2 and only F_2 carries information for place, masking may occur quite readily. However, when in three-formant synthesis, identification fails, upward spread of masking may not be the principal culprit but, rather, poor resolution of the information provided by F_2 and F_3 onset frequencies and formant transitions. In other words, abnormal masking spread occurs in hearing impaired listeners and is of sufficient magnitude to affect phonetic perception in cases of minimal information for place, but it is not of sufficient magnitude to affect phonetic identification when more than minimal information for place is presented.

On this view we might expect to find a beneficial effect of reducing F_1 amplitude in the situation when a stimulus is presented at such a low level that F_2-F_3 and burst are near threshold but F_1 is greatly suprathreshold. In this circumstance the masking effect of F_1 may be maximized. We have tested this hypothesis by presenting "bay," "day," and "gay" to hearing impaired listeners at several sound pressure levels and in two stimulus configurations. In one the stimuli were synthesized with a burst and five formants. In another the stimuli were synthesized without a first formant, that is, with burst and F_2 through F_5. The signals were first presented to the listeners at 90 dB SPL and then the level was reduced in steps until chance performance was reached. At the 90 dB level the full-cue stimuli were well identified. As the level was reduced errors at one place of articulation and then the others occurred. Presumably the point at which errors occurred was the point at which the relevant information from place of articulation became unavailable for use by the listeners. Since the stops were well identified at the highest level, errors in identification as signal level was reduced were due not to distortion but rather to attenuation of information or possibly to masking of the burst and F_2-F_3 information by F_1. Although the familiar variability in performance found with hearing impaired listeners was found here also, the most general interpretation of the data was that the elimination of F_1 in the signal did not reduce errors in identification. Moreover, for many listeners the elimination of F_1 actually *reduced* intelligibility. This set of results and the preference hearing listeners show for signals that include significant low-frequency information (Punch and Beck, 1980) lead us to believe that it is more important to leave F_1 in the signal (at some level) in order to provide "spectral balance" in the frequency domain than to remove it on the grounds that it may mask F_2-F_3.

The Too-Brief Cue Hypothesis

In 1978 Yokkaichi and Fujisaki presented the results of an identification test with vowels, semivowels, and stop consonants which they believed supported the hypothesis that the poor recognition of stop consonants is due to the brief duration of the formant transitions. Normal and mildly to severely hearing impaired listeners were the subjects. Three sets of stimuli were used in the identification tasks: an /i/ to /u/ continuum in which F_2 ranged from 2100 Hz to 1200 Hz, a /wa/ to /ra/ continuum in which transition duration was approximately 150 ms and the onset of F_2 ranged from 930 Hz to 1650 Hz, and a /ba/ to /da/ continuum in which the transition duration was approximately 50 ms and F_2 ranged from 970 Hz to 1690 Hz. The results indicated that all nine hearing impaired listeners could identify the vowels (though not as accurately as normal individuals), six of nine listeners could identify the /wa/ to /ra/ stimuli, but only one of the nine listeners could identify the /ba/ to /da/ stimuli. Since the /ba/ to /da/ and /wa/ to /ra/ stimuli differed only in duration of the formant transitions, this outcome was interpreted as indicating that brief formant transitions are more difficult to process than longer formant transitions.

A similar concept has been advanced, independently, by Godfrey and Millay (1980). In this experiment 15 hearing impaired listeners were presented two vowel identification tasks, two stop semivowel identification tasks, and a stop consonant place of articulation identification task. The outcome was that "all listeners consistently identified the vowels, some could not identify the stop vs. glide series and all but two had difficulty with the stop consonant identification" (p. 200). Given the nearly identical outcome of the two studies cited above, using subjects with hearing impairment ranging from mildly to severely impaired and speaking two different languages (English and Japanese), the "brief duration" hypothesis must be given serious consideration.

There is, however, a major difficulty in comparing the recognition of stop consonants and semivowels in these experiments. In the Japanese study the semivowels were synthesized with a full complement of normal cues. The stop consonants were synthesized without a major cue—the release burst. The difference in outcome may reflect only the difference in intelligibility of signals that have a full or partial complement of cues. A similar objection can be made of the study in English. In this experiment the stop to semivowel continuum was anchored on one end by a semivowel with a full set of cues. The signals at either end of the place of articulation continuum possessed only a partial complement. Again, the relative intelligibility could be attributed to the presence or absence of cues.

At all events the "brief cue" hypothesis would be on firmer ground if it could be demonstrated that lengthening the cues for the stop consonants aided listeners in identification. Two such tests have been conducted. Stewart (1980), borrowing from earlier research with normal listeners by Dechovitz and Mandler (1977), synthesized one /b d g/ continuum in which the duration of all three formant transitions was 30 ms and another in which F_1 remained at 30 ms duration but F_2 and F_3 were stretched to 140 ms. Because F_1 was rapid in both continua, the stimuli in both were heard as stop consonants. When the results from subjects who showed ceiling effects were removed from the data pool (since the subjects could not improve in the "long" transition condition) the remaining listeners with mildly to moderately severe hearing impairment showed a significant increase in /b/ and /g/, but not /d/, identification accuracy. The magnitude of the increase was quite small for /b/ (11%) but was respectable for /g/ (25%). Unfortunately, the gain in identification accuracy afforded by lengthening the transitions of F_2-F_3 has not proved reliable. Hannley and Dobbins (1981) presented /b d g/ synthesized with normal and lengthened transitions to young and elderly hearing impaired listeners. For /b/ and /d/ no increase in identification accuracy was afforded by the lengthened transitions. For /g/ a small gain (10%) was recorded for the elderly hearing impaired listeners in the lengthened transition condition. The young hearing impaired listeners showed no gain.

If upward spread of masking accounts for errors only in two-formant synthesis and if the brief cue duration hypothesis fails to accrue substantial empirical support, what accounts for the poor recognition of voiced stops, especially /g/, when synthesized without a burst? Data from Dobbins (1981) provide the basis for another hypothesis. Dobbins presented his presbycusic listeners with stops synthesized in four configurations: with two formants; with two formants and a burst; with three formants; and with three formants and a burst. Recognition of /b/, even in the two-formant synthesis, was accurate. Recognition of /d/ was poor in the two-formant and two-formant plus burst synthesis but reached normal when a third formant was added. For /g/, recognition was poor in the two-formant synthesis (67%), was normal for the two-formant plus burst synthesis (100%), was again poor in the three-formant synthesis (42%), and was again normal for the three formants and burst synthesis (100%).

We can account for the patterns in Dobbins' data in the following manner. The increase in identification accuracy for /d/ when synthesized with a third formant can be viewed as a consequence of the increase in high-frequency energy at signal onset. A signal with an "up-tilted" spectrum at onset is more appropriate for /d/ than a signal with a "peaked" spectrum in the midfrequencies, which is the result of two-formant synthesis. The failure of the /d/ burst to aid identification when only two formants were synthesized is most likely due to the frequency separation of the burst at 4000 Hz and the onset of F_2 at 1500 Hz, which impaired integration of the cues. The increase in identification accuracy for /g/ when synthesized with a burst can be viewed as a consequence of the increased duration of the midfrequency peak in the running spectrum. A relatively long duration midfrequency peak is more appropriate for /g/ than the very brief peak that results from synthesis without a burst. If our interpretations are correct, there is not a single factor that accounts for errors in stop consonant identification. Rather, errors occur when a portion of the information which normally characterizes a phone, such as an uptilted spectrum for /d/, or a long duration midfrequency peak for /g/, is eliminated from the signal. If so, then hearing impaired listeners can be characterized as needing information for stop consonant recognition that normal listeners usually do not need.

CONCLUDING COMMENT

Experiments using synthetic speech as stimuli have yielded a small but useful body of evidence on phonetic identification by hearing impaired listeners. Two aspects of these data are particularly noteworthy. One is that listeners with mildly through moderately severe hearing loss appear to make normal use of temporal information in the speech signal. This may account, in large measure, for the normal or near-normal phonetic identification scores of listeners with poor frequency selectivity. The other noteworthy aspect is that errors in stop consonant identification are not due to a single factor, such as upward spread of masking. Rather, errors arise at the different places of articulation as a consequence of different factors. An appreciation of this should be useful in designing prosthetic devices with signal processing capabilities.

REFERENCES

Bailey, P. (1983). Hearing for speech: The information transmitted in normal and impaired hearing. In Lutman and Haggard (Eds.), *Hearing science and hearing disorders.* London: Academic Press.

Blumstein, S., Cooper, W., Zurif, E., and Caramazza, A. (1977). The perception and production of voice-onset-time in aphasia. *Neuropsychologia, 15,* 371–383.

Blumstein, S., and Stevens, K. N. (1980). Perceptual invariance and onset spectra for stop consonants in different vowel environments. *Journal of the Acoustical Society of America, 67,* 648–662.

Blumstein, S., Isaacs, E., and Mertus, J. (1982). The role of the gross spectral shape as a perceptual cue to place of articulation in initial stop consonants. *Journal of the Acoustical Society of America, 72*(1), 43–50.

de Boer, E., and Bouwmeester, J. (1974). Critical bands and sensorineural hearing loss. *Audiology, 8,* 205–216.

Bonding, P. (1979). Frequency selectivity and speech discrimination in sensorineural hearing loss. *Scandinavian Audiology, 8,* 205–219.

Bosatra, A., and Russolo, M. (1976). Directional hearing, temporal order and auditory pattern in peripheral and brain stem lesion. *Audiology, 15,* 141–151.

Carney, A., and Nelson, D. (1983). An analysis of psychophysical tuning curves in normal and pathological ears. *Journal of the Acoustical Society of America, 73*(1), 268–278.

Collins, M. J. (in preparation). Tone glide discrimination by normal-hearing and hearing-impaired listeners.

Cooper, F. S., Delattre, P. C., Liberman, A. M., Borst, J. M., and Gerstman, L. J. (1952). Some experiments on the perception of synthetic speech sounds. *Journal of the Acoustical Society of America, 24,* 597–606.

Darwin, C., and Pearson, M. (1982). What tells us that voicing has started? *Speech Communication, 1,* 29–44.

Dechovitz, D., and Mandler, R. (1977). Effects of transition length on identification and discrimination along a place continuum. *Status Report on Speech Research,* SR-51-52, Haskins Laboratories.

Dobbins, E. A. (1982). *Intelligibility of speech varying in acoustic information: Performance of normal and hearing-impaired listeners* (Unpublished master's thesis). Tempe, AZ: Arizona State University.

Dorman, M. F., and Marton, K. (1981). Cochlear frequency selectivity and phonetic identification in aging listeners. *Journal of the Acoustical Society of America, 69,* Supplement 1, S-123.

Dorman, M. F., Studdert-Kennedy, M., and Raphael, L. J. (1977). Stop consonant recognition: Release bursts and formant transitions as functionally equivalent, context dependent cues. *Perception and Psychophysics, 22,* 109–122.

Dubno, J., Dirks, D., and Langhoffer, L. (1982). Evaluation of hearing-impaired listeners using a nonsense syllable test. II. Syllable recognition and consonant confusion patterns. *Journal of Speech and Hearing Research, 25,* 141–148.

Egan, J. (1948). Articulation testing methods. *Laryngoscope, 58,* 955–991.

Erber, N. R. (1972). Auditory, visual, and auditory–visual recognition of consonants by children with normal and impaired hearing. *Journal of Speech and Hearing Research, 15,* 413–422.

Evans, E. F., and Klinke, R. (1974). Reversible effects of cyanide and furosemide on the tuning of single cochlear fibers. *Journal of Physiology, 242,* 129–131.

Festen, J., and Plomp, R. (1983). Relations between auditory functions in unimpaired hearing. *Journal of the Acoustical Society of America, 73*(2), 652–662.

Fitzgibbons, P., and Wightman, F. (1982). Gap detection in normal and hearing impaired listeners. *Journal of the Acoustical Society of America, 72*(3), 761–765.

Florentine, M., Buus, S., Scharf, B., and Zwicker, E. (1980). Frequency selectivity in normal-hearing and hearing impaired listeners. *Journal of Speech and Hearing Research, 23,* 646–669.

Foster, J. R., Glynn, C., Haggard, M., Trinder, J., and Fernandes, M. (1980). Inter-aural spectral differences and spectral slope in intelligibility enhancement. *Journal of the Acoustical Society of America, 68,* Supplement 1, S101.

Ginzel, A., Pederson, C., Spliid, P., and Anderson, E. (1982). The role of temporal factors in auditory perception of consonants and vowels. *Scandinavian Audiology, 11,* 93–100.

Girandi-Perry, D., Salvi, R., and Henderson, D. (1982). Gap detection in hearing-impaired chinchillas. *Journal of the Acoustical Society of America, 72*(5), 1387–1393.

Godfrey, J., and Millay, K. (1978). Perception of rapid spectral change in speech by listeners with mild and moderate sensorineural hearing loss. *Journal of the American Audiological Society, 3,* 200–208.

Godfrey, J., and Millay, K. (1980). Perception of synthetic speech sounds by hearing-impaired listeners. *Journal of Auditory Research, 20,* 187–204.

Hack, Z., and Erber, N. (1982). Auditory, visual, and auditory–visual perception of vowels by hearing-impaired children. *Journal of Speech and Hearing Research, 25,* 100–107.

Hannley, M., and Dobbins, E. (1981). Changes in the identification of full and partial cue syllables by subjects with age-related hearing impairment. *Journal of the Acoustical Society of America, 51*(69), S122.

Hannley, M., and Dorman, M. F. (1983). Susceptibility to intraspeech masking in listeners with sensorineural hearing loss. *Journal of the Acoustical Society of America, 74,* 40–51.

Haas, G. (1982). Impaired listeners recognition of speech presented dichotically through high- and low-pass filters. *Audiology, 21,* 433–453.

Hirsh, I. J., Davis, H., Silverman, S. R., Reynolds, E. G., Eldert, E., and Benson, R. W. (1952). Development of materials for speech audiometry. *Journal of Speech and Hearing Disorders, 17,* 321–337.

Humes, L. (1982). Spectral and temporal resolution by the hearing impaired. In Studebaker and Bess (Eds.), *The Vanderbilt hearing aid report.* Monographs in Contemporary Audiology.

Irwin, R., Hinchcliffe, L., and Kemp, S. (1981). Temporal acuity in normal and hearing impaired listeners. *Audiology, 20,* 234–243.

Ivory, P., and Brandt, J. (1982). Identification of speech and nonspeech cues by hearing-impaired listeners. Paper presented at the Annual Meeting of the American Speech–Language–Hearing Association, Toronto.

Jerger, J., and Jerger, S. (1971). Diagnostic significance of PB word functions. *Archives of Otolaryngology, 93,* 573–580.

Jerger, J., Speaks, C., and Trammell, J. (1968). A new approach to speech audiometry. *Journal of Speech and Hearing Disorders, 33,* 318–328.

Jerger, J., Tillman, R., and Peterson, J. (1960). Masking by octave bands of noise in normal and impaired ears. *Journal of the Acoustical Society of America, 32,* 385–390.

Johnson, D., Whaley, P. and Dorman, M. (1984). The processing of cues for stop consonant voicing by young hearing-impaired listeners. *Journal of Speech and Hearing Research, 27,* 112–118.

Kaplan, H., and Pickett, J. M. (1982). Differences in speech discrimination in the elderly as a function of type of competing noise: Speech-babble or cafeteria. *Audiology, 21,* 325–333.

Kewley-Port, D. (1982). Measurements of formant transitions in naturally produced stop consonant–vowel syllables. *Journal of the Acoustical Society of America, 72,* 379–382.

Kewley-Port, D. (1983). Time-varying features as correlates of place of articulation in stop consonants. *Journal of the Acoustical Society of America, 73*(1), 322–335.

Kiang, N. Y. S., Liberman, M. C., and Levine, R. A. (1976). Auditory nerve activity in cats exposed to ototoxic drugs and high frequency sounds. *Annals of Otology, Rhinology, and Laryngology, 75,* 752–768.

Kiang, N. Y. S., Moxon, E. C., and Levine, R. A. (1970). Auditory nerve activity in cats with normal and abnormal cochleas. In G. W. Wolstenholme and J. Knight (Eds.), *Sensorineural hearing, Ciba Foundation Symposium.* London: Churchill.

Liberman, A. M., Delattre, P. C., Cooper, F. S., and Gerstman, L. J. (1954). The role of consonant vowel transitions in the perception of the stop and nasal consonants. *Psychological Monographs, 68* (8, Whole No. 379), 1–13.

Lisker, L., and Abramson, A. (1964). A cross-language study of voicing in initial stops: Acoustical measurement. *Word, 20,* 384–422.

Martin, E., and Pickett, J. (1970). Sensorineural hearing loss and upward spread of masking. *Journal of Speech and Hearing Research, 13,* 426–437.

Millay, K., and Godfrey, J. (1980). The discrimination of formant frequency differences as a function of duration by hearing-impaired listeners. *Journal of the Acoustical Society of America, 68,* Supplement 1, S113.

Nelson, D. A., and Turner, C. (1980). Decay of masking and frequency resolution in sensorineural hearing-impaired listeners. In G. van der Brink and F. A. Bilsen (Eds.), *Psychophysical, physiological and behavioral studies in hearing.* Delft: Delft U. P.

Owens, E., and Schubert, E. D. (1977). Development of the California Consonant Test. *Journal of Speech and Hearing Research, 20,* 463–474.

Owens, E., Talbott, C., and Schubert, E. (1968). Vowel discrimination of hearing impaired listeners. *Journal of Speech and Hearing Research, 11,* 648–655.

Parady, S., Dorman, M. F., Whaley, P., and Raphael, L. J. (1981). Identification and discrimination of a synthesized voicing contrast by normal and sensorineural hearing-impaired children. *Journal of the Acoustical Society of America, 63*(3), 783–790.

Pick, G. F., Evans, E. F., and Wilson, J. P. (1977). Frequency resolution of patients with hearing loss of cochlear origin. In E. F. Evans and J. P. Wilson (Eds.), *Psychophysics and physiology of hearing.* London: Academic Press.

Pickett, J. M., and Danaher, E. M. (1973). On discrimination of formant transitions by persons with severe sensorineural hearing loss. In G. Fant and M. A. A. Tatham (Eds.), *Proceedings of the symposium on auditory analysis and perception of speech, Leningrad.* London: Academic Press.

Punch, J., and Beck, E. (1980). Low frequency response of hearing aids and judgements of aided speech quality. *Journal of Speech and Hearing Disorders, 45,* 325–335.

Raphael, L. J. (August, 1971). Vowel duration as a cue to the perceptual separation of cognate sounds in American English. *Supplement to: Status Report on Speech Research,* Haskins Laboratories.

Raz, I., and Noffsinger, D. (November, 1979). Perception of voiced stop consonants by hearing-impaired listeners. Paper presented at the Annual Meeting of the American Speech-Language-Hearing Association, Atlanta.

Revoile, S., Pickett, J., Holden, L., and Talkin, D. (1982). Acoustic cues to final stop voicing for impaired- and normal-hearing listeners. *Journal of the Acoustical Society of America, 72*(4), 1145–1154.

Revoile, S., Pickett, J. M., and Wilson, M. P. (1981). Masking of noise bursts by an adjacent vowel for hearing-impaired listeners. *Journal of Speech and Hearing Research, 24,* 576–579.

Rittmanic, P. (1962). Pure tone masking by narrow noise bands in normal and impaired ears. *Journal of Auditory Research, 2,* 287–304.

Schwab, E., Sawusch, J., and Nusbaum, H. (1981). The role of second formant transitions in the stop-semivowel distinction. *Perception and Psychophysics, 29,* 121–128.

Stevens, K. N., and Blumstein, S. (1978). Invariant cues for place of articulation in stop consonants. *Journal of the Acoustical Society of America, 64,* 1358–1368.

Stewart, B. (1980. Normal and hearing-impaired listeners' identification and discrimination of synthetic /bdg/: The effect of transition duration (unpublished master's thesis). Tempe, AZ: Arizona State University.

Stoker, R. G. (1978). Auditory temporal acuity of the hearing impaired and its relationship to speech intelligibility. *Journal of the American Auditory Society, 4,* 24–29.

Summerfield, Q. (1982). Differences between spectral dependencies in auditory and phonetic temporal processing: Relevance to the perception of voicing in initial stops. *Journal of the Acoustical Society of America, 72*(1), 51–61.

Thornton, A. R., and Abbas, P. (1980). Low frequency hearing loss: Perception of filtered speech, psychophysical tuning curves and masking. *Journal of the Acoustical Society of America, 67,* 638–643.

Tillman, T., and Carhart, R. (1966). An expanded test for speech discrimination utilizing CNC monosyllabic words (Northwestern University Auditory Test No. 6). Technical Report, SAM-TR-66-55, USAF School of Aerospace Medicine, Aerospace Medical Division, Brooks Air Force Base, TX.

Trinder, E. (1979). Auditory fusion: A critical interval test with implications in differential diagnosis. *British Journal of Audiology, 13,* 143–147.

Turek, S. v. de G., Dorman, M. F., Franks, J. R., and Summerfield, A. Q. (1980). Identification of synthetic /bdg/ by hearing impaired listeners under monotic and dichotic formant presentation. *Journal of the Acoustical Society of America, 67,* 1031–1040.

Turner, C., and Nelson, D. (1982). Frequency discrimination in regions of normal and impaired sensitivity. *Journal of Speech and Hearing Research, 25,* 34–41.

Tyler, R., Summerfield, A. Q., Wood, E., and Fernandes, M. (1982). Psychoacoustic and phonetic temporal processing in normal and hearing impaired listeners. *Journal of the Acoustical Society of America, 72*(3), 740–752.

Tyler, R.,. Wood, E., and Fernandes, M. (1982). Frequency resolution and hearing loss. *British Journal of Audiology, 16,* 45–63.

Tyler, R., Wood, E., and Fernandes, M. (1983). Frequency resolution and discrimination of constant and dynamic tones in normal and hearing impaired listeners. *Journal of the Acoustical Society of America, 74,* 1190–1199.

Van Tassel, D. (1980). Perception of second-formant transitions by hearing-impaired persons. *Ear and Hearing, 1*(3), 130–136.

Van Tassel, D., Hagen, L., Koblas, L., and Penner, S. (1982). Perception of short-term spectral cues for stop consonant place by normal and hearing impaired listeners. *Journal of the Acoustical Society of America, 72*(6), 1771–1780.

Verbrugge, R., Strange, W., Shankweiler, D., and Edman, T. (1976). What information enables a listener to map a talker's vowel space? *Journal of the Acoustical Society of America, 60,* 198–212.

Walley, A., and Carrell, T. (1983). Onset spectra and formant transitions in adult's and child's perception of place of articulation in stop consonants. *Journal of the Acoustical Society of America, 73*(3), 1011–1022.

Wightman, F., McGee, T., and Kramer, M. (1977). Factors influencing frequency selectivity in normal and hearing-impaired listeners. In E. F. Evans and J. P. Wilson (Eds.), *Psychophysics and physiology of hearing.* London: Academic Press.

Williams, S., Whaley, P., and Dorman, M. F. (November, 1981). *Identification of /s/ by hearing impaired and normal hearing children.* Paper presented at the Annual Meeting of the American Speech–Language–Hearing Association, Los Angeles.

Yokkaichi, A., & Fujisaki, H. (1978). Identification of synthetic speech stimuli by hearing impaired subjects. Paper presented at the Joint Meeting of the Acoustical Society of America and the Acoustical Society of Japan, Honolulu, Hawaii.

Zwicker, E., and Schorn, K. (1978). Psychoacoustical tuning curves in audiology. *Audiology, 17,* 120–140.

Zwicker, E. and Schorn, K. (1982). Temporal resolution in hard-of-hearing patients. *Audiology, 21,* 474–492.

CHAPTER 5

Structure and Function of the Lateral Precentral Cortex: Significance for Speech Motor Control

James H. Abbs
Carol Welt

Over 100 years ago, based upon clinical observations, Jackson pointed out that dysfunctions following damage to a certain part of the brain cannot be interpreted as indicative of what the normal function of that part might be. After a century of animal research, the testimony is much the same; Glassman (1978) noted that, "brain lesions do not show you what the region in question does, but rather what the rest of the whole complex brain does *without* the part in question" (p. 8). Apparently, even if lesions are introduced under controlled circumstances and verified histologically, great caution must be taken in interpreting normal brain function from the lesion induced deficits (Finger and Stein, 1982; Norrsell, 1978; Wolf, Stricker, and Zigmond, 1978). These interpretive problems are difficult particularly if one analyzes lesion recovery only in terms of performance *goals* without parallel physiological and morphological analyses of the *means* by which those goals are achieved. As pointed out by Laurence and Stein (1978), "A combination of means and ends analyses is crucial if recovery is to be used either as a method for studying nervous system organization or as part of any debate concerning localization." Attempts to discern function from human lesion data particularly reflect these difficulties. As an extreme example, in many cases of verified brain lesions there are few long-lasting behavioral manifestations. Obviously, such behavioral data alone are not viable as evidence for or against particular views on the localization of brain function. Rather, such phenomena as functional substitution, reorganization, behavioral compensation, neuron regeneration, collateral sprouting, utilization of residual synapses, and denervation supersensitivity may be operating to various degrees to yield "normal" performance ends (Finger and Stein, 1982; Laurence and Stein, 1978; Marshall, 1984). These considerations raise serious questions as to how our understanding of the brain functions underlying speech motor behavior can be enhanced. Also apparent are the difficulties of clinical assessment. For example, in a patient with a computed tomographic (CT) scan indicating a left hemisphere cortical infarct in the lateral precentral region, deviation of the tongue to the left is generally interpreted as evidence of a second lesion in the right hemisphere. However, neurophysiological observations in nonhuman primates indicate that the lower face, tongue, and jaw muscles are activated ipsilaterally as well as contralaterally from the motor cortex (Lauer, 1952; Sirisko and Sessle, 1983a; Welt, Abbs, and Gracco, unpublished observations). As such, deviation of the tongue to the left also may be symptomatic of a left cortical lesion to the ipsilateral tongue representation. As an alternative to exclusive reliance on human cortical lesion data, it obviously is useful to incorporate information obtained with other techniques in nonhuman primates.

In attempts to discern the nature of the peripheral neural mechanisms underlying speech motor behavior, some investigators have incorporated basic neuropathological and neuroanatomical information from animal studies. Based on data from nonhuman primates and even nonprimates, several authors have proposed specific hypotheses concerning peripheral reflex contributions to speech motor control (Abbs and Cole, 1982; Zimmermann, 1980). By contrast, there has been greater reluctance to draw on data even from nonhuman primates in attempting to interpret the higher level control of complex orofacial movements for speech (however, see Armstrong and Falk, 1982; Noback, 1982). This is unfortunate. In the last decade there have been important advances in our knowledge of the anatomy and physiology of the central nervous system, many of which have significant implications for understanding complex speech motor processes and aberrations thereof. One of the most active research efforts has been on the role of the cerebral cortex in the voluntary control of movement. Several cortical regions are involved in the control of movement, including primary motor, premotor, supplementary motor, and somatic sensory areas, in ways that are beginning to be distinguished. Given the extreme difficulty of understanding the functions of the cortex from data on human lesions alone, this chapter is an attempt to summarize some recent advances in our understanding of the precentral motor-sensory cortex as these may be relevant to the neural processes of speech motor control. We consider both lesion studies and more recent neuroanatomical and neurophysiological data. Specifically, this review focuses on select areas of the precentral neocortex, with emphasis on (1) the organization and function of the output of these areas, (2) the types, distribution, and contribution of somatic sensory input, (3) the connections with other cortical areas and to the periphery, and (4) the functional significance of these organizational patterns to speech motor control.

Our current knowledge concerning the organization and functions of the primate motor-sensory cortex has advanced the most from general mapping studies of the entire motor field and from specific analyses of cortical regions related to motor control of the limbs. For this reason, we first consider some of these general advances on motor cortex function and then turn to work on regions of the lateral precentral cortex specialized for orofacial functions. An obvious issue for this chapter is the extent to which the data from animal preparations are valid in highlighting speech functions in human subjects. The present authors are sensitive to these comparative issues (Carlson and Welt, 1981) and, as is apparent in discussions that follow, there are a number of significant parallels between the orofacial cortical organization in human and nonhuman primates.

GENERAL ORGANIZATION OF THE MOTOR-SENSORY NEOCORTEX

Principles of Topographical Organization

Careful observations of motor involvement in human epileptic seizures led to the first proposal of an orderly topographical representation of the parts of the body in the cerebral cortex (Jackson, 1864 [cited in Jackson, 1875]). This clinical inference was confirmed in 1870 by Fritsch and Hitzig who elicited movements of the contralateral limbs by electrically stimulating the frontal cortex of cats and dogs. Further details of the concept of cortical localization followed shortly with Ferrier's map of the electrically excitable area of the monkey's cortex. Ferrier (1876) showed that the different parts of the body are represented in an organized sequence in the precentral gyrus just rostral to the central sulcus.

In a series of experiments between 1888 and 1917, relatively precise localization patterns were defined in the precentral gyrus of the macaque monkey, chimpanzee, gorilla, orangutan, and gibbon by electrical stimulation of the cortical surface (Beevor and Horsley, 1888; Leyton and Sherrington, 1917; Mott, Schuster, and Sherrington, 1917). The topographical pattern was similar in all primates, but more detailed in the apes. Individual movements of the eyelid, nose, pinna, lower lip, upper lip, angle of the mouth, cheek, jaw, and tongue were produced. The figurine map shown in Figure 5–1 shows the relatively extensive and detailed

Figure 5-1. Figurine map showing the location, relative size, and topographical organization of the precentral motor cortex in the orangutan. An orderly and detailed sequence of orofacial and laryngeal responses was elicited by electrical stimulation of the contralateral cortical surface. The drawings of the dorsal and dorsolateral aspects of the left hemisphere show the points where stimuli were applied in relation to the surrounding sulcal pattern. This figure was prepared from Leyton and Sherrington's (1917) published protocols (Welt, 1962).

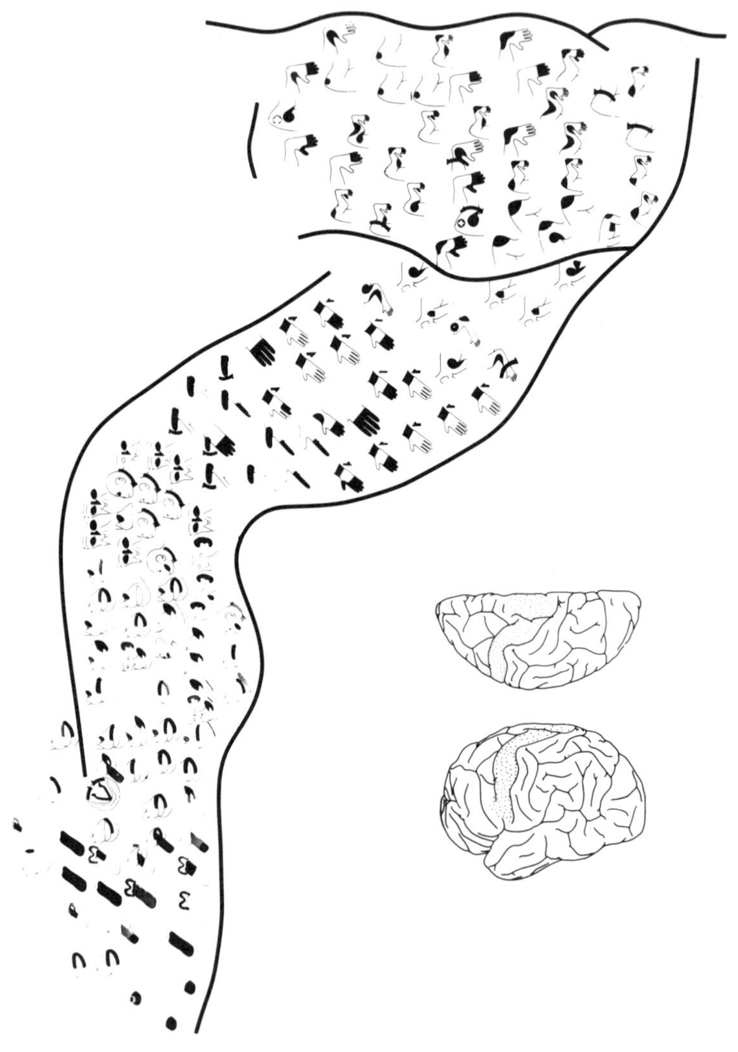

topographical pattern observed by Leyton and Sherrington (1917) in the orangutan (Welt, 1962; Woolsey and Welt, in preparation).

This same time period marked the beginning of anatomical analyses of cortical cytoarchitecture. In a study of the precentral motor region in the dog and monkey and later in humans, Betz (1874) described a special class of large pyramidal cells. Lewis and Clarke (1878), working at the same institution as Ferrier, focused their studies on the precentral gyrus and concluded that the giant Betz cells had "motor significance" (Brazier, 1978). The first three decades of the twentieth century witnessed a proliferation of detailed cytoarchitectonic parcellations of the cerebral cortex in a variety of mammals. Based upon the relative size and number of cell types and their distribution in different layers, the precentral cortex was divided into a caudal area 4 and a more rostral area 6 (Brodmann, 1909; Bucy, 1933; Campbell, 1905; Economo and Koskinas, 1925; Vogt and Vogt, 1919). The boundary between area 4 and area 6, as well as the number of subareas, varied considerably in these early studies. In a later series of comparative cytoarchitectural studies of the precentral cortex in primates, however, Bonin (1938, 1949) and Bonin and Bailey (1947) consistently distinguished three cytoarchitectonic areas in the lateral precentral cortex. These areas are designated 4, 6, and 44 according to Brodmann's nomenclature, or areas FA, FB, and FCBm of Economo and Koskinas (1925). The surface location of these three areas in the cerebral cortex of the human and macaque are shown in Figure 5-2.

Ensuing attempts to understand the role of these cortical areas in motor control involved primarily clinical and experimental lesion studies (Fulton, 1934; Tower, 1940; Travis and Woolsey, 1956; Walshe, 1935). Fulton and his co-workers described different functions for the rostral and caudal portions of the precentral gyrus based upon human lesion data and ablation experiments in animals. They strongly supported the concept of a functionally distinct premotor area rostral to the primary motor cortex. Work in other laboratories, however, questioned these results (Travis and Woolsey, 1956; Walshe, 1935). There was little agreement among these studies on the effects or significance of the lesions in different cortical areas. Although much of the disagreement can be attributed to different experimental conditions such as size of the lesions and methods of analyzing behavioral deficits, one of the most significant factors was the lack of consistency in defining the location and extent of the lesioned cortical areas. In addition, intended lesions of area 4 may have involved area 6 or undercut connections between them and surrounding cortical areas. Recent attempts to define the premotor area using microelectrode and anatomical methods indicate that this area is a functionally distinct

Figure 5–2. The surface location of the precentral cytoarchitectonic areas 4, 6, and 44 in the human and macaque monkey are shown on drawings of the left hemisphere. Only the fissures in the orofacial region including the sulcus subcentralis anterior (SCA) are labeled. Horizontal bar is 2.0 cm; note that the macaque brain is enlarged approximately 3.5 times compared with the human brain. The cytoarchitectonic area 1 representations were adapted from Bonin (1949).

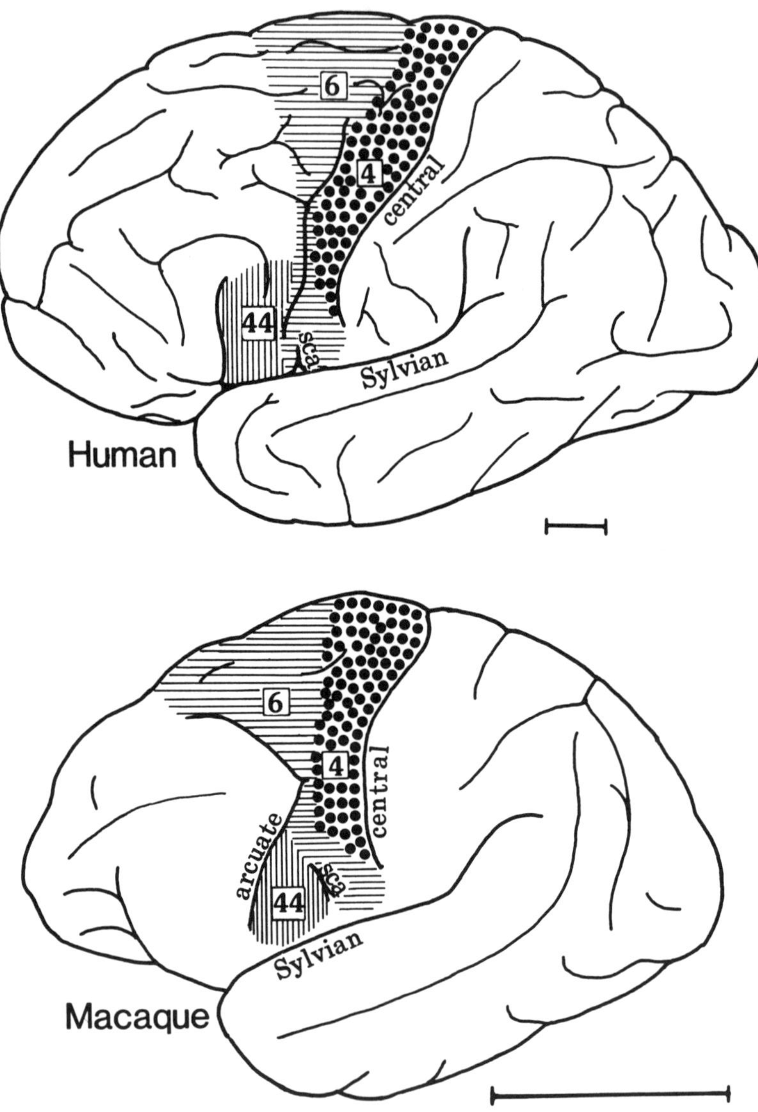

region of motor cortex (Wise, 1984). The recent criteria and evidence for distinguishing the primary and secondary motor areas also have been reviewed by Wiesendanger (1981). He indicates that it is current practice to equate primary motor cortex or precentral motor cortex with area 4, premotor cortex with the dorsolateral and lateral parts of area 6, and supplementary motor area (SMA) with the mesial surface of area 6. It must be emphasized, however, that precise boundaries and exact correlations between the functional and cytoarchitectonic areas have not been established. The recent anatomical, electrophysiological, and connectivity studies suggest that the premotor cortex and SMA are "centers executing higher order control" (Wiesendanger, 1981). Wise (1984) also has carefully reviewed the distinguishing features of the nonprimary cortical areas in the control of movement, and he concluded that these areas may play an important role in the preparation for and the sensory guidance of complex movements.

The concept of somatotopic localization and the basic plan of organization of cortical motor areas was elaborated in an extensive series of mapping studies by Woolsey and co-workers (Woolsey, 1958; Woolsey et al., 1951). Using electrical stimulation of the cortical surface, they found a complete and continuous pattern of motor representation on the precentral gyrus, extending from the depths of the central sulcus to the posterior bank of the arcuate sulcus, and from the anterior subcentral sulcus laterally to the cingulate sulcus medially. In these studies, no single cytoarchitectonic area coincided with the complete precentral motor map. The topographical relations of individual motor foci paralleled the arrangement of body segments at the periphery. Woolsey emphasized, however, that there is "very extensive overlap in the cortical motor patterns" (Woolsey et al., 1951).

With the introduction of microelectrode recording and stimulating techniques and of more precise anatomical methods, issues related to functional localization patterns and correlated cytoarchitecture have been reexamined. In addition, new questions concerning the activity of individual cortical neurons during voluntary movement have been investigated. These approaches, especially when used in combination, offer new perspectives on motor cortex function.

Microelectrode Mapping of Motor Cortex

An advance in the study of cortical motor organization was achieved with the technique of intracortical microstimulation (ICMS). By inserting a microelectrode into the depths of the cortex, Asanuma and

Sakata (1967) found that electrical stimulation with very low currents (less than 10 μA) of relatively short duration was effective in eliciting body movements as well as contractions of individual muscles. Topographical localization patterns could be determined with finer resolution because ICMS influences a more restricted focus of cortex than does surface stimulation. The initial ICMS studies, carried out by Asanuma and co-workers in cats and monkeys, activated individual muscles from relatively small cortical foci of about 1 mm^2; these foci overlapped at the fringes. The discrete character and short latency of the movements (Sakata and Miyamoto, 1968) elicited by ICMS indicate that the pyramidal tract is the corticofugal pathway. Much wider, extensively overlapping cortical efferent zones have been described in other studies using different stimulus parameters (Phillips, 1973). Asanuma and colleagues (Asanuma and Arnold, 1975; Asanuma, Arnold, and Zarzecki, 1976) presented some evidence that the stimulus parameters were responsible for the larger foci, but the effects of systematically varying these parameters have not yet been determined. Other methodological issues that remain to be resolved in regard to ICMS include (1) determining the exact influence of long duration stimulus trains on the excitation of neurons; (2) identifying the intracortically activated (or inhibited) neuronal elements and their corticofugal pathways; and (3) determining the extent to which ICMS induces local synaptic activation of neurons. These technical considerations serve as a reminder that electrical stimulation does not initiate spatiotemporal sequences of neuronal activity that are characteristic of the normal, intact animal. Nevertheless, in cases in which ICMS and cortical single neuron unit recording in awake animals have been used in parallel, comparable topographical patterns of output organization have been observed (Humphrey, 1982). ICMS studies in different laboratories have confirmed several principles of organization of the motor cortex and suggested hypotheses on functional localization (Kwan, MacKay, Murphy, and Wong, 1978; Sessle and Wiesendanger, 1982). Organizational features of motor cortex that have been consistently demonstrated with ICMS include:

1. Discrete movements of a single joint, an individual muscle, or a fascicle of a muscle are elicited with microstimulation presumably localized to a few pyramidal cells (threshold currents). Increasing stimulus intensity produces more complex responses.
2. Most responses, as well as the lowest threshold responses, are elicited from cortical layers V, III, and VI.
3. Cortical excitability is influenced by limb position, peripheral cutaneous stimulation, and the arousal state of the animal.

4. Distal muscles are activated by lower stimulation currents than are more proximal muscles, on the average. The caudal part of area 4 is more excitable than the rostral regions of area 6.

5. The topographical pattern consists of semicircular or horseshoe-shaped cortical zones for arm and shoulder, elbow, wrist, and digits; within this organization, the cortical zone controlling a more distal joint is partially enclosed by zones controlling successively more proximal joints, resulting in a pattern with finger zones at the center and shoulder at the periphery.

6. Foci for adjacent joints or muscles overlap extensively, whereas nonadjacent joints show minimal or no overlap; movement of a single joint or a single muscle is often elicited at multiple noncontinguous sites.

These studies have also shown that neurons in multiple, discontinuous cortical areas converge on individual motoneuron pools. For example, using ICMS techniques in acute mapping experiments, Strick and Preston (1978a, 1982a) delineated *two* spatially distinct representations of the hand and wrist in area 4 of squirrel monkeys. Correlated cytoarchitectural studies placed both of these zones entirely within area 4. Strick and Preston (1978a, 1982a) view these two outputs as parallel pathways influencing the same lower motoneuron pools. It is not known, however, if identical motor units are activated by these parallel pathways. On the other hand, neurons in one cortical locus can activate more than one motoneuron pool. Collaterals from single corticospinal axons have been shown to innervate different motor nuclei (Shinoda, Zarzecki, and Asanuma, 1979). Asanuma, Zarzecki, Jankowska, Hongo, and Marcus (1979) have shown that adjacent pyramidal tract cells within area 4 often distribute collaterals to separate motor nuclei. Taken together, the evidence indicates that at least some of the motor cortex neurons involved in the control of movement have multiple muscle targets. *Presumably, these various patterns of muscle activation from the cortex have functional significance.* For example, in natural motor behaviors certain muscles, while physically separate at the periphery, often are coupled in multimovement tasks. Such coupling would appear critical to the obligatory multimovement gestures of human speech (Abbs, Gracco, and Cole, 1984).

Organization of Somatic Sensory Input to Motor Cortex

The functional organization of the motor cortex in the control of movement has been further revealed by analyses of sensory inputs from various peripheral sites. In contrast to the relatively indirect visual, auditory, and vestibular pathways to precentral cortex, somatic sensory afferents reach the motor cortex through direct, short-latency afferents from the periphery (Malis, Pribram, and Kruger, 1953). Projections from deep somatic structures to individual neurons in motor cortex have also been confirmed (Albe-Fessard and Liebeskind, 1966; Hore, Preston, Durkovic, and Cheney, 1976; Wiesendanger, 1973). The sensorimotor input–output characteristics of motor cortex sites have been studied by using the same microelectrode for ICMS and also for recording the discharges of cortical neurons in response to sensory stimulation.

In New World *Cebus* monkeys, Rosén and Asanuma (1972) recorded discharges of individual neurons in the forelimb area elicited by natural somatic sensory stimulation and then determined the motor response produced by ICMS at the same cortical site. All receptive fields were located in or around the joint movement activated by ICMS, suggesting that the somatic sensory input plays a "feedback" role for modulating the output of efferent zones (Rosén and Asanuma, 1972). In this type of study it is not known if the cortical neurons responding to sensory input and those activated by ICMS are identical; certainly they are in proximity. These initial studies showed that vertical aggregates of cells with similar input–output properties were aligned in a columnar fashion with the radially oriented fiber bundles. In subsequent studies, Wong, Kwan, MacKay, and Murphy (1978) found that neurons with similar receptive fields (RFs) also occurred at several different sites, providing evidence for multiple representations of tightly coupled input–output units. For the two spatially separate motor representations of the hand within area 4 of the squirrel monkey, Strick and Preston (1978b, 1982b) found that motor cortex neurons in the caudal hand area received primarily cutaneous input, whereas neurons in the rostral hand area 4 received mainly deep input. Strick and Preston concluded that within cytoarchitectonic area 4 there are two functionally distinct areas that can be defined on the basis of different input–output coupling. The concentration of deep RFs in the rostral zone suggests that this hand representation may be preferentially involved in movements using kinesthetic feedback such as load compensation, whereas the caudal zone is preferentially involved in movements using cutaneous feedback as in tactile exploration (Strick and Preston, 1982b). In the more dorsal motor cortex region of awake rhesus monkeys, Tanji and Wise (1981) found rostral and caudal representations of the hindlimb which also received projections from cutaneous and deep receptors, respectively.

Most of the above studies that focused on sensory mapping of a relatively large region of motor cortex were conducted in anesthesized or passive animals. However, it might be expected that somatic sensory input to motor cortex in influenced by active motor behaviors. Some investigators have used awake, behaving animals to examine the influence of natural peripheral stimulation on cortical neurons that discharge in association with a particular limb movement. Using this approach, Lemon (1981) found that the overall somatotopy of the sensory input was similar to that previously reported by Wong and co-workers (1978) and by Sessle and Wiesendanger (1982). In addition, however, he found that some cell groups with similar movement-associated activity and afferent input were found at separate locations in the motor cortex. Lemon suggested that this multiple representation reflects the participation of different cortical cells in a particular movement under different circumstances; ti parthat is, one cortical subarea may be involved when a movement is executed in isolation, and a second subarea takes part when that movement co-occurs with movements at other joints. For example, some hand units fire only when the wrist is in a particular position. Lemon concludes that "it is important to examine area 4 neurons during movements which call up different strategies of muscular coordination to determine whether the fine organization of the motor cortex is designed to make such strategies possible" (Lemon, 1981, p. 538).

The apparent tight coupling of peripheral sensory fields to motor cortex output illustrates the seemingly obligatory utilization of afferent information in motor control. The powerful input to motor cortex from cutaneous as well as deep receptors is particularly significant in relation to motor control of the orofacial system, given the dense cutaneous receptive fields of the lips and tongue. Recent estimates suggest that over 50% of motor cortex neurons receive cutaneous input (Tanji and Wise, 1981). The observations by Lemon in behaving animals also suggest a labile linking of various inputs and outputs via the motor cortex, dependent upon moment-to-moment changes in motor goals. As noted previously, these kinds of sensorimotor processes, operating among multiple muscles and movements, may be of substantial significance in the coordination and control of speech-motor actions.

Single Unit Activity in Motor Cortex During Voluntary Movement

The activity patterns of cortical neurons associated with voluntary movement also have been examined, permitting evaluation of specific hypotheses concerning control contributions of the motor cortex. In the middle 1960s, Evarts (1964, 1966) adapted a technique from Jasper (1958) and Hubel (1959) that permitted the recording of discharge patterns of individual motor cortex neurons associated with movement in awake monkeys. In conjunction with these recordings, Evarts took special care to train the animals to generate a stereotypic movement with which to correlate observed cortical activity. Although it is beyond the scope of this chapter to discuss the many observations made with this technique over the last 20 years, certain general observations and precautions are warranted. Early analyses focused primarily on the distal upper limbs and included simultaneous observations of pyramidal tract neurons (PTNs) along with muscle activity, the generated force, or the associated movement (Evarts, 1966, 1968, 1969), or a combination of these. Current work similarly is aimed with particular emphasis on primary motor cortex control of fine force and movement of the distal upper limb (Evarts, 1981; Evarts, Fromm, Kröller, and Jennings, 1983). In addition, several investigators have recorded cortical cell activity in premotor cortex, supplementary motor area, and/or sensorimotor cortex during voluntary movement (Wise, 1984; Wiesendanger, 1981).

Early observations indicated that PTN firing changes in response to a peripheral "perturbation" in a performing animal and that EMG changes occurred at a latency appropriate to consider this a "transcortical reflex" (Conrad, Matsunami, Meyer-Lohmann, Wiesendanger, and Brooks, 1974; Conrad, Meyer-Lohmann, Matsunami, and Brooks, 1975; Evarts, 1973). Many subsequent studies have focused on this issue, with particular emphasis on the ascending sensory pathways that might underlie these PTN responses and the cortical cell input–output response characteristics (Evarts, 1974; Evarts and Fromm, 1977, 1978; Lucier, Ruegg, and Wiesendanger, 1975; Wiesendanger, Seguin, and Künzle, 1973). As noted previously, parallel studies were aimed at the specificity of the various receptor sites from which PTNs could be driven, using both quantitative and qualitative techniques (Fetz, Finocchio, Baker, and Soso, 1980; Lemon and Porter, 1976). These analyses also were extended to include longer latency PTN responses to peripheral loads, including a class of sensorimotor actions referred to as reaction time responses (Evarts and Tanji, 1974, 1976). *The powerful afferent drive to the motor cortex reflected in these various studies further emphasizes the importance of these sensory signals to motor control.*

An early issue also arising in these studies was whether the particular PTN being recorded was in fact directly "causing" the voluntary movement or muscle contraction, or rather was involved in an indirect way (e.g., providing the tonic background for a phasic movement). Fetz, Cheney, and German (1976), Cheney and Fetz (1980), and Fetz and colleagues (1980) used the PTN spikes as triggers for averaging the electromyogram (EMG) associated with the voluntary movement (spike-triggered averaging, STA).

They reported that between 25% and 40% of their recorded cortical units manifested time-locked changes (i.e., post-spike facilitation) in the associated EMG. Those PTNs showing post-spike facilitation (PSF) were considered to have a monosynaptic drive to lower motoneurons. From these analyses it was posssible to discern several different kinds of PTN–muscle contraction patterns (e.g., phasic-tonic, tonic, phasic-ramp). Additionally, Fetz and co-workers (1976) and Fetz and Cheney (1978) showed that the discharge of single cortical neurons sometimes yielded PSF in the activity of multiple muscles.

One methodological problem with cortical cell recording relates to sampling bias: large pyramidal tract (PT) cells appear to be sampled disproportionately. It is estimated that only 10% to 20% of the efferent projecting cells in the layer V of the motor cortex are large PT cells (Humphrey and Corrie, 1978; Towe, Patton, and Kennedy, 1963). Given these considerations, it is apparent that PTN recording in awake animals may reflect only a subset of the cortical activity involved in motor control. It is heartening, however, to recognize the likelihood that the discharge of large PTs may underlie the most precise, fractionalized control of muscles and movements (Evarts, 1981). It is also argued that the motor behaviors involving most direct pyramidal cell projections are executed in the "least automatic" fashion, especially for systems like the digits and the orofacial region where pyramidal cells make monosynaptic connections (Denny-Brown, 1960; Evarts, 1981).

Corticocortical and Subcortical Patterns of Connectivity

The question of how motor output from multiple precentral cortex areas is regulated by different sensory submodalities provided the impetus for determining the pathways by which this information gains access to the motor cortex. Equally important for understanding cortical motor control mechanisms was the delineation of the corticofugal pathways and the interconnections among various cortical regions. These issues have motivated neuroanatomists and neurophysiologists in the last 25 years to investigate the interconnections among the cortical and subcortical regions involved in motor control. One of the most significant advances for tracing fiber pathways and terminations in the central nervous system has been the development of axonal transport methods, using enzyme tracers and radioactive proteins. The principal advantages of the axonal transport approach include its reliance on basic physiological processes of nerve cells and avoidance of the tissue destruction and pathological processes inherent in degeneration methods. This technique has led to a more detailed and quantitative evaluation of the complex patterns of cortical connectivity and correlated neuronal architecture (Jones and Hartman, 1978).

The principal *thalamic relays* to motor cortex from the brainstem, cerebellum, basal ganglia, and spinal cord have been well documented in monkeys (Berrevoets and Kuypers, 1975; Strick, 1976; Tracey, Asanuma, Jones, and Porter, 1980). Recently, Schell and Strick (1984) separately injected an enzyme tracer into three precentral cortical areas (primary motor—area 4; arcuate premotor—lateral area 6; and supplementary motor—medial area 6) and found differential projections to these areas from subnuclei of the thalamus; this finding in turn indicates differential projections to these three precentral areas from cerebellar and striatal sites. These observations point to the functional significance of the cytoarchitectonic classification of these precentral cortex subareas. The specific ascending routes by which various somatic sensory submodalities reach the motor cortex, however, have not been unequivocally established (Jones, 1982).

In an extensive series of degeneration studies, Kuypers (1964) and co-workers described the *descending pathways* from the cerebral cortex. In higher primates and humans some corticospinal axons terminate directly on motoneurons of the distal upper limb (Kuypers, 1960; Kuypers and Brinkman, 1970). Kuypers (1964) has also shown that neurons in the lateral precentral cortex terminate directly on motoneurons in the facial, trigeminal, and hypoglossal motor nuclei. Unfortunately, these studies have not been replicated using the more specific and sensitive axoplasmic tracing techniques.

The intra- and interhemispheric connections of primary motor and somatic sensory cortex also have been studied extensively in the macaque with degeneration (Jones, 1969; Pandya, Gold, and Berger, 1969; Pandya and Küypers, 1969), autoradiographic (Künzle, 1976, 1978), and combined autoradiographic and enzyme tracing methods (Jones, Coulter, and Hendry, 1978). Pandya and Vignolo (1971) examined the corticocortical projections of the precentral and premotor areas of macaques, specifically using the cytoarchitectural designations of Bonin and Bailey (1947) and the physiological maps of Woolsey (1958). Major subdivisions for each body part were connected with surrounding subdivisions in both hemispheres. Precentral cortical efferents were traced bilaterally to somatic sensory areas I and II, to the supplementary motor area to area 5 in parietal cortex, into the ventral bank of the cingulate sulcus, and to area 6. For area 6, Pandya and Vignolo (1971) showed reciprocal connections with the caudal precentral gyrus, the supplementary motor area, and the prefrontal cortex. The source of the cutaneous inputs to multiple areas within primary motor cortex described by Strick and Preston (1978a) and Tanji and Wise (1981) remains undetermined.

Use of axoplasmic tracing techniques also has further indicated that within precentral cortex a given body part is represented at more than one site. Muakkassa and Strick (1979) showed that there are four spatially separate regions in the superior frontal gyrus that project bilaterally to the arm, leg, and face subdivisions of the area 4 motor cortex. For example, to the primary motor face area 4 there are separate projections from the inferior precentral sulcus (lateral area 6 and area 44), the inferior limb of the arcuate sulcus (area 44), rostral SMA (medial area 6), and rostral cingulate sulcus. These latter observations indicate a functional distinction among the areas of the precentral gyrus and, as is discussed subsequently, a possible sequence of cortical actions preceding from a "higher level" (areas 44 and 6) to a "lower level" (area 4) of control.

A Multiple Perspective Approach to Motor Cortex Function

With the exception of a few investigations, attempts at relating precentral cortical organization to detailed aspects of the motorsensory periphery have been limited. Of particular interest is the question of what functionally distinct roles might be played by the multiple representations of a given body part. In a series of related studies, Humphrey and Reed (Humphrey, 1982; Humphrey and Reed, 1981, 1983) sought to distinguish the roles of two adjacent areas of precentral cortex—a caudal wrist area and a rostral wrist area—in their differential control of two wrist actions. Humphrey and Reed identified two different wrist actions that they termed "reciprocal" and "coactivation" which correspondingly appeared to be controlled by these caudal and rostral hand areas. Reciprocal actions were phasic movements of the wrist—either flexion or extension. Coactivation gestures, as implied, involved fixing the wrist by cocontraction of wrist flexor and extensor muscles. These two adjacent cortical wrist areas manifested several distinguishing functional characteristics, including differences in (1) sensitivity to peripheral cutaneous stimuli applied to the hand, (2) modulation of cortical unit discharge by forces applied to the wrist, (3) muscle activation via ICMS, and (4) cortical unit activation during voluntary reciprocal and coactivation gestures. Humphrey and Reed were also able to determine that the caudal cortical area, apparently specialized for "reciprocal" actions, had four times as many PTNs as the rostral area specialized for "coactivation" functions.

Effectively, Humphrey and Reed's observations suggest that, while a given muscle may be represented at more than one site on the motor cortex, each representation may be associated with different uses (tasks) of those muscles. In this context, Humphrey and Reed's observations suggest an important hypothesis concerning the differential actions of the various orofacial structures in speech articulation. It might be speculated that certain basic actions of a particular speech articulator (e.g., protrusion and occlusion of the lips) are controlled by different motor cortex centers, which can be activated separately or independently in time to generate their observed overlapping manifestations.

It is apparent that combining multiple techniques permits us to investigate the functional organization of the motor cortex and its peripheral motor-sensory manifestations in a manner that was not possible just a few years ago. Simply being able to experimentally consider motor task subdivisions of the precentral gyrus offers a substantially increased possibility of gaining insight into cortical contributions to the process of motor control. Clearly, the goal of these investigations was to discern some of the basic organizational principles of precentral cortex function in relation to their peripheral actions. Given the power of such multiple analysis techniques, it is apparent why these new approaches have largely replaced lesion studies, especially with the inherent difficulty of interpreting the lesions' results in relation to cortical functions. As was noted, these general motor-sensory cortical processes provide a perspective for examining parallel mechanisms in the control of the orofacial region. The following section deals with those orofacial mechanisms.

THE LATERAL PRECENTRAL MOTOR-SENSORY CORTEX

The objective in this section is to consider the cortical regions involved with orofacial motor-sensory function that lie within and around the *lateral precentral gyrus*. Although many other cerebral cortex regions are involved in human communication, the lateral precentral region is particularly important to the motor control of expressive communication; many large pyramidal cells in lateral precentral cortex make monosynaptic connections to the facial, hypoglossal, and masticatory motor nuclei. We have chosen to focus on the three classic cytoarchitectonic areas—4, 6, and 44 (Figure 5-2). In this second section of the chapter we review observations from both normal and brain damaged human subjects and then evaluate these observations in relation to findings on lateral precentral cortex function in nonhuman primates.

Precentral Cortex Anatomy: Human and Nonhuman Primates

Three distinct cytoarchitectonic areas (4, 6, and 44) have been described in the lateral precentral cortex of primates, including humans. The distinctions among these areas, however, may be manifest as gradual changes in various features of the cortical layers as one proceeds rostrally and laterally from area 4 to 6 to 44, rather than as sharply bounded regions. For example, although the size and number of pyramidal cells is greater in area 4 than in areas 6 and 44, all of these areas have some large pyramidal cells. In the discussions that follow, we use the cytoarchitectonic designations of Brodmann (1909), partly as a matter of convenience and partly because many experiments on the lateral precentral cortex have been based on these designations.

The distinctions among precentral orofacial areas 4, 6, and 44 are based on size and density of cell bodies and the distribution of these various cell types in the layers of the cortex. Area 4 is described as agranular cortex, with a thick layer of gray matter and very large pyramidal cells (or Betz cells) in layer V. Area 6 lacks Betz cells, but the other pyramidal cells in area 6 are only slightly smaller than those in area 4. Layer V of area 6, as well as the gray matter itself, is somewhat thinner than in area 4. Area 44 is different from areas 4 and 6 in several major respects: (1) the gray matter layer is thinner, (2) there is a greater degree of stratification, and (3) layers II and IV are distinct. These cytoarchitectonic features appear to characterize both the human and the nonhuman primate lateral precentral cortex, with some species differences (Bailey and Bonin, 1951). For example, the cortical surface area designated as area 4 is smaller, relatively, in humans than in Old World monkeys. Quantitative studies of cell size, number, and density, especially in relation to their laminar distributions, are needed to confirm and refine these interareal distinctions.

The functional significance of cortical cytoarchitectonic distinctions has long been a matter of controversy (Lashley and Clark, 1946). However, more recent neuroanatomical studies indicate differential patterns of afferent and efferent connectivity for these subareas, thus supporting their functional distinctions. For example, as noted previously, axoplasmic tracing methods indicate three separate face representations in lateral precentral cortex, one each in areas 6, 44, and 4 (Muakkassa and Strick,

1979). The descending projections from these three precentral motor areas also differ. Area 4 projections include dense monosynaptic connections to brainstem motor nuclei of the fifth, seventh, and twelfth cranial nerves in macaque, chimpanzee, and humans (Kuypers, 1958a, b, 1960). These data suggest that area 4 acts like an "upper motoneuron pool" (Phillips and Porter, 1977) (i.e., a near final stage of the motor execution process). By contrast, descending projections from lateral area 6 to the brainstem motor nuclei are indirect, with a much greater percentage of connections to adjacent rechicular regions, such as the supratrigeminal nucleus (Kuypers, 1958b; Kuypers and Lawrence, 1967; Watson, 1975). Reticular regions like the supratrigeminal nucleus are thought to be interneuronal pools that integrate multiple peripheral and central influences upon the cranial motoneurons. In comparison to areas 4 and 6, descending pathways from area 44 are both less dense and more diffuse in their termination in the regions "adjacent" to the cranial motor nuclei (Kuypers and Lawrence, 1967; Watson, 1975). Area 44 and lateral area 6 also receive projections from posterior temporal regions in Old and New World monkeys (Galaburda and Pandya, 1982; Forbes and Moskowitz, 1977; Jürgens, 1982) and projections from lateral posterior parietal face area, 7b (Godschalk, Lemon, and Kuypers, 1983). Finally, there is some suggestion that the density of projections to the ventrolateral subnucleus of the pars paricellularis in the red nucleus in greater from face area 4 than from 44 (Kuypers and Lawrence, 1967; see also Kohlerman, Gibson, and Houk, 1982; Larson and Yumiya, 1980).

The functional implications of these anatomical observations are that (1) *area 4* is involved directly in activating muscles for individual movements and (2) *areas 6 and 44* provide inputs to area 4 and to subcortical regions in controlling the "macroprogramming" of more global motor actions or multiple movements. Projections from posterior parietal and temporal cortical regions to areas 6 and 44 also are comparable to the posterior to anterior anatomical cortical connections thought to underlie human language and speech (Galaburda and Pandya, 1982). These posterior perietal and temporal regions appear to be of special importance to intended motor goals in humans, possible including the motor goals for speech (Abbs, 1984). Unfortunately, many of these important connectivity data have been obtained with degeneration methods that may have involved lesions that crossed functional boundaries. As noted recently by Kuypers, many of these observations are likely to be "dramatically expanded" by utilization of axonal fiber tracing techniques (Kuypers, 1982, pp. 381, 394). Also, the cortical areas examined in many of these studies were not identified with respect to the representations of individual orofacial structures, such as the lips, tongue, or jaw. The use of axonal tracing procedures in conjunction with micromapping identification of the separate lip, jaw, and tongue cortical areas should allow us to address specific questions more directly (e.g., are orofacial cortical projections to the supratrigeminal nucleus exclusively from the jaw areas?).

Human Lateral Precentral Cortex Function

In considering the motor-sensory cortical mechanisms underlying the execution of complex orofacial movements and speech, some information is found in reports dealing with the influences of cortical lesions. However, as noted above, interpretation of cortical lesions with regard to orofacial motor functions must be undertaken with great caution. Postmortem confirmation of the suspected brain lesions is rare, and even when these are conducted, subtle damage, such as remote loss of blood supply, may not be detected (Mohr, 1976). Even modern brain imaging techniques are subject to serious errors in not revealing certain lesions, especially early following onset. Also, in most reports on human cortical lesions the alleged aberrations in speech motor behavior have not been subjected to quantitative physiological analysis. This general absence of interpretable data on cortical deficits is serious; the clinical labels often used to describe these speech motor aberrations (e.g., aphemia, apraxia, dysarthria) have not been standardized, and disagreement is common.

Despite these problems, the clinical literature on the role of precentral cortical areas in speech motor behavior provides certain provocative "clues." In general, patients with lesions to the precentral cortical region (lateral areas 4, 6, and 44) that spare the most rostral portion of area 44 exhibit a variety of aberrations in speech motor control (Barlow and Abbs, 1983; Benson, 1967; Darley, Aronson, and Brown, 1975; Fromm, 1981; Fromm, Abbs, McNeil, and Rosenbek, 1982; Mohr, 1976; Mohr et al., 1975, 1978). Of interest in this chapter are circumstantial data suggesting differential functions for the three lateral precentral areas.

Lesions confined to motor-sensory face area 4 yield a pattern of aberrations different from lesions that include the more lateral and rostral cortical areas 6 and 44. For example, lesions to area 4 appear to yield weakness and some loss of motor dexterity in the contralateral orofacial regions. Usually for unilateral lesions a mild dysarthria is in evidence, with little or no loss of normal speech. By contrast, if the lesion is more extensive, especially in the left hemisphere (encompassing areas 4, 6, and 44) or confined to areas 6 and 44, the speech patterns are often grossly abnormal. Symptoms range from muteness (early following onset) to disintegration of the multiple speech movement patterns, including effortful orofacial struggle, major sound distortions, groping, and a general disruption of fluent speech, particularly for multisyllabic, multiword utterances, albeit of a transient nature (Mohr, 1976; Mohr et al., 1975, 1978; Roch-LeComs and Lhermitte, 1976; Schiff, Alexander, Naeser, and Galaburda, 1983). As Mohr and co-workers (1978) point out, a "restricted" lesion to these areas leads us to view their function as *"mediating a more traditionally postulated role as a premotor association cortex region concerned with acquired skilled oral, pharyngeal, and respiratory movements, involving speaking as well as other behaviors but not essentially language or graphic behavior, per se"* (p. 22, italics added).

Recent EMG and movement investigations in the so-called "apraxia of speech" population (presumably due to lesions "anterior" to the central sulcus in the lateral precentral region) reveal that the speech sound substitutions, sometimes interpreted as evidence for a "linguistic selection" disorder, (1) almost exclusively co-occur with significant movement and muscle activity aberrations, and (2) are better characterized as sound "distortions" (Fromm, 1981; Fromm et al., 1982; Itoh, Sasanuma, Hirose, Yoshioka, and Ushijima, 1980; Itoh, Sasanuma, and Ushijima, 1979). These speech movement observations suggest that a major aspect of the speech motor problem in this population is one of breakdown in multiple speech movement coordination and sequencing. Corroborative evidence for the importance of this lateral precentral region to speech motor control is apparent from surface stimulation of the human cortex, even when that stimulation is applied to the nondominant hemisphere (Ojemann, 1983; Penfield and Rasmussen, 1950; Penfield and Roberts, 1959).

Other evidence for the importance of motor-sensory cortical areas for speech movement coordination is provided from studies with unanticipated perturbations of speech movements in normal human subjects. Those studies show that the compensatory sensorimotor actions elicited by unanticipated perturbation operate at latencies consistent with suprabulbar and possibly "transcortical" pathways. These perturbation analyses have also provided some suggestions as to the task-oriented cortical control of human perioral muscles (Abbs and Gracco, 1983). Abbs, Gracco, and Blair (1983) also observed task-dependent part-muscle compensatory responses to perturbations at latencies characteristic of cortical pathways. Some limited data on intracortical microstimulation of motor cortex reveal submuscle activation of some of the same facial muscles in nonhuman primates (McGuinness, Siversten, and Allman, 1980).

Nonhuman Primate Precentral Cortex Function

Our knowledge of the motor-sensory cortical organization underlying control of orofacial movements is relatively limited. However, the dozen or so studies variously employing lesion, fiber tracing, stimulation, chronic recording, and sensory mapping techniques in several different primate species offer some intriguing hypotheses regarding lateral precentral cortical areas and their peripheral actions. The picture that emerges is surprisingly consistent with observations in human subjects and provides some insights concerning the differential role of lateral precentral subregions in the control of the orofacial system.

Lesion Studies

Cortical areas 4, 6, and 44, separately or together, have been lesioned separately, sequentially, or both (Luschei and Goodwin, 1975; Larson, Byrd, Garthwaite, and Luschei, 1980; Rizzolatti, Matelli, and Pavesi, 1980; Watson, 1975) in macaque monkeys. A representative finding is that of Luschei and Goodwin (1975), who contrasted the effects of lesions to area 4 with lesions in area 44 and lateral area 6. Prior to lesioning, all animals were trained to produce a low-level biting force. Postoperatively, animals with area 4 lesions were not able to generate the steady, low-level biting forces but could manipulate food and feed themselves without major problems. By contrast, an animal with a lesion to areas 6 and 44 (sparing area 4) was able to perform the controlled force biting task, *but was not able to adequately feed itself.* Luschei and Goodwin's findings are consistent with other investigations (Larson et al., 1980; Walker and Green, 1938; Watson, 1975) using larger numbers of animals. As noted by Larson and co-workers (1980), coordination and integration of the "more complex" lip, tongue, and jaw movements necessary for food manipulation, chewing, and swallowing were impaired specifically with lateral area 6/area 44 lesions.

Results of a more extensive investigation (Watson, 1975) involving lesions to areas 4, 6, and 44 (both separately and in combination) are in agreement with the studies cited above and support functional distinctions among orofacial areas 4, 6, and 44. The unique deficits consistently manifest with area 6 lesions were in the organization of "the complex sequence of movements of the facial, jaw, and tongue musculature which normally occur during mastication, deglutition, and sucking" (Watson, 1975, p. 95). *These observations are strikingly similar to those made by Mohr (1976), noted earlier, regarding the interpretations of comparable lesions in human cortex.* Lesions restricted to area 44, by contrast, revealed only minor deficits, one of which noted by Watson (1975) was a "neglect" of the orofacial region contralateral to the lesion. The absence of obvious functional deficits following circumscribed lesions to area 44 are consistent with the results of Sutton, Larson, and Lindeman (1974), who reported no influence of such lesions on simple conditioned vocalizations in rhesus monkeys. These lesional effects are paralleled by differences in descending projections from these two areas (Kuypers, 1958a; Watson, 1975). However, inasmuch as the inclusion and exact location of area 44 in the genus Macaca is not without controversy (Galaburda and Pandya, 1982), additional information on the physiological and anatomical distinctions between area 6 and area 44 would be of particular value.

Sensory Mapping of Lateral Precentral Cortex

Electrophysiological recording of single- and multicell discharges in areas 4, 6, and 44 suggest that these cortical regions are differentially activated by sensory input. Direct comparisons among these areas in the same experiment, however, have generally not been done. In the one study involving sensory mapping of more than one orofacial cortical area, observations were made under alpha-chloralose anesthesia (O'Brien, Pimpaneau, and Albe-Fessard, 1971), which enhances cortical responsiveness to sensory input. O'Brien and co-authors reported that multiple orofacial afferents converged over a larger cortical area and with greater magnitudes on areas 6 and 44 as compared to area 4. Their results agree with more recent observations in awake animals. Rizzolatti, Scandolara, Gentilucci, and Camarda (1981) and Rizzolatti, Scandolara, Matelli, and Gentilucci (1981) likewise reported that cutaneous and joint afferents from multiple peripheral sites (ipsi- and contralateral) converged on individual cells in lateral area 6. Rizzolatti, Scandolara, Matelli, and Gentilucci (1981) emphasize particularly that the nature as well as the complexity of sensory inputs to area 6 are different from those typically observed for area 4. That is, instead of the close, single movement, input–output coupling described earlier for area 4 (Rosen and Asanuma, 1972), area 6 appears to receive an afferent drive that is related to multimovement goals such as finger–mouth interactions. Rizzolatti, Scandolara, Gentilucci, and Camarda (1981) interpret the difference in afferent projections to area 6 versus area 4 as reflecting the importance of area 6 in "programming" complex, multiaction motor behaviors. Unfortunately, Rizzolatti and his colleagues recorded only in area 6 and relied on published studies from other laboratories as a basis for their comparison to recordings in area 4.

A close anatomical input–output coupling in area 4 is supported by other studies. In their recordings from cortical units in area 4, Hoffman and Luschei (1980) modulated the unit discharge patterns with imposed jaw stretch, indicating a direct input–output coupling to neurons that was preferentially active during conditioned jaw biting. In contrast, Zealear and Hast (1982), working in awake animals, found both closely coupled *and* more complex sensory projections in an area rostral and lateral to face area 4 (around the subcentral anterior sulcus—SCA).

These differential patterns of sensory projection to *areas 6 and 4* reflect the functional differences between these cortical regions. One interesting hypothesis is that the autogenic and nonautogenic (intermovement) responses to perturbations during speech (Abbs and Gracco, 1984; Abbs et al., 1984) could be mediated differentially via areas 4 and 6, respectively. Inasmuch as the control of multiple movement coordination is the essence of speech control, the functions of area 6 (and 44) would appear very important. The lesion data cited above support this hypothesis.

Chronic Recording

Recording of cortical cell activity in awake, behaving animals has also revealed some functional differences between cytoarchitectonic areas 4 and 6 of lateral precentral cortex. Specifically, for a simple conditioned movement of a single structure (a jaw biting task), cortical cell discharge in area 4 correlated with the force of the jaw closing (Hoffman and Luschei, 1980; Luschei, Garthwaite, and Armstrong, 1971). By contrast, during more complex movements involving orofacial food manipulation and chewing, area 4 cell activity was not related to jaw movements (Hoffman and Luschei, 1980; Luschei et al., 1971). *A different pattern appears to be manifest in the discharge patterns of single units in the region described as lateral to area 4 (presumably corresponding to area 6).* Both Kubota and Niki (1971) and Lund and Lamarre (1974) recorded cortical units in this region of "lateral precentral cortex" and found cell discharges that related to natural jaw or tongue movements in a consistent manner. These apparent area 6 neurons also were sensitive in some cases to sensory inputs from the jaw and tongue (Lund and Lamarre, 1974). Antidromic activation from the cerebral peduncle was utilized by Kubota and Niki (1971) to distinguish direct corticobulbar tract pyramidal cells from cells projecting indirectly; the former cells were relatively rare (10%) in lateral area 6 (in contrast to observations in area 4) and consistent with cytoarchitectonic differences between these areas. Although Hoffman and Luschei (1980) used spike-triggered averaging to verify the connections between the cortical cells in area 4 and the jaw muscles, investigators recording in area 6 did not.

The correlation between single unit discharge in area 6 and parameters of jaw and tongue movement reported by Lund and Lamarre is difficult to reconcile with the reported small percentage of direct projections to the brainstem motoneurons from this area. A route through area 4 is unlikely inasmuch as firing of single neurons in that area does not relate to jaw movements during chewing (Hoffman and Luschei, 1980). Although the exact contributions of area 6 (and possibly area 44) are ambiguous, these data suggesting its (their) general involvement with complex multiple movement actions of the orofacial region are consistent with the animal and human lesion studies cited earlier. Unfortunately, as in some of the previous comparisons, most of these area 4 area 6 comparisons were not systematically documented in a single study using similar techniques. Furthermore, it is difficult without histological studies, verification via cortical stimulation, or more detailed information on standard cortical landmarks to determine the exact sites within area 6, area 44, or both, of Kubota and Niki's or Lund and Lamarre's recordings.

Surface Stimulation Studies

Further distinctions among areas in lateral precentral cortex have been demonstrated with surface electrical stimulation. Numerous investigators have noted that electrical stimulation of primary motor cortex (area 4) yields semidiscrete activation of individual orofacial muscles or small groups of muscles. By contrast, stimulation of lateral area 6 premotor cortex has been reported to elicit rhythmical, coordinated movement of the jaw, characterized as "chewing" (Beevor and Horsley, 1884; Grunbaum and Sherrington, 1901, 1904; Hines 1940; Lund and Lamarre, 1974; Walker and Green, 1938). These results have been uniformly interpreted as evidence of an area 4–area 6 distinction (Larson et al., 1980; Lund and Lamarre, 1974; Watson, 1975). Lauer (1952) also applied surface stimulation to various sites in the lateral precentral cortex in monkeys under light ether anesthesia (Lauer, 1952). Lauer's brief report described a second facial muscle representation immediately medial and caudal to the subcentral anterior sulcus (SCA) where stimulation primarily yielded ipsilateral facial muscle responses. Lauer's results with light ether anesthesia are interesting, particularly inasmuch as early surface stimulation studies conducted in animals under sodium pentobarbital (Nembutal) indicated that area 44 was not excitable. Additionally, Lauer reported tongue and jaw responses from an area lateral and rostral to SCA. Lauer notes that these responses were obtained in area 6 and perhaps the superior part of area 44. Lauer's observations also confirmed a short report by Sugar, Chusid, and French

(1948) of a far lateral area of excitable cortex yielding facial and laryngeal movements. Interestingly, Hast, Fischer, Wetzel, and Thompson (1974) elicited discrete activation of individual contralateral laryngeal muscles of rhesus monkeys (under alpha-chloralose anesthesia) in the regions rostral to the SCA (area 44). These earlier reports, using surface stimulation, indicate that in addition to complete contralateral representation of the lips, jaw, and tongue in area 4, there may be separate ipsilateral and contralateral representations caudal and rostral to SCA. Additionally, it is apparent from these reports that portions of 6 and 44 are excitable, yielding orofacial and laryngeal responses. Obviously, these multiple lateral regions of excitable cortex yielding orofacial responses have not been adequately delineated, especially given their potential importance in understanding cortical mechanisms for orofacial and laryngeal control. Although these studies utilizing surface stimulation in these regions are intriguing, the picture that emerges is incomplete, and additional work in this area, using modern techniques (e.g., ICMS), is sorely needed.

Intracortical Microstimulation

Several recent investigations have used the more precise intracortical microstimulation (ICMS) technique in the orofacial regions of the lateral precentral gyrus. The first such investigation of orofacial precentral area 4 (Clark and Luschei, 1974) is difficult to interpret inasmuch as the stimulation currents and pulse train durations were much greater than desirable for restricting activation to a single functional field (Asanuma and Arnold, 1975; Asanuma et al., 1976). Of interest in this initial study, however, was the report of latencies from the motor cortex to the jaw muscles as short as 8 to 10 ms. Sirisko, Lucier, Wiesendanger, and Sessle (1980) subsequently confirmed these latencies using much lower currents. Other than some initial work by the present authors (Welt, Abbs, and Gracco, unpublished observations) in monkeys under ketamine anesthesia, there have been no studies in which ICMS has been used to map lateral area 6 or area 44. In our study we found areas 4, 6, and 44 to be excitable, all with short latency projections to orofacial sites.

The most complete ICMS investigation of the orofacial cortical area 4 reported to date is that of McGuinness, Siversten, and Allman (1980). Other recent ICMS studies of the area 4 face representation have been reported only in brief form (Sirisko and Sessle, 1981, 1983a, b; Sirisko et al., 1980; Zealear and Hast, 1982), or were focused primarily on the upper limbs (Sessle and Wiesendanger, 1982). The results from these latter studies are in most respects consistent with the findings of McGuinness and colleagues (1980), who focused specifically on the primary motor regions of orofacial precentral cortex using awake animals quieted with small doses of ketamine. Their findings were remarkable in several respects. These authors found that the largest number of responses were from the muscles of the lower face for the perioral region, with fewer responses from the tongue and jaw, in that order. Also, there appeared to be at least two cortical motor fields for the facial muscles; individual muscles or parts of muscles were represented in several noncontiguous foci. In particular, muscles of the lower face were represented in both the caudal and rostral regions of the primary motor area, with a tongue muscle representation in between (see also Sirisko et al., 1980; Zealear and Hast, 1982). McGuinness and associates also observed a notable discreteness of the responses; they commented that the "usual response was a discrete focus in part of a muscle" (p. 594) and that moving the electrode commonly revealed a second, but different, response in another part of the same muscle or a contiguous muscle.

The cortical fractionalization of the facial muscles observed by McGuinness and colleagues was based on visual inspections rather than analyses of EMG responses. Their interpretations of these discrete, part-muscle responses are, however, significant. They suggest that "it may be appropriate to consider cortical representation of the face as organized by groups of neurons projecting to a facial nucleus motor neuron pool innervating a specific [intramuscular] branch of facial nerve *rather than a specific muscle*" (italics added) (p. 606). These observations indicate the importance of the fine motor mapping available using ICMS for delineating organizational patterns of the motor cortex devoted to orofacial function. Since McGuinness and colleagues did not examine sensory input to these cortical sites, it is not known if the caudal and rostral perioral zones they reported are analogous to the dual representation reported for the forelimb (Strick and Preston, 1982b) and the hindlimb (Tanji and Wise, 1981).

To obtain a more complete documentation of the structural and functional characteristics of lateral precentral multiple orofacial cortical representations, we have undertaken a series of studies of areas 4, 6, and 44 using combined recording, stimulation, and anatomical methods. In the initial ICMS study of areas 4, 6, and 44 (Welt et al., unpublished observations) we confirmed the presence of relatively small cortical foci where low-current stimulation produced a discrete muscle responses (McGuinness et al., 1980). Multiple, noncontiguous fields were found for the lips, tongue, and jaw. In a region rostral to the SCA we obtained low-threshold responses in the tongue, face, and velum. In terms of the cytoarchitectonic areas, these penetrations apparently were in both areas 6 and 44 (Bonin, 1949; Figure 5–2). Orofacial responses in these areas have not been reported previously with ICMS. Perhaps the most complex response was a combination of perioral, tongue, and velar movements obtained from a penetration that was the most lateral and clear in area 44. Finally, we observed a number of ipsilateral tongue and lip movements from stimulation in a region caudal and medial to the subcentral dimple, most probably in area 6. This location is similar to the ipsilateral orofacial area reported by Lauer (1952). The ability to elicit orofacial motor responses with ICMS applied to lateral cortical areas 6 and 44 under ketamine supports the importance of these regions to orofacial motor control. Further studies are needed to determine if these multiple orofacial regions are comparable to those in the distal upper limbs, which would indicate that such representations in motor cortex may underlie multiple, but functionally distinct, actions of the same muscles. Thus, while these results are preliminary, they indicate the importance of carefully and systematically studying the lateral precentral cortex as a further basis for delineating the role of this area in orofacial motor control.

IMPLICATIONS FOR SPEECH MOTOR CONTROL

The foregoing review provides a number of intriguing hypotheses concerning some specific cortical mechanisms that might underlie the control of complex motor actions for human speech. For example, documenting the short latency outputs from the motor cortex to the orofacial structures allows us to consider, in a concrete manner, the powerful and direct influence of cortical outflow on moment-to-moment control of the orofacial system. As reported by Clark and Luschei (1974) and Sirisko and co-workers (1980), the latencies of these corticofugal pathways are in the 7 to 10 ms range. Similarly, determining the projections of sensory afferents from the various orofacial structures to the motor cortex output cells indicates the important contribution of these inputs to the control of speech movements. The observations by O'Brien and colleagues indicate that tongue, lip, and laryngeal afferents project to areas 4, 6, and 44 with latencies that are commonly less than 12 ms. Moreover, based upon the observation of several investigators (Lemon, 1981; Zealear and Hast, 1982), the inputs from a particular peripheral site are enhanced by voluntary movement at that same site. In this light, and given the documented influence of pyramidal cell discharge on lower motoneurons in the orofacial region, the long-standing debate concerning whether afferent input is involved in speech motor control becomes moot. This interpretation, of course, is consistent with observed compensatory responses at latencies of 25 to 40 ms in the speech muscles to unanticipated perturbation (Abbs and Gracco, 1984).

The motor output and sensory input characteristics of the three precentral cortical areas discussed earlier (4, 6, and 44) suggest further that the coordinative coupling among the multiple muscles and movements of the orofacial region for speech may be reflected in the actions of these cortical areas. All three cytoarchitectonic areas appear to contain at least a partial representation of the lips, tongue, and jaw; the interconnections among these areas seem particularly significant given the data from human and nonhuman primates indicating their differential contributions to complex orofacial movement control. That is, there appears to be cortical involvement of areas 7b, 5, 44, 6, and 4, perhaps in that order, with the former areas being involved in the higher level planning or programming and the latter areas more closely coupled to the periphery in carrying out the actual motor-sensory execution. In that vein, the fact that perturbations of a given speech movement yield both intra- and intermovement compensatory adjustments (Abbs et al., 1984) may reflect input-output actions of both lower level cortical regions (area 4) and higher level regions (areas 6 and 44), respectively. Needless to say, the consideration of these multiple areas, their interconnections, the cortical activity associated with voluntary movement, and responses to sensory stimulation substantially augment the more limited perspectives offered by cortical lesion deficit data.

Perhaps the most intriguing hypothesis that might be offered involves extrapolation of the work in the limbs by Humphrey (1982), Strick and Preston (1982a, b), and Tanji and Wise (1981) to control of the orofacial system for speech. As described, these investigators provided evidence for the parcellation of the precentral cortex into multiple task-dependent representations of each body part. The implication of this work was that while one precentral cortical subarea is involved for certain actions of the hand (or leg or wrist), and adjacent but separate subarea primarily controls actions for a different motor task. As described earlier, within the lateral precentral cortex there are multiple, separate representations of the tongue, lips, and jaw. The influence of sensory input, the degree of control precision, the duration and speed of movement, the degree of synergistic and antagonist muscle activation, and other factors, are likely to vary with the motor actions of a given articulator for different speech sounds (e.g., lip actions for vowels versus stop consonants). It might thus be hypothesized that different motor cortical representations underlie the motor executions in a given articulator for different speech motor tasks. Such multiple, task-dependent representations would be consistent with empirical observations of such phenomena as coarticulation; perhaps the timing of lip rounding and lip elevation for speech appear independent (even though contraction of some of the same muscles are involved) because they are controlled from different cortical foci. Given the observations of Lemon, the task-dependent sensorimotor actions in speech motor control recently reported (Abbs and Gracco, 1983; Abbs et al., 1983; Kelso, Tuller, and Fowler, 1982) would also be consistent with this view. This hypothesis also may address the reasons that certain individuals with speech disorders have greater difficulty with some classes of speech sounds than with others. This hypothesized process of motor-sensory cortical control of speech movements is subject to the criticism that it is not parsimonious; seemingly such a model would require a separate cortical representation for each articulator for each distinct speech sound. However, an elemental set of muscle contractions (apparently few in number) could, in various combinations, account for an almost infinite number of distinct configurations. As noted by Phillips (1973), in a parallel interpretation of motor cortex organization, "many chords, musical expressions, and tunes can be made out of a few notes" (p. 36).

Obviously, the final limitation on our understanding of the apparently elegant cortical functions underlying speech motor control is an inability to undertake detailed physiological and anatomical investigations in the human animal who exhibits this important behavior naturally. However, as is apparent from this review, certain valuable insights are available from work with nonhuman primates. Moreover, the principles of motor-sensory cortex organization and function being revealed by ongoing work in the limbs is likely to be of continuing importance in broadening our horizons regarding cortical functions for speech. In parallel, with increasing focus upon the lateral regions of the cortex underlying orofacial control, we can expect that future research also will provide us with a more substantive neurophysiological and neuroanatomical base for understanding human oral communication.

REFERENCES

Abbs, J. H. (1984). Invariance and variability in speech production: A distinction between linguistic intent and its neuromotor implementation. In J. Perkell and D. Klatt (Eds.), *Invariance and variability of speech processes.* Hillsdale, NJ: Lawrence Erlbaum Associates.

Abbs, J. H., and Cole, K. J. (1982). Consideration of bulbar and suprabulbar afferent influences upon speech motor coordination and programming. In S. Grillner, B. Lindblom, J. Lubker, and A. Persson (Eds.), *Speech motor control* (pp. 159–186). New York: Pergamon.

Abbs, J. H., and Gracco, V. L. (1983). Sensorimotor actions in the control of multimovement speech gestures. *Trends in Neuroscience, 6*(9), 391–395.

Abbs, J. H., and Gracco, V.L. (1984). Control of complex motor gestures: Orofacial muscle responses to load perturbations of the lip during speech. *Journal of Neurophysiology, 51*(4), 705–723.

Abbs, J.H., Gracco, V. L., and Blair, C. (1983). Intramuscular partitioning of the facial muscles during speech movements: Possible cortical correlates. *Society for Neuroscience, 9*(Part 1), 178 (Abstract).

Abbs, J. H., Gracco, V. L., and Cole, K. J. (1984). Control of multimovement coordination: Sensorimotor mechanisms in speech motor programming. *Journal of Motor Behavior, 16* (No. 2).

Albe-Fessard, D., and Liebeskind, J. (1966). Origine des messages somatosensitifs activant les cellules du cortex moteur chez le singe. *Experimental Brain Research, 1,* 127–146.

Armstrong E., and Falk D. (Eds.). (1982). *Primate brain evolution. Methods and concepts.* New York: Plenum.

Asanuma, H., and Arnold, A. P. (1975). Noxious effects of excessive currents used for intracortical microstimulation. *Brain Research, 96,* 103–107.

Asanuma, H., Arnold, A., and Zarzecki, P. (1976). Further study on the excitation of pyramidal tract cells by intracortical microstimulation. *Experimental Brain Research, 26,* 443–461.

Asanuma, H., and Sakata, H. (1967). Functional organization of a cortical efferent system examined with focal depth stimulation in cats. *Journal of Neurophysiology, 30,* 35–54.

Asanuma, H., Zarzecki, P., Jankowska, E., Hongo, T., and Marcus, S. (1979). Projection of individual pyramidal tract neurons to lumbar motor nuclei of the monkey. *Experimental Brain Research, 34,* 73–89.

Bailey, P., and Bonin, G. von (1951). *The isocortex of man* (Vol. 6). Urbana, IL: University of Illinois Press.

Barlow, S. M., and Abbs, J. H. (1983). Force transducers for the evaluation of labial, lingual, and mandibular function in dysarthria. *Journal of Speech and Hearing Research, 26*(4), 616–621.

Beevor, C. E., and Horsley, V. (1888). A further minute analysis by electrical stimulation of the so-called motor region of the cortex cerebri in the monkey *(Maccus sinicus). Philosophical Transactions, 179B,* 205–256.

Benson, F. D. (1967). Fluencey in aphasia: Correlation with radioactive scan localization. *Cortex, 3,* 373–394.

Berrevoets, C. E., and Kuypers, H. G. J. M. (1975). Pericruciate cortical neurons projecting to brainstem reticular formation, dorsal column nuclei and spinal cord in the cat. *Neuroscience Letters, 1,* 257–262.

Betz, V. (1874). Anatomischer nachweis zweier gehirnzentra. *Zentralblatt Med. Wiss., 12,* 578–580, 595–599.

Bonin, G. von (1938). Studies of the size of the cells in the cerebral cortex. II. The motor area of man, cebus, and the cat. *Journal of Comparative Neurology, 69,* 381–390.

Bonin, G. von (1949). Architecture of the precentral motor cortex and some adjacent areas. In P. C. Bucy (Ed.), *The precentral motor cortex* (pp.7–82). Urbana, IL: University of Illinois Press.

Bonin, G. von, and Bailey, P. (1947). *The neocortex of Macaca mulatta.* Urbana, IL; University of Illinois Press.

Brazier, M. A. B. (1978). *Architectonics of the cerebral cortex:* Research in the 19th century. In M. A. B. Brazier and H. Petsche (Eds.), *Architectonics of the cerebral cortex* (International Brain Research Organization Monograph Series, Volume 3, pp. 9–29). New York: Raven Press.

Brodmann, K. (1909). *Vergleichende Lokalisationslehre der Grosshirnrinde in ihren Prinzipien dargestellt auf Grund des Zellenbaues.* Leipzig, Germany: Barth.

Bucy, P. C. (1933). Electrical excitability and cytoarchitecture of the premotor cortex in monkeys. *Archives of Neurology and Psychiatry, 39*, 1205-1224.

Campbell, A. W. (1905). *Histological studies on the localisation of cerebral function.* Cambridge: Cambridge University Press.

Carlson, M., and Welt, C. (1981). The somatic sensory cortex: SmI in prosimian primates. In C. N. Woolsey (Ed.), *Cortical sensory organization, Vol.1: Multiple somatic areas* (pp. 1-27). Clifton, NJ: Humana Press.

Cheney, P. D., and Fetz, E. E. (1980). Functional classes of primate corticomotoneuronal cells and their relation to active force. *Journal of Neurophysiology, 44*, 773-791.

Clark, R. W., and Luschei, E. S. (1974). Short latency jaw movement produced by low intensity intracortical microstimulation of the precentral face area in monkeys. *Brain Research, 70*, 144-147.

Conrad, B., Matsunami, K., Meyer-Lohmann, J., Weisendanger, M., and Brooks, V. B. (1974). Cortical load compensation during voluntary elbow movements. *Brain Research, 71*, 507-514.

Conrad, B., Meyer-Lohmann, J., Matsunami, K., and Brooks, V. B. (1975). Precentral unit activity following torque pulse injections into elbow movements. *Brain Research, 94*, 219-236.

Darley, F. L., Aronson, A. E., and Brown, J. R. (1975). *Motor speech disorders.* Philadelphia: Saunders.

Denny-Brown, D. (1960). Motor mechanisms—Introduction: The general principles of motor integration. In H. W. Magoun (Ed.), *Handbook of physiology, Section 1* (pp. 781-796). Washington, DC: American Physiological Society.

Economo, C. von, and Koskinas, G. N. (1925). *Die cytoarchitectonik der hirnrinde des erwachsenen menschen.* Berlin: Springer.

Evarts, E. V. (1964). Temporal patterns of discharge of pyramidal tract neurons during sleep and waking in the monkey. *Journal of Neurophysiology, 27*, 152-171.

Evarts, E. V. (1966). Methods for recording activity of individual neurons in moving animals. In R. F. Rushmer (Ed.), *Methods in medical research* (Vol. 2, pp. 241-250). Chicago: Year Book Medical Publishers.

Evarts, E. V. (1968). Relation of pyramidal tract activity to force everted during voluntary movement. *Journal of Neurophysiology, 31*, 14-27.

Evarts, E. V. (1969). Activity of pyramidal tract neurons during postural fixation. *Journal of Neurophysiology, 32*, 375-385.

Evarts, E. V. (1973). Motor cortex reflexes associated with learned movement. *Science, 179*, 501-503.

Evarts, e. V. (1974). Precentral and postcentral cortical activity in association with visually triggered movement. *Journal of Neurophysiology, 37*, 373-381.

Evarts, E. V. (1981). Role of motor cortex in voluntary movements in primates. In V. B. Brooks (Ed.), *Handbook of physiology, Section 1* (Vol. II: Motor control, Part 2, pp. 1083-1120). Bethesda, MD: American Physiological Society.

Evarts, E. V., and Fromm, C. (1977). Sensory responses in motor cortex neurons during precise motor control. *Neuroscience Letters, 5*, 267-272.

Evarts, E. V., and Fromm, C. (1978). The pyramidal tract neuron as summing point in a closed-loop system in the monkey. In J E. Desmedt (Ed.), *Cerebral motor control in man: Long loop mechanisms* (Vol. 4, pp. 56-69). Basel: Karger.

Evarts, E. V., Fromm, C., Kröller, J., and Jennings, V. A. (1983). Motor cortex control of finely graded forces. *Journal of Neurophysiology, 49*(5), 1199-1215.

Evarts, E. V., and Tanji, J. (1974). Gating of motor cortex reflexes by prior instruction. *Brain Research, 71*, 479-494.

Evarts, E. V., and Tanji, J. (1976). Reflex and intended responses in motor cortex pyramidal tract neurons of monkey. *Journal of Neurophysiology, 39,* 1069–1080.

Ferrier, D. (1876). *The functions of the brain* (pp. 1–323). London: Smith, Elder & Co.

Fetz, E. E., and Cheney, P. D. (1978). Muscle fields of primate corticomotoneuronal cells. *Journal de Physiologie (Paris), 74,* 239–245.

Fetz, E. E., Cheney, P. D., and German, D. C. (1976). Corticomotoneuronal connections of precentral cells detected by postspike averages of EMG activity in behaving monkeys. *Brain Research, 114,* 505–510.

Fetz, E. E., Finocchio, D. V., Baker, M. A., and Soso, M. J. (1980). Sensory and motor responses of precentral cortex cells during comparable passive and active joint movements. *Journal of Neurophysiology, 42,* 1070–1089.

Finger, S., and Stein, D. G. (1982). *Brain damage and recovery. Research and clinical perspectives.* New York: Academic Press.

Forbes, B. F., and Moskowitz, N. (1977). Cortico-cortical connections of the superior temporal gyrus in the squirrel monkey. *Brain Research, 136,* 547–552.

Fritsch, G. T., and Hitzig, E. (1870). Über die elektrische Erregbeit des Grosshirns. *Arch. Anat. Physiol. Wiss. Med., 37,* 300–332.

Fromm, D. (1981). *Investigation of movement/EMG parameters in apraxia of speech.* Unpublished master's thesis, University of Wisconsin-Madison.

Fromm, D., Abbs, J. H., McNeil, M., and Rosenbek, J. C. (1982). Simultaneous perceptual–physiological method for studying apraxia of speech. In R. Brookshire (Ed.), *Proceedings of the Annual Clinical Aphasiology Conference.* Minneapolis: BRK Publishers.

Fulton, J. F. (1934). Forced grasping in relation to the syndrome of the premotor area. *Archives of Neurology and Psychiatry, 31,* 221–235.

Galaburda, A. M., and Pandya, D. N. (1982). Role of architectonics and connections in the study of primate brain evolution. In E. Armstrong and D. Falk (Eds.), *Primate brain evolution* (pp. 203–216). New York: Plenum.

Glassman, R. B. (1978). The logic of the lesion experiment and its role in the neural sciences. In S. Finger (Ed.), *Recovery from brain damage. Research and theory* (pp. 4–31). New York: Plenum.

Godschalk, M., Lemon, R. N., and Kuypers, H. G. J. M. (1983). Afferent and efferent connections of the postarcuate region of the monkey cerebral cortex. *Society for Neuroscience, 9* (Part 1), 490 (Abstract).

Grunbaum, A. S. F., and Sherrington, C. S. (1901). Observations on the cerebral cortex of some of the higher apes. *Proceedings of the Royal Society of London* (Series B), *69,* 206–209.

Grunbaum, A. S. F., and Sherrington, C. S. (1904). Observations on the physiology of the cerebral cortex of the anthropoid apes. *Proceedings of the Royal Society of London* (Series B), *72,* 152–155.

Hast, M. H., Fischer, J. M., Wetzel, A. B., and Thompson, V. E. (1974). Cortical motor representation of the laryngeal muscles in *Macaca mulatta. Brain Research, 73,* 229–240.

Hines, M. (1940). Movements elicited from precentral gyrus of adult chimpanzees by stimulation with sine wave currents. *Journal of Neurophysiology, 3,* 442–466.

Hoffman, D. S., and Luschei, E. S. (1980). Responses of monkey precentral cortical cells during a controlled jaw bite task. *Journal of Neurophysiology, 44,* 333–348.

Hore J., Preston, J. B., Durkovic, R. G., and Cheney, P. D. (1976). Responses of cortical neurons (areas 3a and 4) to ramp stretch of hindlimb muscles in the baboon. *Journal of Neurophysiology, 39,* 484–500.

Hubel, D. H. (1959). Single unit activity in the striate cortex of unrestrained cats. *Journal of Physiology, 147,* 226–238.

Humphrey, D. R. (1982). Separate cell systems in the motor cortex of the control of joint movement and of joint stiffness. In P. A. Buser, W. A. Cobb, and T. Okuma (Eds.). *Kyoto Symposia* (EEG Suppl. No. 36) (pp. 393–408). Amsterdam: Elsevier Biomedical Press.

Humphrey, D. R., and Corrie, W. S. (1978). Properties of pyramidal tract neuron system within a functionally defined subregion of primate motor cortex. *Journal of Neurophysiology, 41,* 216–243.

Humphrey, D. R., and Reed, D. J. (1981). Separate cortical systems for the control of joint movement and of joint stiffness. *Society for Neuroscience, 7,* 740 (Abstract).

Humphrey, D. R., and Reed, D. J. (1983). Reciprocal and coarticulation of antagonist muscles. New evidence for separate cortical systems in the control of joint movement and of joint stiffness. In J. Desmedt (Ed.), *Motor control in health and disease.* New York: Raven Press.

Itoh, M., Sasanuma, S., Hirose, H., Yoshioka, H., and Ushijima, T. (1980). Abnormal articulatory dynamics in a patient with apraxia of speech: X-ray microbeam observation. *Brain and Language, 11,* 66–75.

Itoh, M., Sasanuma, S., and Ushijima, T. (1979). Velar movements during speech in a patient with apraxia of speech. *Brain and Language, 7,* 227–238.

Jackson, J. H. (1875). *Clinical and physiological localization of movements in the brain.* (Selected Writings, Vol. 1, pp. 37–76). London: Churchill.

Jasper, H. H. (1958). Recent advances in our understanding of ascending activities of the reticular system. In H. H. Jasper, L. D. Proctor, R. S. Knight, W. C. Noshay, and R. T. Costello (Eds.), *Reticular formation of the brain* (pp. 423–434). Boston: Little, Brown.

Jones, E. G. (1969). Interrelationships of parieto-temporal and frontal cortex in the rhesus monkey. *Brain Research, 13,* 412–415.

Jones, E. G. (1982). Pathways for short latency afferent input to motor cortex in monkeys. In P. A. Buser, W. A. Cobb, and T. Okuma (Eds.), *Kyoto Symposia* (EEG Suppl. No. 36, pp. 367–374). Amsterdam: Elsevier Biomedical Press.

Jones, E. G., Coulter, J. D., and Hendry, S. H. C. (1978). Intracortical connectivity of architectonic fields in the somatic sensory, motor and parietal cortex of monkeys. *Comparative Neurology, 181,* 291–348.

Jones, E. G., and Hartman, B. K. (1978). Recents advances in neuroanatomical methodology. In W. M. Cowan, Z. W. Hall, and E. R. Kandel (Eds.), *Annual review of neuroscience* (pp. 215–296). Palo Alto, CA: Annual Reviews, Inc.

Jürgens, V. (1982). Afferents to the cortical larynx area in the monkey. *Brain Research, 239,* 377–389.

Kelso, J. A. S., Tuller, B., and Fowler, C. (1982). The functional specificity of articulatory control and coordination. *Journal of the Acoustical Society of America, 72,* S103 (Abstract).

Kohlerman, N. J., Gibson, A. R., and Houk, J. C. (1982). Velocity signals related to hand movements recorded from red nucleus neurons in monkeys. *Science, 217,* 857–860.

Kubota, K., and Niki, H. (1971). Precentral cortical unit activity and jaw movement in chronic monkeys. In R. Dubner and Y. Kawamura (Eds.), *Oral-facial sensory and motor mechanisms* (pp. 365–379). New York: Appleton.

Künzle, H. (1976). Bilateral projections from the precentral motor cortex in Macaca fascicularis. *Brain Research, 105,* 253–267.

Künzle, H. (1978). Cortico-cortical efferents of primary motor and somatosensory regions of the cerebral cortex in *Macaca fascicularis. Neuroscience, 3,* 25–39.

Kuypers, H. G. J. M. (1958a). Corticobulbar connections to the pons and lower brainstem in man: An anatomical study. *Brain, 81,* 364–388.

Kuypers, H. G. J. M. (1958b). Some projections from the pericentral cortex to the pons and lower brain stem in monkey and chimpanzee. *Jounal of Comparative Neurology, 110,* 221–256.

Kuypers, H. G. J. M. (1960). Central cortical projections to motor and somato-sensory cell groups (an experimental study in the rhesus monkey). *Brain, 83,* 161–184.

Kuypers, H. G. J. M. (1964). The descending pathways to the spinal cord, their anatomy and function. In J. C. Eccles and J. P. Schade (Eds.), *Progress in brain research, organization of the spinal cord* (Vol. II, pp. 178–200). Amsterdam: Elsevier.

Kuypers, H. G. J. M. (1982). A new look at the organization of the motor system. In H. G. J. M. Kuypers and G. F. Martin (Eds.), *Progress in brain research, Vol. 57: Anatomy of descending pathways to the spinal cord* (pp. 381–403). New York: Elsevier Biomedical Press.

Kuypers, H. G. J. M., and Brinkman, J. (1970). Precentral projections to different parts of the spinal intermediate zone in the rhesus monkey. *Brain Research, 24,* 29–48.

Kuypers, H. G. J. M., and Lawrence, D. G. (1967). Cortical projections to the red nucleus and the brain stem in the rhesus monkey. *Brain Research, 4,* 151–188.

Kwan, H. C., MacKay, W. A., Murphy, J. T., and Wong, Y. C. (1978). Spatial organization of precentral cortex in awake primates. II. Motor outputs. *Journal of Neurophysiology, 41*(5), 1120–1131.

Larson, C. R., Byrd, K. E., Garthwaite, C. R., and Luschei, E. S. (1980). Alterations in the pattern of mastication after ablations of the lateral precentral cortex in rhesus macaques. *Experimental Neurology, 70,* 638–651.

Larson, K. D., and Yumiya, H. (1980). The red nucleus of the monkey. *Experimental Brain Research, 40,* 393–404.

Lashley, K. S., and Clark, G. (1946). The cytoarchitecture of the cerebral cortex of *Ateles:* A critical examination of architectonic studies. *Journal of Comparative Neurology, 85,* 223–306.

Lauer, E. W. (1952). Ipsilateral facial representation in motor cortex of macaque. *Journal of Neurophysiology, 15,* 1–4.

Laurence, S., and Stein, D. G. (1978). Recovery after brain damage and the concept of localization of function. In S. Finger (Ed.), *Recovery from brain damage. Research and theory* (pp. 369–407). New York: Plenum.

Lemon, R. N. (1981). Variety of functional organization within the monkey motor cortex. *Journal of Physiology, 311,* 521–540.

Lemon, R. N., and Porter, R. (1976). Afferent input to movement-related precentral neurones in conscious monkeys. *Proceedings of the Royal Society of London* (Series B), *194,* 313–339.

Lewis, W. B., and Clarke, H. (1878). The cortical lamination of the motor area of the brain. *Proceedings of the Royal Society, 27,* 38–49.

Leyton, A. S. F., and Sherrington, C. S. (1917). Observations on the excitable cortex of the chimpanzee, orang-utan and gorilla. *Quarterly Journal of Experimental Physiology, 11,* 135–222.

Lucier, G. E., Ruegg, D. C., and Wiesendanger, M. (1975). Responses of neurones in motor cortex and in area 3A to controlled stretches of forelimb muscles in *Cebus* monkeys. *Journal of Physiology (London), 251,* 833–853.

Lund, J. P., and Lamarre, Y. (1974). Activity of neurons in the lower precentral cortex during voluntary and rhythmical jaw movements in the monkey. *Experimental Brain Research, 19,* 282–289.

Luschei, E. S., Garthwaite, G. R., and Armstrong, M. E. (1971). Relationship of firing patterns of units in face area of monkey precentral cortex to conditioned jaw movements. *Journal of Neurophysiology, 34,* 552–561.

Luschei, E. S., and Goodwin, G. M. (1975). Role of monkey precentral cortex in control of voluntary jaw movements. *Journal of Neurophysiology, 38,* 146–157.

Malis, L. I., Pribram, K. H., and Kruger, L. (1953). Action potentials in "motor" cortex evoked by peripheral nerve stimulation. *Journal of Neurophysiology, 16,* 161–167.

Marshall, J. F. (1984). Brain function: Neural adaptations and recovery from injury. *Annual Review of Psychology, 35,* 277–308.

McGuinness, E., Siversten, D., and Allman, J. M. (1980). Organization of the face representation in macaque motor cortex. *Journal of Comparative Neurology, 193,* 591–608.

Mohr, J. P. (1976). Broca's area and Broca's aphasia. In H. Whitaker & H. Whitaker (Eds.), *Studies in neurolinguistics* (Vol. 1, pp. 201–236). New York: Academic Press.

Mohr, J. P., Funkenstein, H., Finkelstein, S., Pessin, M., Duncan, G. W., and Davis, K. (1975). Broca's area infarction versus Broca's aphasia. *Neurology, 25,* 349.

Mohr, J. P., Pessin, M. S., Finkelstein, M. D., Funkenstein, S., Duncan, G. W., and Davis, K. R. (1978). Broca aphasia: Pathologic and clinical. *Neurology, 28,* 311–324.

Mott, F. W., Schuster, E., and Sherrington, G. S. (1917). Motor localization in the brain of the gibbon, correlated with a histological examination. *Proceedings of the Royal Society of London, 84B,* 67–74.

Muakkassa, K. F., and Strick, P. L. (1979). Frontal lobe inputs to primate motor cortex: Evidence for four somatotopically organized 'premotor' areas. *Brain Research, 177,* 176–182.

Noback, C. R. (1982). Neurobiological aspects in the phylogenetic acquisition of speech. In E. Armstrong and D. Falk (Eds.), *Primate brain evolution. Methods and concepts* (pp. 279–289). New York: Plenum.

Norrsell, U. (1978). Testing procedures and the interpretation of behavioral data. In S. Finger (Ed.), *Recovery from brain damage. Research and theory* (pp. 199–216). New York: Plenum.

O'Brien, J. H., Pimpaneau, A., and Albe-Fessard, D. (1971). Evoked cortical responses to vagal, laryngeal and facial afferents in monkeys under chloralose anesthesia. *Electroencephalography and Clinical Neurophysiology, 31,* 7–20.

Ojemann, G. A. (1983). Brain organization for language from the perspective of electrical stimulation mapping. *Behavioral and Brain Sciences, 2,* 189–230.

Pandya, D. N., Gold, D., and Berger, T. (1969). Interhemispheric connections of the precentral motor cortex in the rhesus monkey. *Brain Research, 15,* 594–596.

Pandya, D. N., and Kuypers, H. G. J. M. (1969). Cortico-cortical connections in the rhesus monkey. *Brain Research, 13,* 13–36.

Pandya, D. N., and Vignolo, L. A. (1971). Intra- and interhemispheric projections of the precentral, premotor and arcuate areas in the rhesus monkey. *Brain Research, 26,* 217–233.

Penfield, W. R., and Rasmussen, T. (1950). *The cerebral cortex of man.* New York: Macmillan.

Penfield, W., and Roberts, L. (1959). *Speech and brain mechanisms.* Princeton, NJ: Princeton University Press.

Phillips, C. G. (1973). Cortical localization and 'sensorimotor processes' at the 'middle level' in primates—Hughlings Jackson Lecture. *Proceedings of the Royal Society of Medicine, 66* (Section of Neurology), 987–1002.

Phillips, C. G., and Porter, R. (1977). *Corticospinal neurones: Their role in movement.* London: Academic Press.

Rizzolatti, G., Matelli, M., and Pavesi, G. (1980). Neurological deficits following postarcuate lesions in monkeys. *Society for Neuroscience, 6,* 675 (Abstract).

Rizzolatti, G., Scandolara, C., Gentilucci, M., and Camarda, R. (1981). Response properties and behavioral modulation of 'mouth' neurons of the postarcuate cortex (area 6) in macaque monkeys. *Brain Research, 255,* 421–424.

Rizzolatti, G., Scandolara, C., Matelli, M., and Gentilucci, M. (1981). Afferent properties of periarcuate neurons in macaque monkeys. 1. Somatosensory responses. *Behavioral Brain Research, 2,* 125–146.

Roch-LeComs, A., and Lhermitte, A. R. (1976). The 'pure form' of the phonetic disintegration syndrome. *Brain and Language, 3,* 88–113.

Rosén I., and Asanuma, H. (1972). Peripheral afferent inputs to the forelimb area of the monkey motor cortex: Input-output relations. *Experimental Brain Research, 14,* 257–273.

Sakata, H., and Miyamoto, J. (1968). Topographic relationship between the receptive fields of neurons in the motor cortex and the movements elicited by focal stimulation in freely moving cats. *Japanese Journal of Physiology, 18,* 489–507.

Schell, G. R., and Strick, P. L. (1984). The origin of thalamic inputs to the arcuate premotor and supplementary motor areas. *Journal of Neuroscience, 4*(2), 539–560.

Schiff, H. B., Alexander, M. P., Naeser, M. A., and Galaburda, A. M. (1983). *Archives of Neurology, 40,* 720–727.

Sessle, B. J., and Wiesendanger, M. (1982). Structural and functional definition of the motor cortex in the monkey *(Macaca fascicularis). Journal of Physiology, 323,* 245–265.

Shinoda, Y., Zarzecki, P., and Asanuma, H. (1979). Spinal branching of pyramidal tract neurons in the monkey. *Experimental Brain Research, 34,* 59–72.

Sirisko, M., Lucier, G., Wiesendanger, M., and Sessle, B. (1980). Multiple representation of face, jaw, and tongue movements in *Macaca fascicularis* as revealed by cortical microstimulation. *Society for Neuroscience, 6,* 157 (Abstract).

Sirisko, M., and Sessle, B. J. (1981). Intracortical microstimulation and single neurone recording data related to face, jaw, and tongue representations in sensorimotor cortex of *Macaca fascicularis. Society for Neuroscience, 7,* 564 (Abstract).

Sirisko, M., and Sessle, B. J. (1983a). Primate face motor cortex: Representation of ipsilateral and complex orofacial movements. *Society for Neuroscience, 9* (Part 1), 490 (Abstract).

Sirisko, M., and Sessle, B. J. (1983b). Corticobulbar projections and orofacial and muscle afferent inputs of neurons in primate sensorimotor cerebral cortex. *Experimental Neurology, 82,* 716–720.

Strick, P. L. (1976). Anatomical analysis of ventrolateral thalamic input to primate motor cortex. *Journal of Neurophysiology, 39*(5), 1020–1031.

Strick, P. L., and Preston, J. B. (1978a). Multiple representation in the primate motor cortex. *Brain Research, 154,* 366–370.

Strick, P. L., and Preston, J. B. (1978b). Sorting of somatosensory afferent information in primate motor cortex. *Brain Research, 156,* 364–368.

Strick, P. L., and Preston, J. B. (1982a). Two representations of the hand in area 4 of a primate I. Motor output organization. *Journal of Neurophysiology, 48*(1), 139–149.

Strick, P. L., and Preston, J. B. (1982b). Two representations of the hand in area 4 of a primate II. Somatosensory input organization. *Journal of Neurophysiology, 48*(1), 150–158.

Sugar, O., Chusid, J. G., and French, J. D. (1948). A second motor cortex in the monkey *(Macaca mulatta). Journal of Neuropathology and Experimental Neurology, 7,* 182–189.

Sutton, D., Larson, C., and Lindeman, R. C. (1974). Neocortical and limbic lesion effects on primate phonation. *Brain Research, 16,* 61–75.

Tanji, J., and Wise, S. P. (1981). Submodality segregation in the sensorimotor cortex of the unanesthetized monkey. *Journal of Neurophysiology, 45,* 467–481.

Towe, A. L., Patton, H. D., and Kennedy, T. (1963). Properties of the pyramidal system in the cat. *Experimental Neurology, 1963, 8,* 220–238.

or real, associated with a view that at some point in a chain of events underlying speaking, the events cease to be cognitive and representational and become motor instead.

One problem, of course, is the deep philosophical puzzle of how mental and physical events are related (or of whether it is even sensible to address the puzzle couched in this way [Ryle, 1949]). Largely, this difficulty is handled in language and speech production models by a kind of sleight of hand. The final stage in the model of language production in Figure 6-1 and an intermediate stage in the model of speech production is a bridging stage, in which "motor commands" are sent out to the vocal tract. Proposing this bridging stage is a sleight-of-hand maneuver because, whereas "commands" are things that arise in the mental or cognitive domain, the presumed recipients of the commands, motoneurons or muscles, exist in the physical realm. In other usages, motoneurons and muscles are not seen as the kinds of things that obey commands; rather, they respond to release of transmitter substances. The kinds of things that can obey commands are sentient, sapient beings. Therefore, the concept of motor command (or the like) is a metaphor for which there may or may not exist a real-world interpretation.

There are other, less abstruse difficulties with the practice of assuming without study that control of speaking involves a sequence of cognitive–representational events followed by a sequence of motor events. For example, researchers have not typically asked explicitly which issues and which phenomena require explanation in cognitive or linguistic terms and which require explanation in motor process terms. One consequence of neglecting careful consideration of these questions is that some issues and phenomena may be addressed and given incompatible accounts in both realms and others may be left aside. The large number of hypothetical processing stages underlying speaking that emerge from an attempt to interface extant models of speech and language production (as in Figure 6-1) suggests that there may indeed be some redundancy with respect to the production events for which each presumed phase takes responsibility. Other events or issues may be neglected. For example, the second global stage in MacKay's model is the domain of the phonological system. The model is laid out as if this stage stands in a hierarchical relation both to the conceptual stage and the motor stage. That is, it appears as if relatively large units of the syntactic structure of a sentence (clauses, words) are *partitioned* into relatively smaller phonological units (syllables, syllable constituents, phonological segments, land features) that in turn are partitioned into constituent motor commands. But this layout is somewhat misleading. In fact, the units of the "metrical structure" of an utterance are not just syllable constituents and syllables, but in addition are stress feet (e.g., Liberman and Prince, 1977) and possibly "prosodic words, " phonological phrases, and intonational phrases as well (e.g., Selkirk, 1980a, b). These structures emerge as relevant and necessary to attempts to capture systematic differences in the relative prominence of syllables in an utterance and also, perhaps, to rationalize talkers' pausing patterns in speech (Gee and Grosjean, 1983). The metrical structures are not *constituents* of syntactic units. Rather, syllables, stress feet, phonological phrases, and intonational phrases are similar in size, respectively, to morphemes, words, syntactic phrases, and clauses, but they may be different in domain. For example, the utterance "Omaha Nabraska" consists lexically of two words, but metrically of three stress feet, "Ohma," "haNe," and "braska," which violate the lexical structure of the utterance. Instead of standing in a subordinate—superordinate relationship to syntactic units, then, metrical structures appear to relate to syntactic units as one perspective on a Necker cube relates to the other. That is, they emerge from different perspectives on approximately the same grain-size of analysis of the language. (It may still be the case, however, as MacKay intends, that, in a sequence of events preceding articulation, a talker's specification of the phonological [and metrical] structure of an utterance is temporally later than his or her specification of the syntactic structure.)

Metrical structures apparently stand in a closer relation to articulatory performance than do syntactic units. Whereas syntactic units are preserved in written language productions, metrical structures need not be and frequently are not. The metrical structures, then, may have their rationale—and they need one from production theorists—in special characteristics or strategies of the articulatory system that are required when it confronts the task of realizing the syntactic units of language.

The many puzzles to which the existence of these structures gives rise have largely been neglected. Linguists have attempted to capture their systematic properties (Liberman and Prince, 1977; Prince, 1983; Selkirk, 1980a); however, their function in utterance production is unknown. If syntactic units indeed are "packaged" into metrical structures before (or at the same time as) speech is produced, there must be reasons why they are. However, metrical structures have no discernible role in MacKay's model and they do not appear in Perkell's. Something important is missing from the models—possibly because of the meager attention devoted to issues surrounding the relationship between the representational–cognitive and motor aspects of speech.

There is a final problematic consequence of dividing the labor of studying spoken language along the lines cognitive and motor. In particular, the partitioning might exacerbate the difficulty of integrating the domains of speech production if such an attempt were to be made. Because the units

Tower, S. S. (1940). Pyramidal lesion in the monkey. *Brain, 63,* 36–90.

Tracey, D. J., Asanuma, C., Jones, E. G., and Porter, R. (1980). Thalamic relay to motor cortex: Afferent pathways from brain stem, cerebellum, and spinal cord in monkeys. *Journal of Neurophysiology, 44*(3), 532–554.

Travis, A. M., and Woolsey, C. N. (1956). Motor performance of monkeys after bilateral partial and total cerebral decortication *American Journal of Physical Medicine, 35,* 273–310.

Vogt, C., and Vogt, O. (1919). Allgemeine ergebnisse unserer Hirnforschung. *Journal of Psychology and Neurology, 25,* 277–462.

Walker. A. E., and Green, H. D. (1938). Electrical excitability of the motor face area: A comparative study in primates. *Journal of Neurophysiology, 1,* 152–165.

Walshe, F. M. R. (1935). On the "syndrome of the premotor cortex" (Fulton) and the definition of the terms "premotor" and "motor": With consideration of Jackson's views on the cortical representation of movements. *Brain, 58,* 49–80.

Watson, C. (1975). *The role of precentral gyrus in the control of facial movement in Macaca mulatta.* Unpublished doctoral dissertation, University of Chicago.

Welt, C. (1962). *Topographical organization of somatic sensory and motor areas of the cerebral cortex of the gibbon (Hylobates) and chimpanzee (PAN).* Unpublished doctoral dissertation, University of Chicago.

Welt, C., Abbs, J. H., and Gracco, V. L. (1984). Unpublished observations.

Wiesendanger, M. (1973). Input from muscle and cutaneous nerves of the hand and forearm to neurones of the precentral gyrus of baboons and monkeys. *Journal of Physiology (London), 228,* 203–219.

Wiesendanger, M. (1981). Organization of secondary motor areas of cerebral cortex. In V. B. Brooks (Ed.), *Handbook of physiology, Section 1* (Vol. II: Motor Control, Part 2, pp. 1121–1147). Bethesda, MD: American Physiological Society.

Wiesendanger, M., Seguin, J. J.. and Künzle, H. (1973). The supplementary motor area—A control system for posture. In R. B. Stein, K. C. Pearson, R. S. Smith, and J. B. Redford (Eds.), *Control of posture and locomotion* (pp. 331–346). New York: Plenum.

Wise, S. P. (1984). Non-primary motor cortex and its role in the cerebral control of movement. In *Dynamic aspects of neocortical function,* G. Edelman, W. M. Cowan, and E. Gall (Eds.), Neurosciences Institute. New York: John Wiley and Sons.

Wise, S. P., and Tanji, J. (1981). Supplementary and precentral motor cortex: Contrast in responsiveness to peripheral input in the hindlimb area of the unanesthetized monkey. *Journal of Comparative Neurology, 195,* 433–451.

Wolf, G., Stricker, E. M., and Zigmond, M. J. (1978). Brain lesions: Induction, analysis, and the problem of recovery of function. In S. Finger (Ed.), *Recovery from brain damage. Research and theory* (pp. 91–112). New York: Plenum.

Wong, Y. C., Kwan, H. C., MacKay, W. A., and Murphy, J. T. (1978). Spatial organization of precentral cortex in awake primates. I. Somatosensory inputs. *Journal of Neurophysiology, 41*(5), 1107–1119.

Woolsey, C. N. (1958). Organization of somatic sensory and motor areas of the cerebral cortex. In H. F. Harlow and C. N. Woolsey (Eds.), *Biological and biochemical bases of behavior* (pp. 63–81). Madison, WI: The University of Wisconsin Press.

Woolsey, C. N., Settlage, P. H., Meyer, D. R., Sencer, W., Hamuy, T., Pinto, T., and Travis, A. M. (1951). Patterns of localization in precentral and "supplementary" motor areas and their relation to the concept of a premotor area. *Association for Research in Nervous and Mental Disease, 30* (Chapter XII), 238–264.

Zealear, D. L., and Hast, M. H. (1982). The organization of the primary motor cortex controlling larynx tongue, jaw, and face in the monkey. *Society for Neuroscience, 8,* 411 (Abstract).

Zimmermann, G. (1980). Stuttering: A disorder of movement. *Journal of Speech and Hearing Research, 23,* 122–126.

CHAPTER 6

Current Perspectives on Language and Speech Production: A Critical Overview

Carol A. Fowler

Speech presents two quite distinct aspects to the researcher. On the one hand, it is a linguistic communication consisting of symbols combined by grammatical rules. On the other hand, it is a complex motor skill in which activities of the respiratory system, the larynx, and the supralaryngeal vocal tract are coordinated at several temporal scales.

These different aspects of speech invite theorizing of distinct types. When linguists, psycholinguists, and cognitive psychologists study speech in its linguistic–representational aspect, they focus on language as a "mental" or cognitive capability and attempt to discover and formalize private representational correlates of articulatory performance. When phoneticians, speech scientists, and students of motor performance study speech, they focus on its physical manifestations and ask how the primitive units of a linguistic description can be realized as coordinated gestures of the vocal tract.

Perhaps because the labor of studying speech is divided in this way, we know very little about the relationships between its two aspects. An assumption reflected in many models of language production (used here to mean putative private mental events occurring prior to and during actual speech utterance) and of speech production (used here to refer to aspects of motor control during speaking) is that the different aspects constitute different *phases* in a speech event; in particular, the output of the representational component serves as the input to the motor component. Indeed, in some instances, models of language production and of speech production appear to dovetail relatively well because the one model leaves off where the other begins.

An example is provided in Figure 6-1. Figure 6-1*a* and *b* are adaptations of recently proposed models of language production (MacKay,

Figure 6–1. Recent models of language production (MacKay, 1982) and speech production (Perkell, 1980).

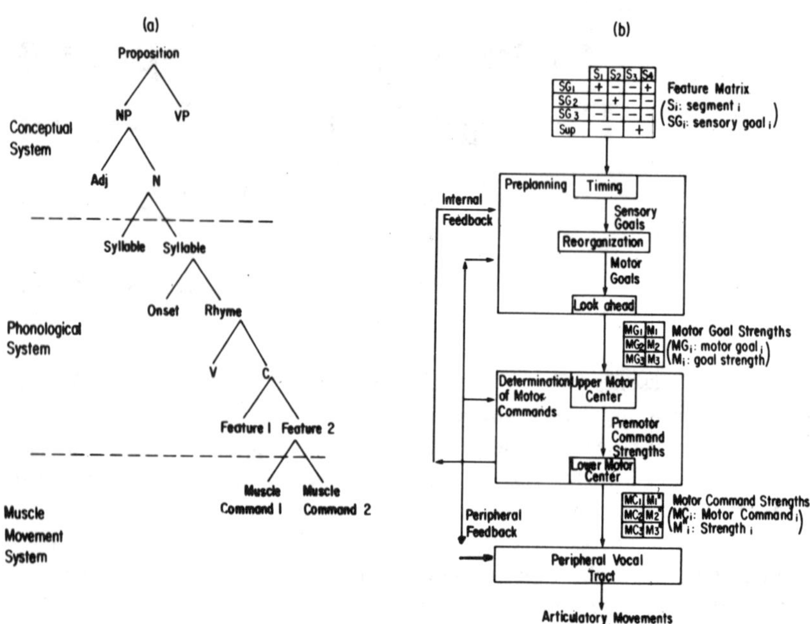

1982) and of speech production (Perkell, 1980). MacKay's model posits three global stages in utterance production: a conceptual stage in which ideas are realized as a grammatical sequence of words, a phonological stage in which words are realized as sequences of phonetic feature specifications for individual phonological constituents of a word, and a motor stage in which feature specifications become motor commands. In contrast, Perkell's model begins with feature specifications and details hypothetical events intervening between those specifications and movements of vocal tract structures. His model also has three global stages, consisting of a preplanning stage, a stage in which motor commands are determined, and one in which movements are produced. Together, then, the two models outline five or six global stages in the process of utterance production. At least the first three of these, and perhaps more, occur in the representational–cognitive phase of language production; the last necessarily is motor.

The assumption that the representational and motor aspects of speech relate sequentially as they do in these models is largely unexamined and should not be accepted uncritically. There are several problems, apparent of articulation do seem different in some ways from those of language viewed as a representational system, investigators in the representational domain feel free to ignore research on articulation. For example, according to Dell (1980), "What we know of production comes from a rather unique source of data—speech errors or slips of the tongue" (p. 1). Similarly, some investigators in the speech production realm are tempted to ignore the units of language's representational aspect. For example, MacNeilage and Ladefoged (1976) recognize, among speech production researchers,

> an increasing realization of the inappropriateness of conceptualizing the dynamic processes of articulation itself in terms of discrete, static, context-free linguistic categories, such as "phoneme" and "distinctive feature." This development does not mean that these linguistic categories should be abandoned as there is considerable evidence for their behavioral reality (Fromkin, 1971). Instead, it seems to require that they be recognized, even more than before, as too abstract to characterize the actual behavior of articulators themselves. They are, therefore, at present better confined to primarily characterizing earlier premotor stages of the production process, as revealed by speech errors, and to reflecting regularities at the message level (Fant, 1962) of the structure of language, such as those noted by phonologists. (p. 90)

Yet it is clear that the separation between the representational and motor aspects of language is not entirely clean. First, as already noted, some of the systematic properties of the phonologies of language—in particular, their metrical structures—apparently must have, at least in part, a rationale in articulatory terms. Second, other aspects of the phonologies of language—the popularity of certain "natural" rule types (Donegan and Stampe, 1979), the segment inventories of languages (Lindblom, 1971), and aspects of their diachronic changes (Ohala, 1981)—reflect fairly clearly the fundamental bond between language, the vocal tract, and the ear. Languages evolved to be spoken and heard. On the other side, the character of speech as a motor skill is affected by the fact that articulation realizes a language. To a large extent, the sequencing of articulatory events in speech is dictated by the language's grammar. A special property of grammars is that the constraints on symbol combination that they impose are arbitrary with respect to vocal tract movement capabilities. (That is, for example, the vocal tract has no preference for subject-verb-object orderings.) Perhaps this arbitrariness explains why ordering errors are so common in speech but are relatively rare in activities in which the sequencing of events is not arbitrary from the perspective of the implementing system. So, for example, we never mistakenly attempt to inhale twice without exhaling in between; and, while walking, we never inadvertently take two steps with our left foot without taking one with the right foot in between. There is, clearly, a serial ordering problem in talking that is diminished in activities in which "cognitive" choices are limited (Dell, 1980).

In the present chapter, some recent accounts of language production are reviewed, followed by some of the evidence and proposals concerning regulation of speech production. The review is intended to make two major points in itself and to serve as the basis for speculation concerning the relationships between language and speech.

One major point to make clear is that when proposals concerning the "mental processing" involved in language and speech production are gathered together, and the talker's many hypothesized processing representations are examined, they loom impossibly large. This is perhaps already evident in Figure 6–1a and b, but the model becomes even more outsized when proposals concerning processing to achieve durational patterns, pausing patterns, and intonation in language production and to achieve durational patterns in speech prooduction are added to the models. Future theoretical efforts will need to be directed toward collapsing and categorizing these different sources of evidence and toward minimizing rather than proliferating hypothetical processing stages.

A second major point, already alluded to, is that despite the size that any integrated model of language and speech would take, it would fail to provide an understanding of the role of speech in language. A realistic model of language production will have to provide that understanding.

LANGUAGE PRODUCTION

In this chapter, issues surrounding the pragmatics of conversation are left aside to focus narrowly on those issues surrounding the production of an utterance by a talker who has already selected its content. That is, only at models that begin more or less where MacKay's model begins are discussed.

An adequate theory of language production, restricting itself to this limited domain, would have to address a variety of issues and account for certain performance measures.

Issues

Two central concerns for language production theories are considered. One is to characterize and explain the capabilities to which linguistic competence gives rise. The other is to rationalize language's multiple levels and kinds of structure.

Capabilities of a Language User. Communications by humans need not, although they can, express emotional states; likewise, they need not, but can, refer to ongoing events. That they need not either express emotional states or refer to events in the here and now probably sets them off from nonlinguistic communications by other species and follows from a great evolutionary discovery of language: the use of rules and representations that are largely conventional in nature, and wholly conventional in function, and that thereby realize a separation at once of function and form and form and substance in language.

The rules and representations of language are conventional in two senses. First, they are largely arbitrary both with respect to the physical system that realizes them (here, the talker, and in particular, his or her vocal tract) and with respect to their significations. This frees utterances from serving only as *signs* either of internal or of external states of affairs. Second, the rules and representations of language are conventional in that they are shared by a linguistic community. Because they are shared, a language user can count on his or her communication being understood even though it consists of symbols rather than signs and of orderings of symbols that are "frozen accidents" (Pattee, 1973).

Two other salient capabilities of language users are those of producing and understanding utterances they have never heard spoken. To theorists, this generativity in language use implies two underpinnings. First, language is "rule governed"; second, spoken utterances are planned. Knowing the rules of a system allows a participant to generate any and only legal instances in the system. However, using the rules of a system—in particular, using the grammatical rules of a language—requires planning. In speech, a plan has to span the domain of a rule, which may be several words in extent. Explaining generativity and planning are central concerns of a theory of language production.

Levels of structure in speech. Another concern of language production theories is to rationalize language's multiple structural aspects. First, as Hockett (1960) has pointed out, languages have "duality of patterning." They consist of meaningless segments and rules for their combination. One reason for duality of patterning in language is fairly uncontroversial. Providing sentences with an internal structure of words makes the class of sentences that can be uttered and understood open rather than closed. Similarly, providing the primitive meaningful units of language—words or morphemes—with an internal structure opens up the lexicon of a language. Were each word or morpheme a unique utterance without internal structure, we would, perhaps, soon run out of words we could coin and remember.

A different perspective on the multiplicity of structured aspects to language has already been alluded to and becomes salient when the interface between language and speech production is contemplated. Languages consist of units that participate in rules for creating sentences and they consist of other units that do not. Units of the first type—phonological segments, morphemes, words, syntactic phrases, and clauses—tend to exist in all human language systems, spoken and signed, and they tend be preserved in derivative writing systems. Units of the second type—syllable constituents, syllables, stress feet, and possibly larger metrical units—apparently do not exist in sign and are not, largely, preserved in writing systems.

Performance Measures

In addition to the issues just considered, the literature offers several performance measures for a theory of language to address. Oldest, and perhaps most productive of research, are speech errors. Errors of spontaneous language production have long been viewed as providing a window to the mind behind an utterance (Freud, 1958; Merringer and Meyer, 1895). Recently, spontaneous error collections have been supplemented by experimentally induced errors (e.g., Baars, 1980; Dell, 1980; Kupin, 1979) and by simulations of error-producing language systems (Dell, 1980), and researchers have begun seeing the whole array of errors as providing a window, specifically, to the cognitive–representational aspects of utterance production.

Similarly, pausing by talkers (or segmental lengthening) has recently been used as an index of planning (Cooper and Paccia-Cooper, 1980) or execution (Gee and Grosjean, 1983) in production. Measures of fundamental frequency declination (Breckenridge, 1977; Cooper and Sorenson, 1981) apparently provide compatible, or even redundant, information.

Two final performance measures used to study language production are less detectable in spontaneously produced speech than in experimentally provoked utterances. They are latency to begin producing a planned utterance and utterance duration. These measures vary in systematic and interesting ways with certain structural properties of an utterance (Sternberg, Monsell, Knoll, and Wright, 1978) and with practice (MacKay, 1982) and are used as the basis for inferences about speech planning and execution.

Models of Language Production

Models of language production, or more loosely, proposals concerning its underpinnings, suffer somewhat from narrowness of scope. With few exceptions, they have been based largely on the patterning of just one dependent measure. The measure for many researchers is speech errors, for others it is pausing, and for a few, utterance latency and duration. This chapter is organized, therefore, primarily around the different dependent measures and secondarily around model types.

Speech Errors

Logic. An utterance contains a speech error if its producer agrees that it deviates from his or her intended utterance. Excluded from consideration, therefore, are productions that other listeners would consider deviant but that conform to what the talker meant to utter.

To a degree, the strategy for drawing inferences from speech errors is similar to that suggested by the Russian theorist and physiologist Bernstein (1967). Bernstein suggested that the design character of an unknown system can be determined by discovering what classes of tasks the system accomplishes with equal ease and what classes it accomplishes with difficulty or not at all. For example, with a compass it is possible to draw circles of many radii with equal ease, but an ellipse or a rectangle only with difficulty; a compass is designed for drawing circles.

The logic behind studying speech errors is similar in part. By discovering the conditions under which errors occur frequently, researchers learn something of the hidden workings of the system behind the verbal output. For example, phonological segments frequently are anticipated, perseverated, or exchanged as in Examples 1 to 3 below. (The errors reported here are either from a small corpus of the author's, or, where noted, from published examples.)

1. tree lined lane—tree laned
2. sore shoulder—sore soulder
3. face painted—pace fainted

Two striking properties of these errors are that the source and destination contexts of the migrating segment or segments are phonologically very similar, and interacting segments themselves are phonologically similar. In Example 1, for instance, the vowel /ey/ occurs in the context /1/—/n/ in both the source and the destination word. Similarly, in Example 2, the segment /s/ occurs in the context #—V in both the source and the destination word. In Example 3, not only are the contexts similar from which and to which the exchanging segments move, but also the exchanging segments themselves are similar. Both /f/ and /p/ are voiceless, labial consonants.

These are well-documented characteristics of sound errors, and presumably they reveal that, for the job of ordering phonological segments, similar segments—particularly in similar contexts—make the ordering job difficult. A model of production that includes an ordering mechanism, then, will have to incorporate a like fallibility.

Examples 1 to 3 are seen as providing evidence not only about the processes underlying utterance production, but also about the structures on which the processes work. That phonological segments move frequently in errors implicates them as discrete units in language production. Indeed, speech errors may provide the strongest behavioral evidence currently available that phonological segments (at some, as yet undetermined, level of abstraction) are "psychologically real."

The errors above also provide information about the "window" of speech on which processes work when phonological segments are being ordered. Anticipation errors indicate that the window extends beyond a word in which segments are being selected or ordered. Perseveration errors indicate that the window also extends backward in articulatory time. According to Garrett's findings (1980a), in approximately 87% of exchange errors the window extends to, but not across, a phrase (e.g., noun phrase [NP] or verb phrase [VP]) boundary. Thus, the range over which speech elements can interact may provide information about the domain of a speech plan.

However, these inferences have to be drawn cautiously. The evidence provided by Garrett's percentages are not taken to signal the window size of *the* speech plan. Different kinds of errors may have different domains, and based on this and other evidence, investigators have tended to posit a variety of plans in utterance production, each with its own window and its own job to perform in constructing an utterance.

Speech errors sometimes suggest inferences about orderings of events in utterance production. In Example 4 (from Garrett, 1980a), a third person singular morpheme shifts from one word to another. (This shift is classified as a morpheme shift rather than a phonological segment shift because word-final segments that are morphemes are vastly overrepresented in word-final segment shifts.)

4. It certainly runs out fast—ran outs fast
                                     /s/

In shifting, the phonological realization of the morpheme accommodates to its new context. Whereas the third person singular morpheme would be realized /z/ in "runs," it is realized as /s/ in "outs." This is interpreted by Garrett and others as revealing that the error occurred prior to a stage of language production in which the phonetic form of morphemes is determined.

Garrett (1980a) proposes two additional guidelines for drawing inferences from speech errors. These take the form of plausible assumptions that reduce the ambiguity associated with drawing inferences. One assumption is that if two elements interact in an error they are elements of the same descriptive type. The second is that the set of conditions underlying the occurrence of a particular kind of error will always be conditions of just one descriptive type.

A final assumption made by error collectors is that, despite being labeled "slips of the tongue," speech errors occur "in the head," not "in the mouth." That is, they are errors of language production, not of speech production. Evidence for this view is that speech errors of approximately the same types and in approximately the same proportions are reported by subjects engaging in internal speech as by subjects talking aloud (Dell, 1980). Additionally, Baars, Motley, and MacKay (1975) elicit slips of the tongue by inducing subjects to develop covert and competing utterance plans and then requiring them to select one plan under time pressure. For example, subjects see and prepare to say one at a time the sequence of word pairs: Ball Doze, Bash Door, Bean Deck, and Bell Dark. The sequence of B—D— items leads subjects to expect another. If, instead, Darn Bore is presented for rapid production, subjects often produce Barn Door erroneously.

The Data. This section presents only as much information as is necessary to motivate the language production models described below. More comprehensive reviews are available in a variety of sources (Dell, 1980; Fromkin, 1980; Garrett, 1980a; Shattuck-Hufnagel, 1979; Stemberger, 1982; see also Cutler, 1982).

Most of the errors made by talkers can be classified as one of the following types: anticipation, perseveration, exchange, substitution, addition, deletion, or shift. The first three error types were illustrated in Examples 1 to 3 for sound errors. Examples 5 to 8 illustrate the remaining error types, also for sound errors.

    5. collect them—correct them   (substitution)
    6. back burner—black burner   (addition)
    7. painstaking—paintaking   (deletion)
    8. slept soundly—sept sloundly   (shift)

Elements of speech that move in errors most commonly are phonological segments, clusters, morphemes, and words. Most researchers agree that errors involving feature movements are rare (but see Stemberger, 1982).

Errors in which syllables move also occur, but they are rare. However, syllables and other metrical structures are involved in the specification of the conditions in which errors—especially sound errors—will occur, and of the ways in which the errors will manifest themselves. For example, consonants that move in an error almost always preserve their original location either before or after a vowel in a syllable. (In addition, vowels interact only with vowels and consonants with consonants.) So, for instance, Examples 9 and 10 (from Garrett) are common error types. Errors such as Example 11 (from Shattuck-Hufnagel, 1979) are rare.

9. Do you know where I can get a clear piece—clear pliece
10. It happened in the first, second, third, and fourth—thirth and fourth
11. Trees—stree

Similarly, interacting sounds tend to occur in metrically similar environments. That is, for the most part stressed segments interact with stressed segments and unstressed segments with unstressed segments. Finally, interacting segments tend to be members of the same phonemic clause (Garrett, 1980a).

Metrical structures do not appear to play a similar role in word or morpheme errors. It is true that, in some cases, the environments for two exchanging words are metrically quite similar (from Garrett, 1980a):

12. You should see the one I kept pinned to the door of my room—to the room of my door

In other cases, however, they are not similar and indeed, the stress patterns and syllable compositions of interacting words may be quite different (from Garrett, 1980a):

13. I left the cigar in my briefcase—I left the briefcase in my cigar
14. Fancy getting your nose remodeled—Fancy getting your model renosed

Words involved in errors do tend to share stress level; that is, a stressed word does not normally exchange with an unstressed word. However, that observation may be a consequence of the confounding of stress level with classification of words as "content" and "function" words.

A major condition on whole-word exchanges is that the interacting words are members of the same grammatical class. This occurs 85% of the time according to Garrett's corpus. Word exchanges tend to occur over longer stretches of speech than sound exchanges. Moreover, in contrast to sound errors, they need not be phonologically very similar or to occur in similar contexts (but see Dell and Reich, 1981, for a qualification).

Garrett, Shattuck-Hufnagel

Garrett (1975, 1980a,b) proposes a fundamental separation in processing type during language production between a "functional" and a "positional" level.

At the functional level, words are selected and their grammatical roles and phrasal memberships are determined. At this level, the phonetic forms of words are unspecified and hence, if an error occurs, it will be unaffected by the phonetic properties of a word. Errors will tend to be substitutions of words or word blends, for example, or exchanges, anticipations, or perseverations of words in which the interactions are among words of the same grammatical form class.

At the positional level, the words selected and organized at the functional level are inserted into a structural frame in which affixes and function words are specified. Stress levels are also part of the structural frame. Errors may occur if lexical items are inserted incorrectly into the frame as in "stranding" errors (from Garrett, 1980b):

15. I went to get a check cashed—cash checked

Alternatively, inflectional affixes may get attached to the wrong content word (from Garrett, 1980b):

16. I'd forgotten about that—I'd forgot abouten that

Notably, errors of both types appear to freely produce ungrammatical forms such as "abouten." The processes appear blind to information about form class or lexicality.

They are not blind to information about phonological realizations of inflections and stems, however. Example 4 reveals that shifts of inflections lead to phonological accommodation.

Sound errors may occur at the positional level. And they may also show accommodation (from Kenstowicz and Kisseberth, 1979):

17. Tail spin ([t^{h}eyl spIn])—pail stin ([p^{h}eyl stIn])

This implies a stage subsequent to the positional level in which the phonetic forms of ordered phonologically specified words are selected. Garrett (1975) includes such a stage in his model followed by one in which instructions to articulators are specified.

An interesting property of Garrett's proposal is its sharp separation of content and frame in sentence production. This separation is an attractive property of the model because it suggests that language production explicitly uses the "great evolutionary discovery" referred to earlier.

This theme is elaborated by Shattuck-Hufnagel (1979). Somewhat in contrast to Garrett's approach, she emphasizes the similarities in the error types characteristic of different linguistic units, especially phonological segments, morphemes, and words. She suggests that because they all participate in the same five basic error types (exchanges, substitutions, additions, omissions, and shifts), "the most parsimonious model...is one in which a single underlying mechanism accounts for all error types across all [types of linguistic units that participate in the error types]" (p. 303). The reason the errors may manifest themselves in somewhat different ways across the different linguistic units—for example, the reason sound errors have phonologically similar source and destination contexts, but word errors do not—is because the mechanism operates at different *levels* of the sentence representation when words and sounds are being ordered and hence it utilizes different information.

The mechanism Shattuck-Hufnagel has in mind incorporates a version of the distinction between functional and positional representations as proposed by Garrett. She lists five linguistic units that participate in the basic error types. They are features, phonological segments, morphemes, words, and sentence constituents. However, apparently, she does not intend that five levels of representation be assumed independently to undergo the serial ordering processes leading to error. In particular, there is some indication (Shattuck-Hufnagel, 1979, p. 313) that, in her view, the morpheme and word levels are not distinct. In any case, at each relevant level of representation, two independent representations of the utterance-to-be are generated. One includes the "content"—that is, the selected linguistic units—the other includes the frame into which they are to be inserted. At the word level, the frame corresponds more or less to Garrett's positional level. At the phonological level, the frame is provided by sequences of canonical syllable structures into which target phonological segments will be inserted.

Insertion of content into frame is achieved by a "scan copier" that selects each appropriate target unit from the content representation and inserted it into its slot in the frame. Two monitors watch over this process. One checks off target segments once they have been selected to prevent their reselection later to fit a similar slot. A second scans the final product for errors.

Justification for separation of content from frame derives most convincingly from exchange errors such as Example 3 above. In these errors, quite remarkably, not only does a segment (/p/ in the example) appear early in a slot similar to its intended slot, but, in addition, the replaced segment (/f/ in the example) shows up in the slot left "empty" by migration of the first segment. In this way, the structure of the utterance is unaffected by the error. Two segments simply changed places. For this to occur requires that the structure of the utterance be, in some way, detachable from the particular segments that realize it.

Shattuck-Hufnagel justifies the two monitors based on occurrence and nonoccurrence of various error types. First, exchange errors suggest a monitor that marks the anticipated segment (the /p/ in Example 3), as already selected, thereby preventing it from occupying its intended slot. If the monitor fails, the error is an anticipation.

The second proposed monitor scans the result of the scan-copy process looking for errors. It may weed out phonotactically improper sequences (for example, word-initial /tl/), or sometimes it may wrongly weed out sequences that look like the kind of error the scan-copy mechanism would make. For example (from Shattuck-Hufnagel, 1979),

18. That would be behaving—That would be having

Here an apparent perseveration may have been "corrected" by an error monitor.

Activation Models

The speech error literature offers a different kind of model from those of Garrett and Shattuck-Hufnagel. Versions offered recently by Dell and Reich (Dell 1980; Dell and Reich, 1980, 1981) and by Stemberger (1982), differ in one (Stemberger) or two (Dell) major ways from the proposals of Garrett and Shattuck-Hufnagel. First, they adopt an old, but currently popular, associationist approach to characterizing mental events. In these modern forms of association theory, a knowledge system (a lexicon, for example), is instantiated as a network of associated "nodes" (see also MacKay [1982], whose model is depicted in part, in Figure 6–1a). In a lexicon, a node may be a concept, a word, a phoneme, or a letter (see, for example, McClelland and Rumelhart, 1981). A node may be activated in comprehension if it is activated directly or indirectly by stimulus input. It may be activated in production if it is associated directly or indirectly with concepts the talker intends to convey. Activation spreads from a "primed" node to any others to which it is associated, and the selection of a word as present in stimulus input or as one to be uttered is based on the relative activation levels of word nodes. "Spreading activation" models instantiate a small number of very general and simple processing assumptions. In relation to the processes discussed by Garrett or Shattuck-Hufnagel (for example, Shattuck-Hufnagel's error monitor), the fundamental processes in these models are low level, lack intelligence, and are very powerful.

Dell's model differs from those of Garrett and Shattuck-Hufnagel not only in respect to its psychological processing assumptions, but also in respect to the linguistic theory that it instantiates. Dell noted the compatibility between the spreading-activation models being developed in psychology and relational-network theories of language (Lamb, 1966; Lockwood, 1972; Reich, 1970). In Sampson's view (1980), relational-network theory is the "most interesting radical alternative on the contemporary linguistic scene to Chomsky's theory of language" (p. 167).

In a review of the theory, Sampson offers the serious criticism that it apparently cannot handle structure-dependent syntactic processes (that is, processes, such as those involved in relative-clause formation, that depend on the whole structure of a sentence). However, in his view, it is "much more plausible than its rivals as a model of how speakers and hearers actually operate" (p. 177). This is because, in the theory, the speaker-hearer's linguistic competence *is* the means by which he or she both produces and understands sentences. This contrasts favorably with Chomsky's theory in which a grammar enumerates sentences of the language and cannot serve by itself as the means by which sentences are either said or understood. Rather, the grammar is held to be a component in a performance model, whose implementation by performance mechanisms is unspecified.

In relational-network theory, linguistic knowledge consists of two tiered components: a realization network and a set of tactic patterns. The realization network realizes the units of the language—its concepts, words, phonemes, and so forth—essentially as convergences of relations. Figure 6–2a, borrowed from Sampson (1980), makes clear this aspect of the theory. The word "under" is nothing other or more than the convergence of a set of concepts (including "lower than"), an ordered sequence of phonemes, and a form class membership enforced by the tactic pattern (see below). Figure 6–2b is meant to show that the label "under" for the word node is redundant with the set of relationships and need not be represented in the model; the convergence of relations *is* the word.

The second component is a network of tiered tactic patterns. The tactic patterns express the internal relations among units at a particular level of the language. For example, the pattern in Figure 6–3 (also from Sampson, 1980) is counterpart to the phrase–structure rules of a generative grammar; it is part of a system that expresses possible sequences of words in a sentence.

Units in the tactic patterns are connected to their counterparts in the realization network. The realization network, then, captures what the linguistic units *are* (content) and the tactics, the structures in which they can participate (frame).

Let us consider how Dell's model marries spreading-activation models and relational-network theory to create a model of language production that makes natural errors.

Figure 6–2. Fragments of a realization network adapted from Sampson, 1980.

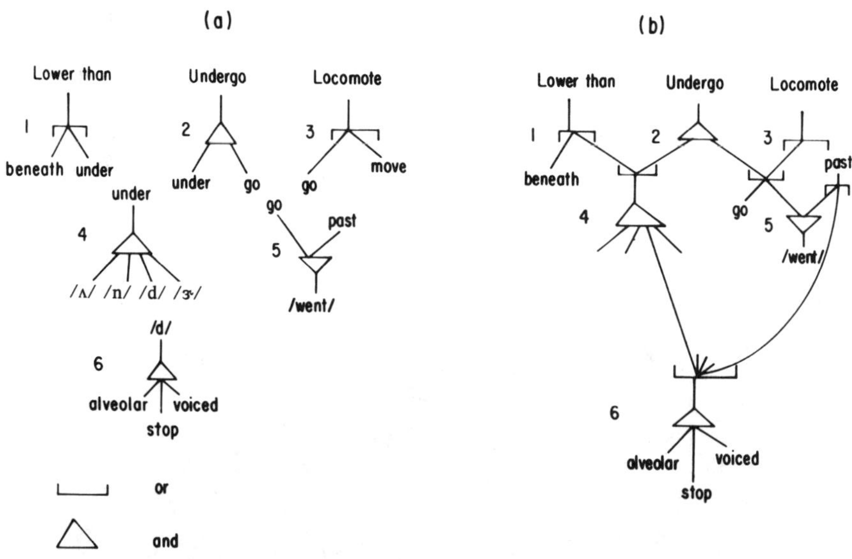

Figure 6–4 (from Dell, 1980) depicts a piece of a realization network. In the network, words are convergences of relations between concepts, phonemes, and tactic patterns. An unusual property of the network is the coding of phonological segments by syllable position. That is, in the model, word-final /t/ in "cat" is a different segment from word-initial /t/ in "tan." As we will see, this property of the network ensures that slipping sounds will retain their intended position within a syllable.

Dell is primarily interested in the patterning of sound errors, and hence, has developed his model largely with reference to utterance realization at the sound level. Sounds are selected for utterance when they are activated in the realization network and selected by the tactic pattern at the sound level, called the "phonotactic selection mechanism."

Dell has realized his model of production as a computer simulation. In Dell's model, a word to be uttered receives some activation; words following it are activated somewhat less. Some proportion of the initial activation then spreads from the word nodes to the concept and phonological segment nodes to which the words are related in the network. In turn, these newly activated nodes send some proportion of their activation to nodes to which they are connected, including the originally activated words themselves.

Figure 6–3. A fragment of a tactic pattern adapted from Sampson, 1980.

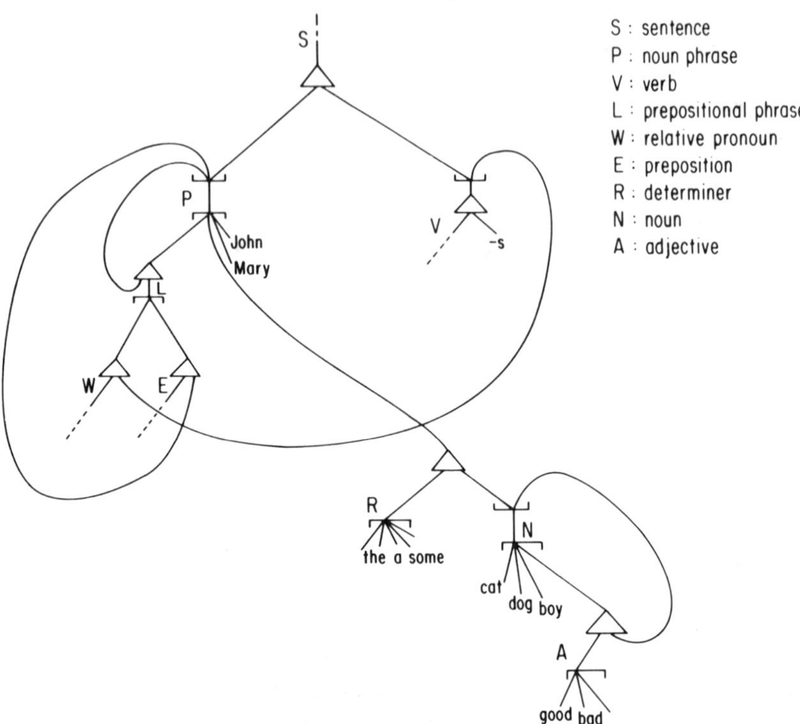

In this way, activation spreads unevenly through the lexicon, with positive feedback relationships being established between nodes of the originally activated words. Periodically, activation decays to some proportion of its current level. This prevents the eventual activation of every node in the lexicon.

The phonotactic selection mechanism allows activation to spread for some period of time. Then it selects the most highly activated of the initial consonants, or it selects more than one highly activated initial consonant if the consonants are phonotactically compatible. The phonotactics order the segments if more than one is selected. For example, if both /t/ and /s/ are activated in prevocalic position, the phonotactics prescribe the ordering /st/ if the language is English. Next, the phonotactic selection mechanism selects the most highly activated vowel and, last, the most highly activated final consonant or consonants. Once a segment has been selected, its activation level in the network is set to zero. However, because its word node is still activated, it is gradually reactivated.

Figure 6–4. A realization network from Dell's (1980) model of language production.

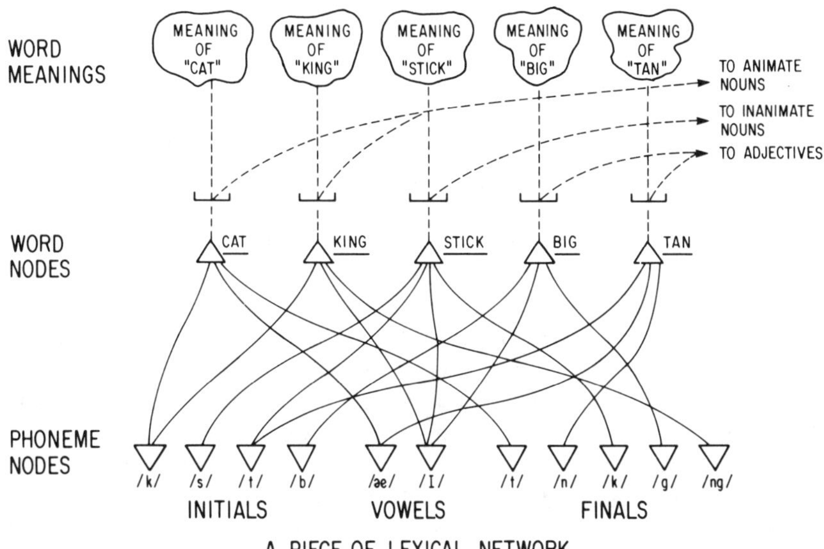

An error occurs if a target segment is not the most highly activated at the time at which selection occurs. This may occur for a variety of reasons. Consider, for example, the error in Example 1 noted earlier. When "lined" is activated, "lane" will get a lesser degree of activation at the same time. "Lined" will activate its component phonemes, two of which, syllable-initial /1/ and postvocalic /n/, are shared with "lane." These phonemes, substantially activated by "lined," will send activation both to "lined" and to "lane." In turn, "lane" will activate its component phonemes. Because of the similarity between "lined" and "lane," as the one grows in activation level, so does the other. Therefore, /ey/ in "lane" will receive more activation than it would in the context of a word less similar to "lane" than is "lined." The existence of words in the lexicon with word-initial /ley/ (for example, "late") or with the rhyme /eyn/ ("mane") will be activated by the corresponding phonemes in "lined" and "lane" and will further boost the activation level of "lane." This pattern of activation, possibly enhanced by noise in the system that boosts the activation level of words at random, may cause /ey/ to be more highly activated than /ay/ when the phonotactic selection mechanism chooses the syllable's vowel. If /ey/ is erroneously selected, its activation level will be set to zero, thereby promoting the occurrence of an exchange error. However, /ey/ will continue to be activated because postvocalic /n/ is activated and because the syntactic selection mechanism will select "lane" as the next word to be said. Whether /ay/ or /ey/ is selected for the vowel in "lane" depends on their relative activation levels when the phonotactic selection device chooses a vowel for "lane." If /ay/ is selected, the error is an exchange; if /ey/ is selected, it is an anticipation.

Dell's model reproduces many of the salient characteristics of sound errors. It produces anticipations, perseverations, and exchanges. The erroneously produced segments preserve their position in the syllable because they are coded for syllable position in the lexicon and the phonotactics select only among segments in the appropriate syllable position. Finally, errors are more likely when the source and destination contexts are similar. The simulation not only produces these error types, but, with appropriate settings of the parameters, it produces them in the relative proportions that they occur in spontaneous-error corpora.

Additionally, the model allows a number of novel predictions, some of which have been tested and confirmed. For example, it predicts a lexical bias in sound errors—that is, a tendency for sound errors to produce real words in the language. In the model, the lexical bias occurs because of the positive feedback relationship that is established between word and segment nodes. If a sequence of phonological segments constitutes a word, then the word will be activated by all of the segments and in turn will activate all of them. A sequence of segments that does not constitute a word has no superordinate node to reinforce it and to be itself reinforced by the sequence. A lexical bias occurs in Dell's simulation. It also occurs in experimentally elicited errors (Baars, 1980) and in corpora of spontaneously produced errors (Dell, 1980; Dell and Reich, 1981). Although other investigators (Fromkin 1973; Garrett 1976) have commented on the large number of nonwords generated by sound errors, analyses by Dell of their corpora as well as his own reveal that words are generated disproportionately. This is not expected in Garrett's model unless it is supplemented by an explicit error monitor, similar to one proposed by Shattuck-Hufnagel, which turns nonwords in the speech plan to words. An elegant feature of Dell's model is that it provides the monitoring function without a homunculus.

In common with Wickelgren's proposals (1969, 1976), Dell's simulation permits the prediction that phonemes shared by neighboring words in a planned utterance will promote errors. In Wickelgren's view, this "repeated phonemes" effect occurs because segments are context sensitive. That is, the /ey/ in "lane" is represented as $_l\text{ey}_n$ and /l/ and /n/ as $\#l_\text{ey}$ and $_\text{ey}n\#$. Errors occur when a serial ordering mechanism attaches a segment to a context that is compatible or partially compatible with its context specifications, but is not the intended context. This serial ordering procedure implies that only segments adjacent to repeated phonemes will slip. Dell's model, however, implies that segments repeated across neighboring words will promote slippage by any other segments in either word. Dell confirmed this prediction in an analysis of spontaneous errors.

Dell has not simulated selection of words by syntactic processes. However, he points out one counterintuitive prediction that such a simulation would provide. Because of the nature of the lexical realization network, not only will sound errors be lexically biased, but in addition word errors will be disproportionately phonologically similar. Phonological similarity between target and error has been noted for one type of word error—namely, malapropisms (e.g., "equivocal" for "equivalent" from Fay and Cutler, 1977), and these have been ascribed to selection errors from a lexicon organized by sound rather than meaning (Fay and Cutler, 1977). However, Dell's model allows the prediction of disproportionate phonological similarity in all word errors including blends (e.g., "class," "course"—"clourse"), so-called meaning errors (e.g., "knee" for "elbow") and even word misorderings within a sentence. Dell has confirmed this in an analysis of word errors in his spontaneous-error corpus.

Commentary

Speech errors probably constitute the richest source of evidence available concerning language production. Not the least of their advantages is that they can be studied both "in the world" and in the laboratory.

Perhaps because the error data are abundant and, in some respects, clear in their patterning, some conclusions can be drawn from the patterns with confidence. These conclusions are common largely to the two model types just described. Both model types capture the distinction between form and function that lies at the heart of language. Similarly, both treat the units of the linguistic message as distinct from their carriers, the syllables of the language. Finally, the models explicitly realize language's duality of patterning by keeping the different levels of structure and the different ordering processes separate.

Both model types also treat the tiered units of a linguistic message as hierarchically organized. Moreover, in these models, speech planning consists of temporally successive phases which respect the hierarachy. Large units are selected and ordered before their realizations as smaller units are determined. The evidence for this notion of speech planning over time is compelling, too. When a talker produces errors such as those in Examples

19 and 20 (from Garrett [1980b]), it is difficult to avoid concluding that two ordered events conspired to generate the error:

19. I don't know that I'd know one if I heard it—I'd hear one if I knew it

20. Even the best teams lost—Even the best team losts.

$$/s/$$

In Example 19, the two words, both verbs, are exchanged. One, "hear," apparently has stranded its tense marker. That marker, attached to "know," is not realized phonologically as /d/ as it would have been in the intended utterance. Rather, remarkably, it is realized as the correct, irregular, past tense of "know." The two ordered events, then, are misordering of words of the same form class and then, *later,* selection of the phonological form of the past tense morpheme.

In Example 20 (see also Example 4 earlier), a morpheme shifts and, in shifting, acquires a new phonological realization. This shift implies two ordered events also, one of which, however, is distinct from the stages inferred in Example 19. When words shift across clauses, as in Example 19, the exchanging words generally share form class. Therefore, when affixes are stranded, they are reattached to a word that can take that affix in some form. In Example 20, however, a bound plural morpheme shifts from a noun to a verb. Verbs do not take the plural {-S} morpheme, and in any case, "lost" can never take any affix realized as an /s/. Despite that, the affix does undergo the voicing assimilation characteristic of the plural morpheme. That is, the plural morpheme, realized as /z/ in "teams" became /s/ in "lost." Two ordered processes are implied here, too, then, and only the second of them may coincide with the two interred from Example 19. In Example 20, a morpheme shifts as if it were blind to form class, and then a phonological voicing assimilation process occurs. One could even argue for four ordered stages based on the errors in Examples 19 and 20. The plural morpheme could not be realized "correctly" as /s/ until "lose" + past (see "know" + past = "knew" in Example 19) became "lost." Hence four ordered events in Examples 19 and 20 are as follows: functional-level word exchange, as in Example 19; past tense realization— still sensitive to lexicality—as in Example 19; affix shift, blind to lexicality and form class, as in Example 20; voicing assimilation of plural morpheme as in Example 20. These kinds of errors strongly imply that speech planning involves some planning events that feed others.

Other properties of the models are less compelling and less attractive. Although appropriately they are models of language production and not of speech errors, nonetheless they have some properties that seem motivated only by the requirement that error patterns be reproduced. Two examples stand out. First, syllables have no role in the models. It is true that Shattuck-Hufnagel has the ordered phonemes of a lexical form read into canonical syllable slots in an output buffer. However, it is not apparent what function the syllable structures serve except to ensure that sound errors will preserve their syllable position. For its part, Dell's model has no syllables at all, but only segments in the lexicon marked for syllable position. This approach is likely to be incorrect for a variety of reasons. First, it fails to motivate the syllabic coding of segments in the first place. Second, it suggests no closer connection for a language user between the /t/ in "tap" and that in "pat" than between the /t/ in "tap" and the /1/ in "pal." Yet alphabetical writing systems in which both versions of /t/ are written with the same letter suggest a close connection. Perhaps from the perspective of the language researcher, it is the speech production theorist's job to motivate the role of syllable structures in speech.

A second feature of both models also seems unmotivated except as a means to generate appropriate error patterns. In both models, words—which are, in part, ordered sequences of segments—are selected and ordered at one stage of the planning process. Even though this should, by implication, order the segments to be produced, in both models a later stage selects and orders the segments of each selected word. As Shattuck-Hufnagel points out, this is difficult to motivate, but it seems necessary to generate sound-ordering errors.

Such an ordered sequence of selections may seem more natural in a spreading activation network in which it takes time to get from a word node to a segment node. However, it would seem that the naturalness is spurious. In relational-network theory a word is nothing other than a convergence of relations between phonological form, form class membership, and semantic usages in the language. The word "node" is just the point of convergence; it is not a thing in itself. Therefore, it still makes little sense to select a word and *then* its component phonemes; the word is, in part, its phonemes. Conceivably, the ordering is not in respect to selection of units of various sizes, but rather in respect to the talker's attention to units of various sizes.

Duration, Pausing, Coarticulation, f₀: Introduction

The literature on errors supports some fairly strong conclusions concerning language production. In particular, it supports a view of language as a tiered structure, apparently constructed over time by sequences of processes each sensitive to linguistic structures at the level on which it is working but relatively blind to those on other tiers.

In this next section, additional theoretical proposals and models of language production are reviewed. These new proposals have been based on a collection of measures other than speech errors. The measures—pausing, segment and word duration, coarticulation and its blocking, and fundamental frequency—provide mutually redundant information and hence are grouped in the review.

For a variety of reasons, proposals concerning language production based on the patterning of these measures are difficult to integrate with those based on speech errors. For one thing, they are proposals of different types than those based on speech errors. Where researchers in the field of speech errors have built models of fallible language production rather than of speech errors per se, researchers studying duration, pausing, and the other measures under review here have modeled the measures themselves. To the extent that they succeed, the models (called "algorithms" by their creators) generate the natural patterning of the measures in an utterance. However, they provide little insight into the means of their generation (or, for that matter, of the wherefores of their generation).

A second difficulty in integrating the findings and proposals based on these new measures with those from the literature on speech errors is that the findings appear to disagree at least with the tenor of those latter proposals. In contrast to the models of Garrett and Dell, in which phonological processes are relatively blind to the syntactic structure of an utterance, the algorithms that generate pausing, duration patterns, and so on, are strongly sensitive to it. Yet these are measures of language *performance* and presumably reflect processes occurring no earlier than those in which the phonological structure of a sentence is realized.

First an overview of the findings based on these measures is provided, then how they may be viewed in relation to theorizing based on speech errors and on the latency measures, which are reviewed next, are discussed.

Duration, Pausing and Coarticulation Blocking: Cooper and Paccia-Cooper and Gee and Grosjean

The basic findings from studies of language production are straightforward (Cooper and Paccia-Cooper, 1980; Gee and Grosjean, 1983). Other things being equal, the duration of a word (or of its final segments), the probability of pausing after a word, the duration of any pause that may occur, and the probability that perseveratory coarticulation will be blocked across the word boundary are all correlated with the "strength" of the boundary following the word. In Cooper and Paccia-Cooper's view, boundary strength is determined by syntactic structure. In Figure 6-5, "leaves" and "Sue" border a major boundary; "will" and "resign" flank a minor boundary. Hence "leaves" is more likely to exhibit

Figure 6–5. A tree-structure representation of a sentence, indicating differences among interword boundaries in "boundary strength" (adapted from Cooper & Paccia-Cooper, 1980).

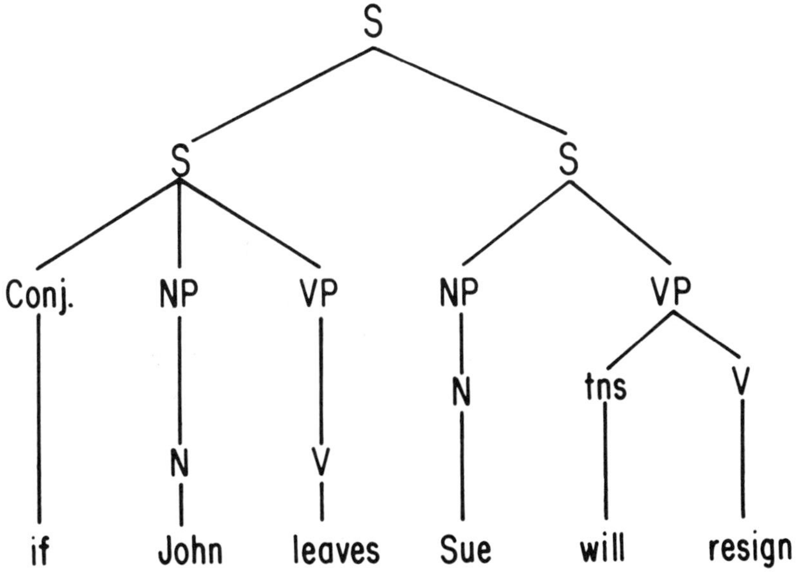

word-final lengthening, a following pause, and blockage of perseveratory coarticulation than is "will."

Measures of pausing and of durational lengthening appear to be quite sensitive to syntactic structure, distinguishing, for example, the two readings of Example 23, at least among readers who are aware of the ambiguity:

23. Lieutenant Baker instructed the troop with a handicap.

The durations of "troop" and of the pause following it are both longer if Lieutenant Baker has a handicap than if the troop has one. This difference between the sentences in duration and pausing mirrors a difference in their syntactic structures, as revealed in Figure 6–6 (from Cooper and Paccia-Cooper, 1980). When the troop is handicapped, "with a handicap" bears a closer syntactic relationship to "troop" than if Lieutenant Baker has the handicap.

In long sentences, the patterning of durational differences and of pauses becomes extremely rich, yet still predictable. Table 6–1 gives most of the steps in an algorithm proposed by Cooper and Paccia-Cooper to reproduce the lengthening and pause structure of sentences.

Figure 6–6. Two readings of an ambiguous sentence represented as differences in phrase-structure representation (adapted from Cooper & Paccia-Cooper, 1980).

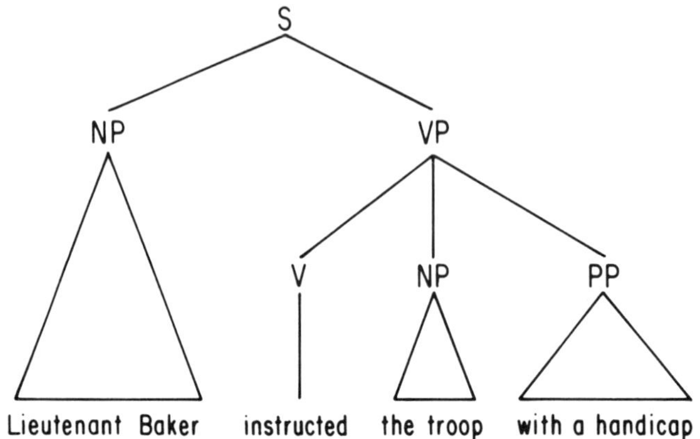

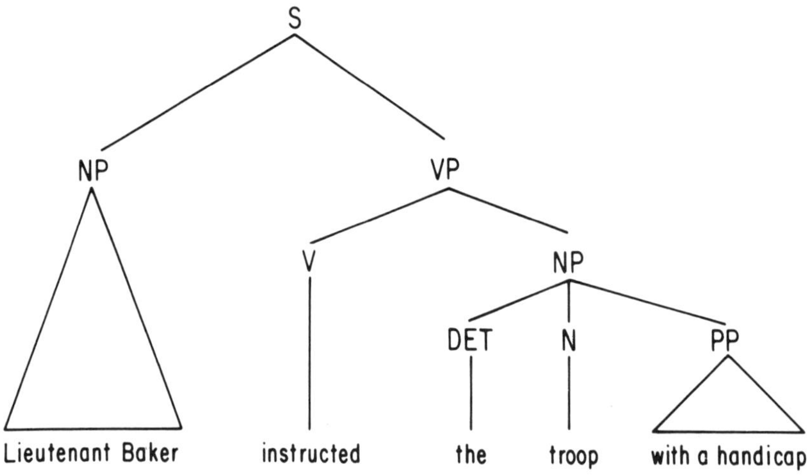

Cooper and Paccia-Cooper point out that they devised the algorithm to generate the patterning of the dependent measures in their experiments and not to mimic, necessarily, the means of its generation by talkers. Indeed, the algorithm has several properties that eliminate it as a candidate

Table 6-1.
Algorithm for Determining Pause Durations.

1. For each critical boundary in a tree-structure representation of a sentence, locate the dominating phrase-structure nodes. These are the highest nodes that do not dominate both the words flanking the critical boundary, but that dominate one or the other.

2. Count the nodes between the nodes just identified and those immediately dominating the words flanking the critical boundary. Discount nodes referring to conjunctions, determiners, and nonlexical prepositions and, on the left side of the boundary, any nonbranching, nonterminal nodes.

3. Increment the count for any branching S node.

4. Multiply by 2 the count for the left side of the boundary.

5. Sum the counts for the two sides of the boundary.

6. Bisection (from Grosjean et al., 1979). Count the number of major grammatical words in the largest constituent being analyzed. Divide by 2. Count the number of major category words from either end of the constituent to the boundary (whichever is less). Divide by the bisection point.

7. Multiply the outputs of steps 5 and 6 for each word boundary. The largest product identifies the major constituent break. Any such boundary retains its product.

8. If the two constituents demarcated by the major break found in the last step contain more than seven major category words, repeat steps 6 and 7.

9. Constituent length—if the largest constituent boundary precedes or follows a constituent including seven or more words belonging to major grammatical classes, add or subtract a percentage amount to the output of the last step for that boundary.

10. Other steps adjust for speaking rate or other prosodic effects.

Adapted from Cooper, W., and Pascia-Cooper, J. (1980). *Speech and syntax.* Cambridge, MA: Harvard University Press.

psychological model of language production. First, the tree structure for an entire sentence is involved in computing measures of word duration, probability of pausing and pause duration, and probability that coarticulation will be blocked at a boundary. Yet is highly implausible that this amount of detail is available before the first word of a sentence is uttered. Second, the algorithm itself is complicated enough to render it implausible that talkers would run through all of the steps before producing an utterance. Third, the algorithm implies that word duration and segment duration are explicitly computed. Yet a large part of the complexity of the algorithm that computes these durations concerns reproducing the complex microstructure of the durational patterns the talker's rationale for which, if any, is obscure. In particular, the full complexity of the durational patterns probably is unappreciated by listeners. Listeners may well hear and use the durational lengthening and pausing at major boundaries, but they are not likely to use, or even to hear, many of the finer aspects of the timing pattern. Nor do the steps in the algorithm typically have an obvious rationale in terms of production. For example, why are left nodes of the tree multiplied by 2? Why do sentences have a bisection point? In short, it is not clear why talkers would bother with the steps of the algorithm if reproducing the microstructure of the durational pattern were an end in itself as the algorithm suggests.

These considerations make clear that, although the algorithm may work to generate the timing pattern of a sentence (in fact, however, it accounts for only 56% of the variance in sentence pauses examined by Gee and Grosjean, 1983), at best it fails to reveal the source and rationale for the pattern, and, at worst, it may obscure it.

Gee and Grosjean (1983) propose a new model designed to overcome the shortcomings of the Cooper and Paccia-Cooper model and similar shortcomings of an earlier model by Grosjean, Grosjean, and Lane (1979). They suggest that two general factors govern the durational structure of a sentence: its syntactic structure and the distinction between content and function words. The latter distinction they see as having two relevent aspects: the different information contents of the two types of words and their different stress levels in production. They suggest, then, that syntactic structure, information load, and stress level all contribute to the durational pattern of a sentence.

To generate the durational patterns of sentences in ways sensitive to the syntactic, informational, and stress patterns of the language, Gee and Grosjean borrowed from the growing literature on prosodic (or metrical) structures in language (Liberman and Prince, 1977; Selkirk, 1980a, b). This literature attempts to characterize and reveal the metrical patterns of language—in particular, the patternings of strong and weak segments and syllables in spoken language. The literature provides perhaps the strongest evidence that sentences have metrical structures—syllables, feet, phonological phrases, and intonation phrases—that are distinct from syntactic units, but are sensitive to them.

Gee and Grosjean use the metrical structures with the largest domain—phonological and intonational phrases—to generate durational patterns in fluent speech. Their algorithm moves left to right through an utterance's surface structure, and determines durational patterns of early sentence constitutents in the absence of a fully specified surface structure for the sentence. In the algorithm, words up to and including the head of syntactic phrase constitue a phonological phrase and are organized together metrically (see also Selkirk, 1980b). Consequently, pausing boundaries within a phonological phrase will be minor boundaries; those across a phonological phrase are more important. Phonolqgical phrases themselves are organized into intonational phrases subject to a few contraints. Two phonological phrases subsumed by the same syntactic phrase (excepting VPs) are organized into a common intonational phrase. A phonological phrase headed by a verb is organized with the following phonological phrase unless the preceding one is less complex. Remaining phonological and intonation phrases are organized left to right in the sentence.

With certain adjustments (for example, nonlexical weak monosyllables are not counted as being followed by a boundary, complex words are flanked by relatively longer pauses than their metrical location would suggest, and sentence-final words are lengthened) this new algorithm can account for 92% of the variance in the pausing data collected by Grosjean. Moreover, it has the advantage over earlier models that it works left to right.

Commentary

There remain three major difficulties with this account of durational lengthening and pausing. It does not explain how the metrical structure gets realized as durational lengthening and pausing. The idea that word and phrase durations are computed and assigned is unattractive because the task of computing and realizing the values would be a big job with no apparent purpose. A more attractive proposal, in my view, would be one in which the metrical structure characterizes some relatively "low-level" organization of the talker's vocal tract achieved to realize the surface structure of the sentence in speech. But we are still far from understanding how such a motor organization would allow or facilitate utterance production.

A related difficulty is that the proposal provides no real insight into why the surface structure of a sentence is realized as a metrical structure. According to Selkirk (1980b):

> [T]his review of prosodic structure has shown quite clearly that prosodic structure is not syntactic structure, nor is it isomorphic to it. The two are quite distinct as formal objects. A mapping from one to the other can, and must, be defined, however, for the prosodic structure reflects syntactic structure in certain ways. We would suggest that the mapping from syntactic to phonological representation of a generative grammar is precisely this mapping—the mapping between syntactic and prosodic structure.
>
> Thinking now in terms of speech production and perception, we would hypothesize that the units of prosodic structure we have discussed here in linguistic terms are indeed the appropriate units in production and perception models, that the effect of syntactic phrasing in reproduction, or access to that phrasing in perception, are crucially mediated by these units of the prosodic hierarchy. (p.29)

But this is not entirely satisfactory. Why cannot a surface structure be produced without introducing metrical structure? Again, perhaps, the rationale may have to be provided by speech production theories.

A final difficulty with the algorithm of durational lengthening and pausing proposed by Gee and Grosjean has been alluded to earlier. It concerns any attempt to integrate the model with those of language production motivated by analyses of speech errors. Why, if the metrical structure is part of the phonological representation of an utterance, as it is presumed to be (for example, in the quotation from Selkirk just cited), is it sensitive to the syntactic structure of a sentence, whereas errors at the phonological level of utterance production (and even "earlier" at Garrett's positional level) are not?

The problem probably cannot be resolved by supposing that the metrical structure is not part of the phonological system and that instead sentence constituents are organized into larger metrical structures early in sentence production—say, at Garrett's functional level of processing. As observed earlier, word exchanges often are not metrically similar. (That is, they differ in number of syllables, as in Example 14, or in stress pattern, as in Example 13.) A careful analysis, analogous to Dell's , revealing lexical bias in sound errors and phonological bias in word errors would possibly reveal a metrical bias in word errors. However, Dell would not expect this because it would signify that metrical structures are embedded somehow in the realization network. Yet if the apparent absence of metrical effects at the word level localizes metrical structures within the phonological phase of sentence production, we are left without an understanding of why they, and not sound errors, are so sensitive to syntactic structure.

Fundamental Frequency

The fundamental frequency (f_0) contour in a speech utterance constitutes a rich source of information for a listener. It provides information about the sex, age, height, and weight (e.g., Lass and Davis, 1976) of a talker and about his or her emotional state (Sherer, 1981, 1982; Tarttar, 1980; Williams and Stevens, 1972). In addition, it provides at least two sources of linguistic information. The global intonation contour distinguishes questions, statements, commands, and more one from the other. In addition, the intonation contour is superimposed on a gradual downdrift in fundamental frequency ("declination") that extends over the course of a major syntactic unit (often a sentence). The downdrift in f_0, then, delimits major syntactic units in an utterance for a sensitive listener.

A theory of language production will have to explain how talkers provide all of the foregoing information in the f_0 contour that is controlled.

So far, however, only the last source of information—f_0 downdrift—has been studied with a view to explaining its regulation. Consequently only declination will be covered in this review.

Declination. Utterances show f_0 peaks and troughs. The peaks correspond largely to prominent syllables in the utterance, and the troughs to less prominent syllables. A curve drawn peak to peak (the "topline" of the declination curve) tends to be negatively accelerated, but linear on a log-linear plot of frequency and time (Cohen, Collier, and t'Hart, 1982). One drawn trough to trough (the "bottomline") is linear with a negative slope. Declination refers to either or both downdrifting tendencies.

Languages typically (but perhaps not universally; see Cooper and Sorenson, 1981, for a brief review) exhibit downdrift. The most studied languages, however, are Dutch (Cohen et al., 1982, and references therein), English (Breckenridge, 1977; Cooper and Sorenson, 1981) and Swedish, (Garding, 1979). In these languages, the fundamental frequency at sentence offset is nearly invariant, while the starting frequency may (Cooper and Sorenson, 1981; Cohen et al., 1982) or may not (Maeda, 1976; Breckenridge, 1977) covary with sentence duration. In any case, the slope of the declination lines decrease with an increase in sentence duration.

Although some investigators have proposed physiological accounts of declination (see Breckenridge for a review), the most comprehensive investigation to date on declination in English (Cooper and Sorenson, 1981) follows conclusions by Breckenridge that the declination topline does not automatically "fall out" of the respiratory and laryngeal events underlying sentence production; rather, it is "programmed" by a talker. Sorenson and Cooper (1980; see also Cooper and Sorenson, 1981) model the declination topline mathematically by fitting a line segment to all f_0 peaks except the first, which lies above the fitted line. The line has the folllowing form (where P_i is the ith f_0 peak; T_i is its time of occurrence relative to sentence onset, and P_n and T_n refer to the final peak and its time of occurrence, respectively):

$$F_0 = P_n + 2/3\,(P_i - P_n/T_i - T_n) \bullet (t - T_n)$$

Using this equation for a line, the "topline rule," an investigator or talker can determine f_0 for a peak occurring at any time "t" in the utterance. The declination curve has as its domain a sentence, or, if it is sufficiently long, a major clause.

Sorenson and Cooper propose that the talker uses the topline rule in the following way:

> How does the speaker program an f_0 declination in fluent speech?...At the beginning of an utterance, the speaker's look-ahead mechanism informs him

> of approximate sentence length, which is somehow used to generate the appropriate f_0 value of the first peak. The approximate value of the last peak is also known to the speaker as evidenced by its constancy across sentences of different length.... Once the speaker begins talking, feedback (auditory or otherwise) informs him of the value of the first peak, which together with the value of the last peak and approximate estimated sentence duration can be used to generate the Topline Rule. The speaker then endeavors to produce those peak values of f_0 based on the rule. (p. 419)

The declination line typically is "reset" at the end of a sentence. However, it may be partially reset at the end of a sentence-internal major clause. In addition, finer marking of syntactic boundaries, compatible with the markings by pausing and word lengthening, is achieved by "fall-rise" patterns—that is, a fall in f_0 at the end of a syntactic unit and a rise at the beginning of the next. These fall-rise patterns do not seem to affect the declination lines and therefore are not identified as resetting.

Commentary. The topline rule and Sorenson and Cooper's proposed psychological implementation of it obviously will generate an f_0 contour that drifts downward over the course of an utterance in approximately the same fashion that the topline drifts downward. It is implausible, however, as a psychological procedure (see also Simon, 1980). In particular, it is another example similar to that of the pausing algorithms in which theorists account for aspects of the superficial form of an utterance by proposing a mechanism to reproduce the aspects explicitly. In essence, the account is that speech exhibits declination in the form that it takes because talkers put it there in that form. But it is not always justified to infer that a particular variable is explicitly controlled in a skilled activity just because it has regular properties, and it may not be wise to assume explicit control as a first hypothesis. Some variables exhibiting regular properties are not the kinds of things that actors *can* regulate. That is, some regularities are not regulated at all. They are in a sense "emergent" in the activity (Kugler, Kelso, and Turvey, 1980), or they are byproducts of other things that the actor is doing. On the surface, the declination lines themselves suggest an account of this sort. As already noted, the vast majority of languages show declination. Moreover, across tone languages, falling tones are more frequent than rising tones. Similarly, (untrained) singers can achieve a fall in f_0 more quickly than a rise (Sundberg, 1979). This suggests that downdrifts are relatively easy and natural to achieve—perhaps because speech is produced on an expiratory airflow. As lung volume decreases, other things equal, subglottal pressure will decrease and f_0 will decline.

Why, then, propose a computational model of declination as Sorenson and Cooper do? There are three reasons. First, it has been argued (Breckenridge, 1977) that physiological accounts cannot handle the magnitude of declination that occurs. These arguments have recently been disputed, however (Cohen et al., 1982). Second, Breckenridge and Sorenson and Cooper appear to assume that declination must be *either* physiologically determined *or* linguistically determined, but cannot have both characteristics. However, declination may be a candidate instance where the form of a linguistic device is explainable in physiological terms (and without reference to linguistic terms), but the deployment of the device, and hence its function, is linguistic.

Alternatively, perhaps even the deployment of declination itself is an automatic more than a "programmed" behavior. In the previous section, research by Gee and Grosjean was described that suggests that speech is packaged for output into metrical rather than syntactic structures. Research has not yet been designed to ask whether these structures rather than syntactic units per se are in fact also the domain of f_0 declination. However, as Cooper and Sorenson point out, a comparison of the pausing data in Cooper and Paccia-Cooper and the f_0 data in Cooper and Sorenson reveals a degree of redundancy in the patterning of major pause boundaries and declination resetting or f_0 fall–rise patterns. This implies that whatever structures, syntactic or metrical, best characterize the packaging of speech involved in generation of pausing patterns, these same structures will characterize that over which f_0 patterns occur. If so, conceivably, declination is not, largely, a contour that a talker programs over a grammatically coherent stretch of speech. It may be a difficult-to-avoid consequence of uttering speech, packaged into metrical structures, and produced on an expiratory airflow.

A third, and perhaps, the main reason why Sorenson and Cooper propose a computational model for declination is that, as a general rule, computational models are the only kinds of models that cognitive psychologists, including psycholinguists, entertain to explain phenomena that they find interesting. The concomitant disinclination to consider accounts whereby the regularities are not explicitly programmed has, possibly, promoted the explosion of variables under review here, which language production theorists, collectively, propose are under programming control.

Latency and Duration

The last model to be considered in this review of language production (Sternberg, Monsell, Knoll, and Wright, 1978; Sternberg, Wright, Knoll, and Monsell, 1980) is distinguished from its predecessors on several counts. First, it is in fact a model of word-string production, not of language production, in that it makes no attempt to explain how grammatical utterances are constructed. Rather it begins with a planned string of words to be produced and it is concerned with their retrieval from a hypothetical output buffer and their execution. (This model in fact might have been included below in the review of speech production theories because it largely concerns itself with execution of a "motor program." It is included here because its explanatory concepts are in the cognitive–representational domain, in contrast, largely, with explanatory concepts invoked by speech production theorists.) Second, the data underlying the model's construction are obtained from utterances that are not naturally produced. Rather, the utterances are produced with as brief a latency as possible after a signal to begin talking and at as fast a rate as possible. This manipulation is meant to force the characters of the retrieval and execution processes to reveal themselves in the durational measures as the processes operate at their upper limits.

In the procedure used by Sternberg and colleagues (1978, 1980), talkers are given an utterance to say. Across trials, the utterances may differ in length (in number of words) or in complexity (in syllables per word or in heterogeneity among words). They are always well-known word strings; they might be the digits from 1 to 3, for example or the five weekdays, or the word "Monday" repeated four times. The talker knows what he or she is to say well in advance of the cue to respond. The cue, then, only signals *when* the talker is to begin talking. The talker is instructed to say the sequence as quickly as possible following the cue to respond. Sternberg and co-workers measure the latency to begin talking and utterance duration, both as a function of sequence length.

The latency and duration data exhibit regular changes with sequence length. In particular, latency is a linear function of utterance length (in number of words), with a slope between 10 and 15 ms. Utterance duration is an accelerating function of length; that is, as utterance length increases, the average word-to-word interval increases. The latency function loses its regularity at utterance lengths of six or more words. Complexity of the words produced (whether the words are monosyllables or disyllables, for example) affects the intercept of the latency function, but not its slope. Comparable words and nonwords have identical latency and duration functions.

Sternberg and associates propose a model of word retrieval and execution to explain these data. In the model, an output buffer for speech holds the motor program for a to-be-produced utterance. Because words and nonwords generate the same latency and duration functions, the buffer is not presumed to have any special connection to the lexicon of the language. The motor program consists of subprograms, one for each production unit in the utterance. To produce an utterance, each unit is retrieved in turn; following retrieval it is "unpacked" into its constituent articulatory units (perhaps syllables or individual articulatory gestures), and finally a command phase executes the unpacked unit.

Latency to begin talking is presumed to include the retrieval and unpacking times for the first unit in the utterance. (The execution interval is supposed to start with vocal tract movement onset.) Latency increases with utterance length because retrieval of a unit is more time consuming the more items there are in the buffer. (This implies that the first thing to be produced does not occupy a slot in the buffer that is first accessed by the retrieval mechanism.) That the slope of the latency function does not increase when disyllables are produced rather than monosyllables, or even when sequences of stressed and unstressed word pairs are produced, implies that the production unit is not the syllable or the word. Sternberg and associates propose, tentatively, that it is the stress foot. That the intercept is larger for disyllables or word pairs than for (stressed) monosyllables suggests that "unpacking" time does increase with complexity of the production unit.

The duration function is modeled as a quadratic function of the number of word-to-word intervals ($n-1$, where n is the number of words in the utterance):

$$D_n = a + b(n-1) + c(n-1)^2$$

The parameter b, but not c, is affected by word complexity (monosyllable or disyllable); c, the rate at which the duration curve accelerates, has a value very similar to the slope of the latency function. Sternberg and co-workers propose that both c and the latency-function slope reflect retrieval time. If they do, then the value of c supports the conclusion that the production unit is the stress group not the syllable or word because, as noted, it is unaffected by word complexity. In addition it suggests that talkers require more time to produce each word in a long string of words than in a short string because, throughout the string, retrieval time is longer in a large than in a small buffer. Finally, because c has the *same* value as the latency slope, and not half of its value, Sternberg and colleagues conclude that the output buffer does not shrink as stress groups are ouput. They propose, then, that retrieval is a serial, self-terminating search through a nonshrinking buffer.

Sternberg and associates (1980) provide two other kinds of information about utterances produced in their experiment. First, the utterances show declination that is very similar in form to declination described for naturally produced grammatical sentences. In particular, across word strings of length two to five, the final f_0 is invariant. The starting f_0 is also invariant;

consequently, as others have observed with natural speech, the slope of the declination function decreases with increases in utterance complexity.

Second, Sternberg and co-authors (1980) provide some information about the durational microstructure of their utterances. Intervals between word onset and the onset of the second syllable in a disyllable ("within-word" duration) increase with serial position in an utterance, but not with utterance length in words. Intervals between onset of the second syllable in a disyllable and onset of the following word ("across-word" durations) show the opposite pattern. This dissociation is not consistent with the idea that serial position and length effects on duration both reflect the operation of the retrieval mechanism.

Commentary. The model of retrieval and execution accounts well for the data on which it was based, with the exception of the within- and across-word durational patterns. Confronted with other data and other models based on them, a number of disagreements arise. These will be described below under "Puzzles and Inconsistencies." One will be considered here.

An unattractive aspect of the model concerns the relationship between the retrieval mechanism and the output buffer. That the mechanism takes longer to select a stress group for output the more stress groups there are in the buffer suggests an unordered collection of stress groups in the buffer—unordered, at least with respect to the behavior of the retrieval mechanism. This is counterintuitive, at least as a general model for buffering syntactically coherent strings. And it is difficult to believe as an explanation for the durational patterns in such sequences as "Monday Monday Monday Monday," in which the order would not seem to matter. In addition, however, the proposal implies that the stress groups themselves are mutually independent. But stress groups are metrical units that participate, allegedly, in larger metrical units. They are not mutually independent in utterances in which there is more than one of them. That they are not independent is revealed in several ways in naturally produced speech: The relative prominences of their component syllables are affected by participation of their stress feet in larger units; the patterns of pausing are affected and so are word and segment durations (e.g., Lindblom and Rapp, 1973).

It is of some interest that both duration algorithms we have examined—those of Cooper and Paccia-Cooper and of Gee and Grosjean—seem to predict that, other things equal, average durations of pauses will grow with utterance length because on the average, more nodes will dominate words flanking a boundary; therefore, boundary strengths can be larger. Perhaps the increases in latency and across-word duration found by Sternberg and colleagues occur because stress groups participate in superordinate metrical units and not because they are harder to find in the output buffer. To reproduce the durational patterning that Sternberg and colleagues report, the word strings would have to have a structure something like the structure in Figure 6–7, with boundary strength increasing left to right.

Language Production: An Attempt at Evaluation, Integration and Reduction

If we try to integrate all of the foregoing proposals, what does the result look like? In particular, how many and which kinds of variables are talkers presumed to control independently? Under the heading "Integration" an attempt is made to suggest one that is as comprehensive as possible. That integration will suggest some puzzles and some disagreements among the foregoing models that research and theorizing will have to resolve. It will also reveal that theorists have collectively given the talker a gargantuan job of planning and regulation. Under "Puzzles and Inconsistencies" are catalogued some of the problems that the attempt at integration suggests. Under "Streamlining a Theory of Language Production," some ways of reducing the talker's hypothetical problem of control are suggested.

Integration

Having decided what message to convey, the talker is required to construct a surface structure of a sentence. This is accomplished, according to Garrett, in two broad phases. One constructs a functional representation of the message and the other inserts this content into a positional frame. Events at the functional level are (relatively) blind to the phonological forms of words. Consequently, Garrett proposes that phonological processes are applied later in the production process. For their part, phonological processes are (relatively) blind to the syntactic form of the utterance and to lexicality. They are assigned to a third stage of sentence generation. A fourth is involved in speech output.

While this sequence of levels captures many properties of speech errors, it does not capture the fact that the functional phase of language production is only *relatively* blind to phonology and the phonological phase only relatively blind to lexicality. Therefore, an instantiation of the phases more or less along the lines simulated by Dell may be required.

Following phonological selection procedures, the talker has, in an output buffer, a sequence of phonemes arranged in canonical syllable structures (Shattuck-Hufnagel), syllabically coded phonemes (Dell), or an array of stress feet (Sternberg et al.). To output the speech (just having

Figure 6–7. A possible tree structure for "Monday Monday Monday Monday Monday" that would give the pattern of increasing duration reported by Sternberg and colleagues (1978).

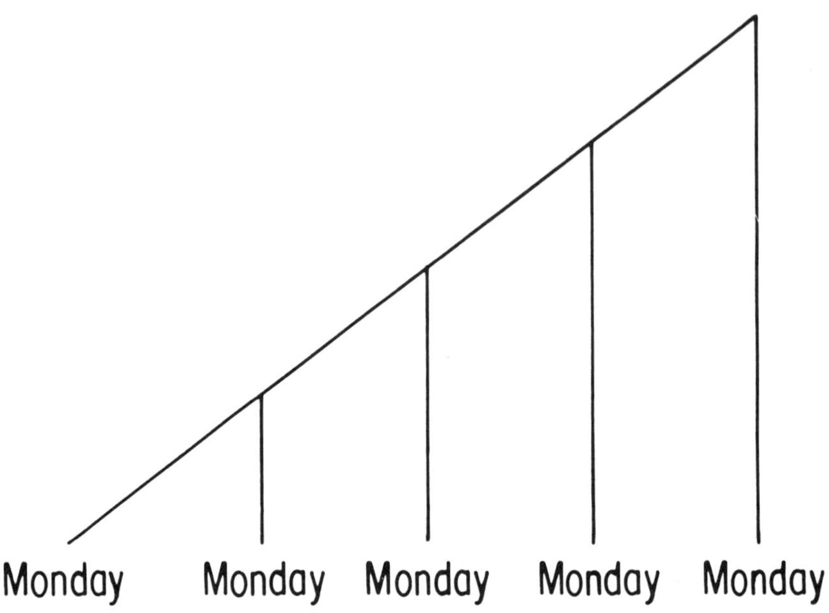

placed them *into* the buffer), the talker retrieves them in foot-sized units using a self-terminating, serial search through an apparently unordered, nonshrinking buffer. (Just having packaged them *into* metrical structures), he or she unpacks them, and executes them as speech. Explaining how the symbols of the linguistic representation are translated into activities that a vocal tract can carry out is the responsibility of a speech production theory.

As yet unordered with respect to the foregoing sequence of events and with each other is the regulation of two other sets of variables. At some time (perhaps as speech is uttered; see the quotation from Sorenson and Cooper [1980] above), the talker applies the topline rule. This involves a close attention to the duration of the utterance on a moment-by-moment basis. If an f_0 peak is to be produced (for reasons not covered in this review, but often corresponding to production of a stressed word), according to the topline rule, the talker needs to know when, in seconds after utterance onset, the peak is occurring and how long in seconds the total utterance duration will be. The result of the computation then has to be translated into effects on subglottal pressure or laryngeal tension, in a way, again, to be explained by a speech production theorist.

In addition, at some time, the talker has to code f₀ fall–rise patterns at syntactic boundaries. Presumably, this happens at the same time that the talker codes the utterance's patterns of pausing, durational lengthening, and coarticulation blocking using the algorithm of Cooper and Paccia-Cooper or that of Gee and Grosjean.

To summarize, then, talkers have independent control over variables of at least five different types. They determine the *syntax* of the sentence and which *words* will be fit into the syntactic structure. Having done that, they select and order the *phonological segments* that will realize the words. Some *metrical structures,* in particular syllables and stress feet, are involved somehow in the packaging of words for output, and other metrical structures—in particular, phonological phrases and intonational phrases— are marked, perhaps, by *acoustic* (and *articulatory) variables* including f₀, pausing, and durational lengthening.

If the separate "mental processes" in which a talker is proposed to engage were counted, the result would be far greater than Figure 6–1*a* would suggest. In Garrett's model there are four broad stages, in Sternberg's three, in Cooper and Paccia-Cooper's up to 14 (*per boundary;* there are somewhat fewer in Gee and Grosjean's), and in Cooper and Sorenson's topline rule there is one per peak.

We could, at this point, sit back and marvel at how wonderful the mind is to be able to keep track of all of these things in the course of language production (all of *these* things and then all of those *other* things that are depicted in Fig 6–1*b* and that get the utterance actually uttered). But instead it seems that something must be wrong with this picture because it gives the talker too much to do. Moreover, some of what the talker has to do (for example, computing the durational microstructure of every interword boundary, or computing the precise form of the declination curve) has no apparent purpose. And some of what the talker does is done in ways that appear somewhat perverse (for example, selecting and ordering words and then later selecting and ordering their [already ordered] phonological segments with the result that ordering errors are made; retrieving components of the output buffer with a mechanism—a self-terminating search through a nonshrinking buffer—that appears blind to the ordering of units in the buffer).

Before examining in detail the problems and puzzles to which the present attempt at integration points, we should briefly consider whether the integration accounts for the performance measures specified earlier as the domain of a language production theory and whether it addresses the issues outlined earlier that a model of language production should address.

Obviously, in a fashion, the integrated model generates the performance measures in its domain. It is worth repeating, however, that it does so in two distinct ways. Its components that are responsible for speech errors and its retrieval and unpacking mechanisms are accounts of language production (or word production) that explain how, in the natural course of production, certain errors or durational patterns occur. In contrast, the components of the model responsible for declination, f_0 fall-rise patterns, durational lengthening, and pausing are devices for producing the measures explicitly. An alternative formulation would be one in which, as a byproduct of the talker's planning and execution of speech, certain f_0 and durational patterns arise.

Three aspects of language production were specified earlier that a theory should address. They were the separation of function and form (and of form and substance) in language and speech, generativity, and the role of metrical structures in language. The first two aspects are realized—potentially, anyway—in the modeling supplied by speech-error researchers. The third is not really addressed by the model.

Puzzles and Inconsistencies

The Output Buffer: an Inconsistency. Based on speech errors, Dell and Shattuck-Haufnagel agree that phonemes are, in some sense, organized syllabically before they are produced. Based on latency and duration data, Sternberg and colleagues (1980) propose an organization in terms of stress feet.

In itself, this does not appear to be a major disagreement, because both conclusions could be true at the same time. Moreover, the observation that sounds that are interacting in an error tend to share level of stress may signify that these errors preserve their intended position not only in the syllable, but also in the foot.

However, there is a more subtle, but real difference between the proposal of Sternberg and co-workers and those of Dell and Shattuck-Hufnagel in terms of how the proposed metrical structure, syllable, or foot, is conceived. For Sternberg and colleagues, the foot is a production unit, or, more specifically, a subprogram of the motor program for an utterance. Stress feet are the things that the retrieval mechanism retrieves. For Shattuck-Hufnagel and Dell, however, the units in the output buffer are phonemes; they are embedded in a syllabic frame, but the syllables are not units themselves.

That there is a distinction between "unit" and "frame" (or at least between conventional linguistic units and metrical structures) is strongly implied by ordering errors in speech. Phonemes and words are misordered in speech; syllables and stress feet rarely are. Rather, syllables and perhaps stress feet provide a frame that constrains how sounds can misorder.

In a short-term memory buffer, as it is conventionally studied, misordering errors are common. Two letters, say, may be recalled correctly, but in the wrong order. It would seem, then, that at least some retrieval mechanisms do make ordering errors and that Sternberg and associates should expect misorderings of the units stored in their output buffer—that is, the stress feet.

That misorderings of these units do not occur suggests that stress feet are not units in an output buffer and hence that the latency and duration data require some other interpretaion. Either the production unit is not a foot or the latency and duration functions are not generated by a process of retrieving and unpacking production units. The first option is possible—Sternberg and co-workers drew their conclusion that the unit is the stress foot only tentatively. However, their data are incompatible with the conclusions that the unit is the phonological segment or that it is the word—the two units that do transpose frequently in speech errors. The second alternative—that the latency and duration functions do not reflect the operations of a retrieval process—is also possible. One hypothesis concerning what they might reflect instead has already been suggested. Perhaps sequences to be produced are metrically structured and have structure similar to that in Figure 6–7. The increasing duration and pausing that occur left-to-right in the data of Sternberg and co-authors, then, reflect that structure. (Although the explanation is contrived, applying the algorithm in Table 6–1 to the structure in Figure 6–7 may even generate the latency function—essentially as a 'pause' before the first word in the utterance. It does so because utterance onset has a high boundary strength owing to the large number of nodes under the node dominating the right side of the boundary—that is, the S node. Moreover, as more words are added to the utterance, the stronger the sentence–initial boundary and hence the longer the latency.)

Unpacking: A Puzzle. Sternberg and associates propose that "unpacking" occurs after a stress foot has been retrieved. The basis for their proposal is that the intercept of the latency function, but not the slope, is affected by the complexity of the production unit. In some respects, this proposal has intuitive appeal. The talker does have to generate the full complement of articulatory gestures that the utterance requires, and articulatory gestures have not yet made an appearance in any of the models of language production under consideration.

What is puzzling is that the phonological segments have just been packaged *into* metrical structures for storage in the retrieval buffer. Why is the structure immediately undone? Put differently, why would a talker have an output buffer requiring a structuring of the language units in a way that they are not structured in early phases of production if the structures have no role to play in articulation?

Durations in Speech: Inconsistencies. Three sources of evidence on durational patterns in speech appear to mutually disagree. Data of Sternberg and colleagues and probably those of Gee and Grosjean and Cooper and Paccia-Cooper suggest a general increase in durations as utterances grow. However, the growth patterns are not alike. This may not be a real inconsistency in view of the fact that Gee and Grosjean and Cooper and Paccia-Cooper ascribe the patterns of durations to syntactic structure (or, in the case of Gee and Grosjean, to syntactic effects on metrical structures). In apparent contrast to these observations, however, are others (see Lehiste, 1980, for a review) in which durations *shrink* as more is said. The bulk of the shrinkage occurs, it is true, as stressed syllables are followed by increasing numbers of unstressed syllables. But shrinkage also occurs as words are added to a sentence. For example, Huggins (1978) provides data showing a 40 ms shortening in the name "Joe" in a five- as compared to a two-word sentence. In the sentences, "Joe took father's shoe bench out," and "Joe called," the key word, Joe, is in both cases at the end of an NP. The boundary strength of "Joe" should be *greater* in the longer sentence, however, and hence "Joe" should be longer in the long than in the short sentence, but it is not.

Streamlining a Theory of Language Production

Clearly, the integrated model—even if all of its parts were compatible—would require streamlining. This will not be attempted here, but two strategies for streamlining are suggested. One is to ask what *minimally* an actor must be assumed to control explicitly in order to explain the dependent measures he reproduces, rather than asking what scheme, however complex, will reproduce the data. This has two corollaries. The first is to look for relationships and dependencies among various measures—that is, to suspect that if four or five measures all exhibit a similar patterning then in some direct or less direct way they are not independently regulated and should not be modeled as if they were five things rather than just one. Prime candidates for reduction in this way are the patternings of f_0, duration, pausing, and blocking of coarticulation, all of which suggest a relaxation of vocal gestures at boundaries (see also Cooper and Sorenson, 1981). A second corollary is that models should be avoided that generate the superficial form of a dependent measure itself without serious attention either to what, if anything, might motivate the talker's imposing the patterning in the measure, or to how little explicit control needs to be assumed to explain the data.

A second strategy is simply to allow the measures from other research domains to limit and guide theorizing based on a particular measure.

SPEECH PRODUCTION

As Studdert-Kennedy (1980) reminds us in his review of *The Signs of Language* (Klima and Bellugi, 1979), language is form, not substance. Quite properly, then, the models of language planning just reviewed focus on providing an account of how language forms are organized to convey an intended message. From that perspective, the job for a speech production theorist seems to be one of explaining how the plan gets translated into action. Indeed, speech production researchers see that task as their job as well; it is the one outlined in Figure 6–8*a*.

As Kent (1983) points out, however, in the translation from planned message to articulation, "a difficult gap has to be bridged" (p. 59) because the things on the two sides of the translation are things of different types. Thinking of a translation like this taking place leads investigators to ask whether it can really be supposed that language forms are *in* vocal gestures (MacNeilage and Ladefoged, 1976). Indeed, some researchers are quite certain that they cannot be (Hammarberg, 1982; Repp, 1981) on grounds that language forms are irretrievably cognitive or mental and *therefore* can exist in the privacy of the minds of talkers and listeners, but can never make a public appearance.

A different way of conceptualizing the relationship between plan and actualization, which to me is more preferable, is schematized in Figure 6–8*b*. This conceptualization makes use of the observation that language forms, whether planned or actualized, are always realized in some physical medium. When they are planned, the medium (that is, the "physical instantiation" of Figure 6–8*b*) is at least neural; when they are uttered it is at least articulatory. In this conceptualization, there is no translation from mental to physical; indeed, there is no change at all at the "mental" or cognitive level of the linguistic message. There is ony a replication of the message across two media, brought about in whatever way that neural activity brings about motor activity.

Few would argue with most of Figure 6–8*b*, although some (Hammarberg 1976, 1982; Repp, 1981) would argue that the articulatory gestures only hint at the linguistic units, but do not in fact realize them.

Figure 6–8. Two views of the relationship between a plan and an utterance. (See the text for elaboration.)

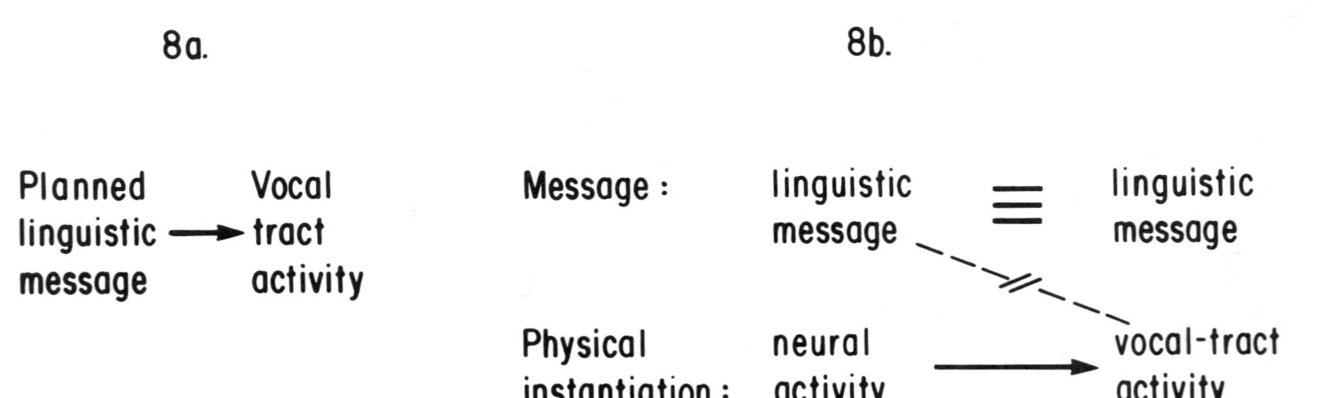

The inclusion of neural underpinnings for the premotor language representation is untendentious, however. Nevertheless, even if it is uncontroversial, investigators still write as if the translation is from the planned message to the activity (that is, along the dashed diagonal of Figure 6–8*b*), not from one physical instantiation to another, and as if the problem of speech production is to explain that translation. (For example, Perkell [1980] states, "With an 'input' in the form of a feature-specified underlying representation, our hypothetical overview must account for the translation into articulatory movements" p. 347.) In Figure 6–8*b*, however, the problem is one of understanding how linguistic messages can be instantiated in physical media, both neural and articulatory, not how they can be translated *into* physical activity; they are already physically realized, and understanding how linguistic messages can be realized in physical activity is no less problematic for the plan than it is for the utterance.

What are the problems in respect to articulation? Consider again the passage from MacNeilage and Ladefoged (1976) cited earlier:

> [Researchers have] an increasing realization of the inappropriateness of conceptualizing the dynamic processes of articulation itself in terms of discrete, static, context-free linguistic categories, such as "phoneme" and "distinctive feature." This development does not mean that these linguistic categories should be abandoned—as there is considerable evidence for their behavioral reality (Fromkin, 1971). Instead, it seems to require that they be recognized, even more than before, as too abstract to characterize the actual behavior of articulators themselves. They are, therefore, at present better confined to primarily characterizing earlier premotor stages of the production process, as revealed by speech errors, and to reflecting regularities at the message level (Fant, 1962) of the structure of the language, such as those noted by phonologists. (p. 90)

MacNeilage and Ladefoged are responding to apparent contrasts between the properties of linguistic units at the message level ("discrete, " "static, ", and "context-free") and those of their realizations or approximations in articulation (coarticulated, dynamic, and context sensitive). These contrasts probably are not unique to articulated language. Presumably, access to the *neural* activity going on as the message plan is constructed would offer no clearer picture of the critical properties of linguistic units than does access to vocal activity. Yet having witnessed the confusing neural activity, we would not conclude that "linguistic units should be recognized as too abstract to characterize the actual behavior of [populations of neurons] themselves" or that linguistic units are "better confined to primarily characterizing the earlier [preneural] stages of the production process." The buck has to stop somewhere.

As an alternative to assuming that phonemes, for example, are not in articulation (or in neural activity) because we cannot see them in it, we need to consider the possibilities that we cannot see them in these media both because we do not know how to look at the media in revealing ways and perhaps also because we are looking for the wrong correlates of linguistic units.

In respect to the latter possibility, we can ask whether the properties of linguistic units that articulated speech does not have—in particular, the properties of being "static, " "discrete, " and "context-free"—*are*, in fact, properties of linguistic units. For example, it can be argued that linguistic units are not static (Fowler, Rubin, Remez, and Turvey, 1980). The dimension of static–dynamic is irrelevant to linguistic units at the message level. At that level, phonemes are symbols engaged in linguistic functions. The critical constraint that linguistic units such as phonemes place on any physical medium that realizes them is not that it realize them as static or as dynamic but that it realize them in *some* way that enables them to perform their linguistic functions.

To serve their functions, phonemes have to be separate one from the other and they have to be serially ordered when they participate in larger linguistic units. To achieve separation and serial ordering, however, phonemes need not be *discrete* if discrete implies nonoverlapping. The separation and ordering of phonemes is preserved in articulation not by discreteness but rather in the order in which each phonological segment predominates over others being coproduced with it, both in the vocal tract and in the acoustic signal (see "Coarticulation as Coproduction" later in this chapter).

Another constraint on a physical realization of linguistic forms is that tokens of a type (e.g., phones of a phoneme) be identifiable as such. The obvious way of ensuring this is to give the tokens of a type some context-free property or properties. Perhaps this is the way the vocal tract realizes this constraint (e.g., Stevens and Blumstein, 1981). We do not yet know, and other ways are possible (Smith and Medin, 1981).

A decision that phonological segments as articulated fail to preserve essential properties of linguistic units commits the theorist to more complicated theories of speech production (because a mind-to-body translation has to be confronted, as in Figure 6–8*a*) and of perception (because the objects of perception are not in the signal) than a decision that the message units are replicated intact across media. It seems to me best to pursue the more straightforward course first. Therefore, although it is a controversial matter, this chapter is written as if the fact that the *linguistic functions* of phonological segments and other linguistic units are preserved in articulation (in that perceivers do extract linguistic messages from acoustic signals) signifies that phonological segments are uttered intact in speech production.

The critical questions on which this focuses are as follows: What are articulated linguistic segments, how are they (here, phonological segments) realized in articulation, and how are vocal structures regulated to realize them?

In contrast to the review of language production in the first part of this chapter, the remainder is not organized around theories of (parts of) speech production because there are relatively few of them. Instead answers to the foregoing questions that have been offered in the literature are presented. Following this, Perkell's (1980) model, which tries to incorporate answers to these questions, is described. Finally, which aspects of the model will need revision or elaboration by future research and theorizing are considered.

What are Articulated Phonological Segments?

MacNeilage (1970) proposed identifying phonological segments with the achievement of spatially defined vocal tract targets. MacNeilage's proposal was based in part on the observation of "motor equivalence" (see later discussion). Talkers produce phonological segments that they and others agree are tokens of the "same" segment in different ways, depending on the context in which the token is produced. To take one of MacNeilage's examples, /t/ after/i/ requires a slight elevation of the tongue tip so that it contacts the alveolar ridge. Producing /t/ after /a/, however, requires closing the jaw and perhaps raising the tongue body in addition to tongue tip movement. All that appears invariant across these productions of /t/ is the spatial target reached by the tongue tip.

Several researchers, including MacNeilage, have pointed out that the proposal that the targets are spatial may be too constraining. For example, when Folkins and Abbs (1975, 1976) apply resistive loading to the jaw during a closing gesture for a bilabial stop, lip closure is achieved, but in a different spatial location from unperturbed closure. Specifically, it is achieved with a more open jaw and with a more extensive excursion of the upper lip than in unperturbed utterances. Possibly something similar happens in normal speech when bilabial closures following or preceding low or high vowels are achieved with relatively lower or higher jaw positions (Sussman, MacNeilage, and Hanson, 1973). In either case, the target is not spatially invariant.

Perkell (1980) has proposed that targets may be "orosensory goals." For example, achievement of bilabial closure, wherever the closure may be absolutely, has similar tactile consequences. Perkell's proposal more generally (see Figure 6–1*b* and later discussion) is that segments are specified as features with both auditory and production correlates. Their production correlates are orosensory goals; they may be proprioceptive or tactile, or they may specify intended air pressure states or airflow characteristics of the vocal tract.

The view of articulated segments as achievements of targets, however defined, captures a central characteristic of the realization of many segments—namely, that of equifinality. However, there is a salient characteristic of articulated segments that the characterizations in terms of targets do not capture well, although with minor modification they could. If segments are only *achievements* of vocal tract states—whether the states are defined spatially or as orosensory goals—then most of the talking process involves getting to segments and less of it is involved in actually producing them. Elsewhere it was proposed (Fowler, 1977) that the phonological segment be seen as the collection of gestures that occur on the way to achieving the equifinal state charcteristic of the segment. In addition to allowing movement to be seen as more than transitional in nature, it allows a conclusion, for example, that vowels that are heard in speech really have occurred even if their "targets" have not been reached.

How are Linguistic Units Realized: Some Measures

One way to examine how linguistic units are realized is to look at the "traces" they leave in various measures investigators take of articulation or of the acoustic signal. Two measures are examined, duration and coarticulation.

Duration

Making durational measurements requires choosing a solution, however temporary or pragmatic, to the "segmentation problem." The segmentation problem in speech is the theorist's problem to extract separate, serially ordered phonological or phonetic segments from an acoustic signal in which acoustic correlates of different segments are interwoven. In studies of duration, typically, the solution is to measure phonological segments as if they were discrete. That is, the signal is segmented by drawing segmentation lines perpendicular to the time axis that serve at once as the "right" edge of one segment and the "left" edge of another. This is not the only way to segment the signal, and as is pointed out later, it implies a particular view of coarticulation that is not the only one possible either. The procedure does, however, reveal some systematic variation in durations of measured segments.

Figure 6-9 shows one of those systematic effects (see also Lindblom and Rapp, 1973). A vowel shortens as preceding or following consonants

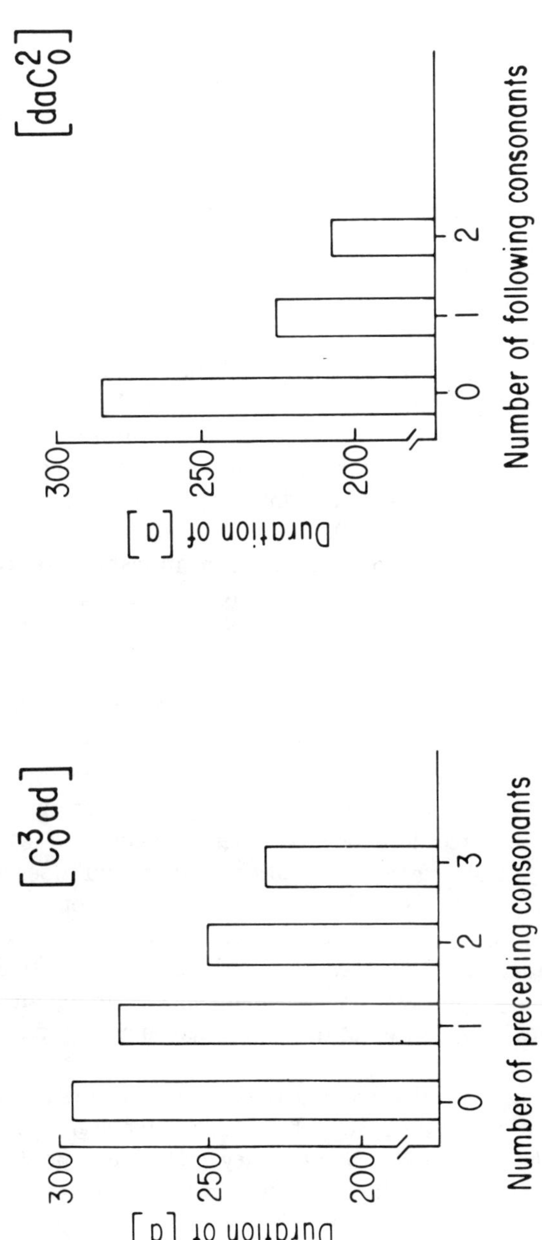

Figure 6–9. Shortening of a vowel as consonants are added to a syllable.

are added to a syllable. Transsyllabic consonants may also shorten a vowel (Lindblom and Rapp, 1973). In the present data, shortening by following intrasyllabic consonants exceeds that by preceding consonants; however, it is not known whether the asymmetry is reliable.

Figure 6–10 shows analogous effects of unstressed vowels on preceding and following stressed vowels. The left side of Figure 6–10*a* shows data from real-word sentences (Fowler, 1977); the data on the right side of Figure 6–10*b* are from reiterant-speech sentences (Fowler, 1981a). In data such as these (see also Huggins, 1975, 1978; Lindblom and Rapp, 1973), effects of preceding syllables are weak and sometimes absent; effects of following syllables are more substantial.

A final, systematic shortening effect occurs on the last stressed vowel of a sentence; this vowel is shortened by the number of stressed words that precede it in the sentence (Lindblom, Lyberg, and Holmgren, 1981; Lyberg, 1981). Analogous effects of preceding and following stressed vowels on nonfinal stressed vowels have been reported using reiterant speech (Lindblom and Rapp, 1973), but not always using real speech (Lyberg, 1981; however, see Huggins, 1978).

As Figures 6–9 and 6–10 reveal, the relationship between duration and number of relevant neighbors is negatively accelerated. It can be described formally (Lindblom, Lyberg, and Holmgren, 1981; see also Klatt, 1976) as follows:

$$D_0 = (D_I - D_{min}) \cdot \alpha^A \cdot \beta^B + D_{min}$$

where D_0 is the measured duration of the vowel, D_I is the "inherent duration" of the segment, D_{min} is the vowel's incompressible duration, α and β are parameters of shortening and A and B are numbers of relevant following and preceding neighbors, respectively.

By itself, of course, the equation describes but does not explain the shortening pattern. Several accounts have been proposed.

One is to relate the shortening effects to alleged syllable and stress timing tendencies in languages (e.g., Abercrombie, 1964). Syllable timing is a tendency for speakers of a language to maintain approximately isochronous syllables; stress timing is a tendency to produce isochronous stress feet.

There are several objections to this account. First, it is incomplete as an explanation. To propose that talkers shorten segments in a syllable as more segments are added because they are trying to produce isochronous syllables leaves unexplained why they are trying to do that. Without some independent motivation for syllable or stress timing, the "explanation" is no more than a crude description of the measurements themselves. Second, the description is very crude. Shortening effects of a syllable or segment are small compared to the added duration of the syllable or segment itself.

Figure 6–10. Shortening effects of unstressed syllables on preceding and following stressed syllables. Data on the left is natural speech from Fowler (1977). Data on the right is reiterant speech from Fowler (1981a).

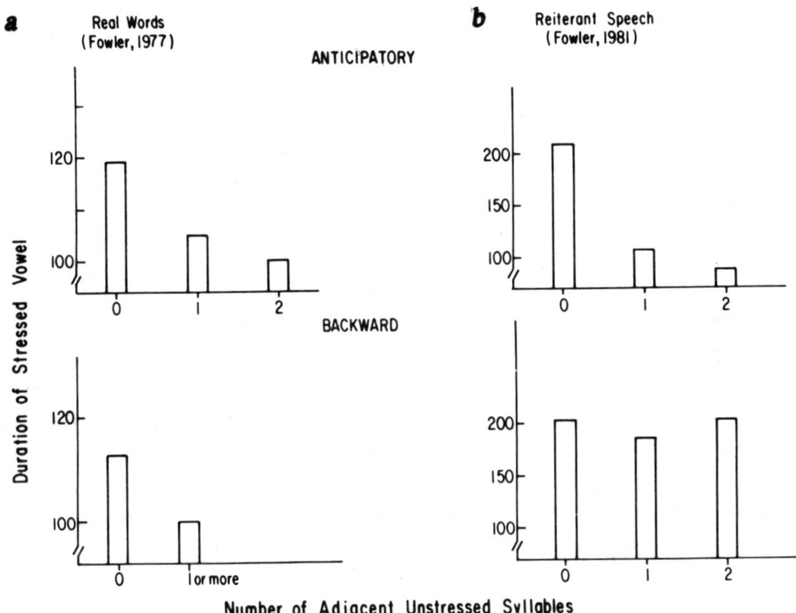

Third, languages are not supposed to be *both* syllable and stress timed, but English and Swedish show both effects.

Lindblom, Lyberg, and Holmgren propose an account in terms of a buffer in which a planned word sequence is stored for outputting. The buffer is seen as analogous to a box with elastic sides. Phonological segments are inelastic, deformable objects that can occupy the box. Shortening economizes on space in the buffer. To explain negative acceleration, Lindblom and colleagues propose that for every added unit in the buffer, a fixed percentage of the segment's compressible duration is given up.

There is one major difficulty with this explanation and one puzzle. The difficulty is in grounding the metaphor of the elastic box. A buffer is an entity at the message level of description of language (and hence, for many researchers, the "premotor" level); consequently, it is difficult to see what the analogue of the elastic walls would be or why segments would occupy space proportional to their uttered duration (that is, why, for example, a 300 ms /a/ would take up more space than a 200 ms /a/). The puzzle is that Lindblom and co-workers invoke an output buffer to explain the shortening they observe, whereas Sternberg and associates invoke one to explain the lengthening they observe. The data bases from which the two sets of investigators make their proposals appear contradictory; this will have to be resolved. However, the disagreement between the proposals reveals something else as well. It is that, if the concept of "output buffer" can handle shortening and lengthening effects just as readily, it has little explanatory value in reference to the physical realizations of utterances.

Other investigators (Bolinger, 1963; Lyberg, 1979, 1981) have explained some of the durational effects in terms of fundamental frequency. In particular, they propose that long stressed vowels—for example, main stressed vowels or vowels in final position—are long to accommodate F_0 excursions that mark main stress or sentence finality. Although this can explain durational effects at the phrase level, it does not seem to address effects at the syllable and foot levels. These latter effects may be distinct in pattern from phrase-level effects (Lyberg, 1981), but they are remarkably similar to each other, as comparison of Figures 6-9 and 6-10 reveals. Presumably, then, they require analogous explanations. It is my belief that they are, in effect, measurement artifacts and reflect coarticulatory patterns (Fowler, 1981a). This viewpoint will be elaborated on after a look at those patterns themselves.

Coarticulation

Coarticulation is an "influence of a phonetic context on a given segment" (Daniloff and Hammarberg, 1973, p. 239) or it is overlapping production of two or more phonetic segments (Fowler, 1980, 1981a, b). First let us examine some of the data giving rise to the view that speech is coarticulated, and then explanations attempting to account for the data.

The Lips and the Velum. Coarticulatory activity by the lips and velum may be special in one or two ways. First, it can range over very long extents; second, it exhibits a large asymmetry in favor of anticipatory coarticulation.

As for the lips, Benguerel and Cowan (1974) report evidence of lip rounding for a rounded vowel among speakers of French as many as six segments in advance of the measured onset of the vowel itself. In particular, they report that lip rounding for a forthcoming rounded vowel begins immediately following a preceding unrounded vowel no matter how many segments intervene between the two vowels.

Bell-Berti and Harris (1979, 1981) provide a different characterization of the extent of rounding anticipation. They report a fixed *temporal* extent of anticipatory coarticulation of lip rounding. In their data, rounding precedes measured /u/ onset by about 200 ms regardless of the number of consonants preceding the vowel either within or across a word boundary.

These different characterizations are, in part, different ways of looking at the same phenomenon, but, in addition, they may rest on contradictory data bases. Benguerel and Cowan do not report the temporal extent of lip rounding in their data, but the implication is there that it increases with the number of consonants preceding the rounded vowel. This finding is present for three speakers of English in research reported by Sussman and Westbury (1981). In contrast, however, Bell-Berti and Harris find a fixed temporal extent. The disagreement in the data is important to resolve because the two descriptions have suggested quite different characterizations of segment production in speech. One has promoted a view of coarticulation as assimilation (e.g., Hammarberg, 1982)—that is, as a spreading of features from one segment to another—while the other suggests that the rounded vowel consists of a temporally extended sequence of gestures, at least one of which overlaps with gestures for other segments.

The observational differences may be resolvable, at least among the English speakers that have been studied. Bell-Berti and Harris do find a shorter anticipation of rounding in a vowel-consonant-/u/ (VCu) context than in a context of two or more consonants preceding the /u/. In their view, this occurs because the talker avoids rounding a preceding phonologically unrounded vowel and would not avoid it with one preceding consonant if the extent of anticipation were as great as it is with two or more preceding consonants. For their part, Sussman and Westbury only compare two contexts for lip rounding: one preceding consonant or three.

As for the velum, lowering the velum for a nasal segment may precede measured onset of a nasal consonant by one segment or two if the segments are vowels (Kent, Carney, and Severeid, 1974; Moll and Daniloff, 1971). Ohala (1971) finds that velum lowering begins as soon as a closed port is no longer needed for production of any obstruent that may precede the nasal consonant. In addition, he finds more extensive anticipatory than carry-over coarticulation.

Bladon and Al-Bamerni (1982a) report two components to many velum-lowering gestures for a nasal consonant. One component increases its anticipatory extent with the number and duration of vowels preceding a nasal consonant. The other, present in about half of the productions, is an additional higher velocity gesture, time-locked to the nasal consonant's oral articulation. The investigators suggest that the second stage may represent onset of palatoglossus activity brought in occasionally to augment the velum-lowering effects of relaxation of the levator palatini.

They provide indirect evidence for this idea in a later study (1982b) in which velar movement is observed in phonological sequences that do not necessarily include a nasal. Utterances, produced by a speaker of Kurdish and a speaker of Arabic, contained vowels surrounding a nasal consonant, or a pharyngeal or glottal fricative. Anticipatory coarticulatory effects of the nasal consonant replicated those of earlier studies, showing earlier anticipation the longer the string of pre-consonantal vowels. Like the nasal consonant, the pharyngeal and glottal consonants were produced with a lowered velum, but in these latter cases, anticipatory velum lowering was time-locked to production of the consonants. Bladon and Al-Bamerni suggest that, in production of pharyngeal consonants at least, the palatoglossus muscle is activated along with other faucial muscles to achieve pharyngeal construction. A byproduct (in this case) of palatoglossus activity is velum lowering. Because activation of faucial muscles achieves the construction that Bladon and Al-Bamerni identify as onset of the fricative, velar lowering here is time-locked to measured consonant onset.

This distinction between types of anticipatory coarticulation seems to imply that some coarticulatory effects are sensitive to the segmental composition of a segment's preceding (and, perhaps following) context (that is, they are context sensitive) while others are involved directly in the realization of the given segment itself (and, relatively speaking, are context-free). If the distinction is real, it may clarify the disagreement between Benguerel and Cowan and Bell-Berti and Harris. The one pair of investigators sees anticipatory lip rounding as a context-sensitive gesture, and the other sees it as a relatively context-free component of rounding a vowel.

Glottal and pharyngeal consonants are not the only oral phonological segments to have characteristic postures of the velum. Velar height in vowels is correlated positively with vowel height, while, among vowels and consonants, obstruents have the most closed velum position. Bell-Berti (1980) has shown that the characteristic velar positions for vowels coarticulate. In particular, she finds that a sequence of obstruents has a higher peak velar position if it is preceded or followed by /i/ than if it is preceded or followed by /a/. Similar to velum lowering for the nasals, there is more anticipatory than carry-over coarticulation of vowel-associated velum height.

Velar gestures show other context effects as well. In a sequence of up to five obstruents, each of which individually has a high position of the velum, Bell-Berti finds that the velum rises throughout the sequence. Therefore, the peak velar position is higher in /ist#ta/ than in /it#ta/ and in /its#sta/ than in /ist#ta/. Bell-Berti suggests that the velum specification for each segment may be a movement relative to the velum's current position rather than a spatial target.

Taken together, these systematic activities of the velum give rise to two related questions. The questions to be asked are to what extent the characteristic velar positions or gestures for oral segments in fact need to be controlled by the talker and to what extent, instead (as in Bladon and

Al-Bamerni's proposal for pharyngeal consonants), they "fall out" of other things that the talker regulates. The second, more general question asks whether phonological segments to be uttered are given values on all possible articulatory dimensions (including velum height for vowels), or whether they are unspecified on certain apparently irrelevant dimensions.

As to the first, more specific, question—whether the velar positions for each oral segment and their anticipatory and carry-over effects are regulated directly—different answers are suggested by different sources of evidence. If it were possible to extrapolate from the findings of Bladon and Al-Bamerni to the vowels and obstruents studied by Bell-Berti by discovering some muscular or mechanical coupling that affects port size, the variability in velar height among vowels and obstruents could be seen as a byproduct of more primary articulatory gestures for the segments. Fujimura (1980) does find that tongue position and velar height are sometimes correlated. In his example, he observes both a higher posterior tongue position and a higher velum in production of the coda in "pence" than in "pens," and suggests that whatever the causal direction of the effect may be, the coupling itself is probably mechanical and perhaps muscular.

However, Bell-Berti (1980) argues that the different velar positions for different oral segments are regulated directly. She cites research showing that velar elevation in oral segments is correlated with activity of the levator palatini whose major action is to raise the velum. She hypothesizes that the port adjustments during vowels are made to prevent nasal coupling. Coupling is less likely at a range of openings during articulation of open than of closed vowels.

The second question becomes important when theories of coarticulation are devised or evaluated (see Explanations of Coarticulation later in this chapter). In some extant theories, that of Henke, for example (1966), anticipatory coarticulation of a "feature" is allowed to range over any segments that are unspecified for that feature. Vowels become nasalized in the context of a nasal consonant because (in English) vowels are unspecified for nasality; chameleon-like, they acquire the properties of their neighbors. However, Bell-Berti interprets her data as evidence that vowels are specified for velum height and she speculates that the specified height is a minimal one for each vowel that will *prevent* nasal coupling. The height specification for a vowel, then, is antagonistic to the nasal feature, and so, according to Henke's theory, it should prevent spread of the nasal feature in vowels. Coarticulatory spreading does occur, however, and, in Bell-Berti's data, it results in something like a vector summation of the different velar heights of neighbors.

Tongue and Jaw. Jaw and tongue movements for a consonant or vowel segment, like the lip and velar movements just described, exhibit both anticipatory and carrry-over coarticulatory spread. The anticipations, however, are less marked than for lip and velum. Indeed, investigators have rarely reported marked asymmetries in direction of tongue and jaw coarticulation, and when they have reported an asymmetry—in particular, for effects of stressed vowels on preceding and following unstressed vowels (e.g., Bell-Berti and Harris, 1976; Fowler, 1977, 1981a, b)—the asymmetry is opposite to that reported for lips and velum: carry-over effects are more substantial and extensive than anticipatory effects.

Sussman and Westbury (1981) suggest that anticipatory coarticulation of tongue gestures is less extensive than lip and velum gestures "for the obvious reason that the tongue is intrinsically involved in all speech segments (except those articulated solely at the glottis)" (p. 16). This conclusion is a little sweeping; the investigators do not defend their implication that the tongue is intrinsically involved in bilabial consonants and labiodentals. More importantly, at least one reading of their proposal does not accurately reflect the full range of coarticulatory interactions in which the tongue does participate. Interactions do occur between tongue gestures of adjacent segments when the tongue, apparently, is "intrinsically" involved in the production of both segments. For example, Perkell's (1969) cineradiographic data show concurrent constricting gestures of the tongue body for /k/ and fronting for /ɛ/ in production of /həkɛ/. During closure for the /k/, the tongue body makes a forward sliding gesture along the palate toward the more front positioning it will take for the /ɛ/. In addition, Kent (1983) reports influences of a /k/ on tongue gestures for a preceding diphthong. Hence, involvement of the tongue in producing a segment does not prevent its being influenced by tongue gestures for neighboring segments.

Sussman and Westbury may have had something else in mind, however. The tongue and jaw are "primary articulators" for many segments, at least in the restricted sense that their movements achieve acoustic consequences that guide researchers' segmentation of the acoustic signal into phonetic segments. That is, investigators do not measure onset of /n/, for example, at the point where nasal coupling for the /n/ is first evident. Instead, they measure its onset from the point where the tongue first makes contact with the palate, thereby initiating the segment's closure phase. Similarly, the onset of /u/, conventionally, is not measured at the point where effects of rounding are first evident in the signal; rather, its onset is located at a point where the jaw and tongue have opened the vocal tract sufficiently to create the voiced formant patterns characteristic of vowels and other sonorants.

Conceivably, then, coarticulation of tongue and jaw gestures is less extensive anticipatorily than lip rounding and nasalization for the same reason that Bladon and Al-Bamerni's high-velocity velar gesture is time-locked to pharyngeal consonant onset. These are gestures that *achieve* the acoustic consequences identified as segment onset. If they were anticipated more, the segment itself would be anticipated.

As for the types of interaction that are achieved, MacNeilage and DeClerk (1969) report less extensive coarticulatory effects of consonants on vowels than the reverse influences in stop-consonant–vowel–stop-consonant (CVC) syllables. In an anticipatory direction, they found the tongue body configuration during the first consonant of a CVC to vary with the identity of the following vowel. Carry-over effects into the second consonant could be detected in the pharyngeal region; the pharynx was narrower following a low than a high vowel.

Many investigators have reported noticeable anticipatory and carry-over effects of vowels on consonants in vowel–consonant–vowel (VCV) productions (Barry and Kuenzel, 1975; Butcher and Weiher, 1976; Carney and Moll, 1971; Kent and Moll, 1972; Ohman, 1966). Ohman characterized the coarticulatory effects in VCV utterances as diphthongal vowel-to-vowel gestures on which consonant gestures are superimposed. Kent and Moll provide limited supportive evidence in a comparison of tongue movement from /i/ to /a/ in the utterances "he honored" and "he monitored." In these productions, the timing and extents of the /i/ to /a/ gestures were identical even though in the one case a consonant intervened and in the other none did.

Carney and Moll (1971) extend Ohman's observations on stop consonants in VCV utterances to fricatives, and again find in cineradiographic vocal tract cross sections, clear evidence of vowel-to-vowel movements of the tongue body during closure for labiodental and alveolar fricatives. In their study, in which both vowels in the VCV utterances were stressed, Carney and Moll found no influence of the second vowel on the steady state configuration of the tongue for the first vowel. They do not discuss carry-over effects on the vowel's steady state. Evidence of vowel-to-vowel coarticulation *is* found when the influencing vowel is stressed and the influenced vowel unstressed (Bell-Berti and Harris, 1976; Fowler, 1977, 1981a, b). These coarticulatory effects are asymmetrical with carry-over effects more extensive and substantial than anticipatory effects.

Explanations for Coarticulation

Several critical reviews of explanations for coarticulation are available in the literature (e.g., Daniloff and Hammarberg, 1971; Kent, 1983; Kent and Minifie, 1977). Only a selective review, therefore, is provided here, focused on three kinds of explanation offered in the literature.

There is no Coarticulation. Wickelgren's proposal (1969; 1976) is that there is no coarticulation. Rather, segments are context sensitive because talkers and listeners store a large inventory of versions of each segment, called "context-sensitive allophones." Talkers pick a version to be uttered according to the context of segments in which it will appear. The stored versions are each adjusted to a unique segmental context of the form X–Y where X and Y are segments that might surround the phoneme in an utterance.

This proposal has not been well accepted in the speech literature. However, as Norman (1980) points out, it has resurfaced in certain machine-based speech-recognition schemes (e.g., Klatt, 1980). In Norman's words:

> I find it somewhat amusing to see this suggestion resurfacing, to see it being taken seriously, and to find that is is perhaps correct. (p. 389)

It is almost certainly not correct, however, and perhaps it is worthwhile to point out some reasons—old and new—why it fails. Criticism of the view has focused largely on the number of allophones that would be required to cover all the ways that a phoneme is produced. When the full range of anticipatory and perseveratory coarticulatory influences is considered as well as the variations in stress and rate of speech that affect segment production, the number of context-sensitive allophones needed to be stored could be very large indeed.

But, of course, so is our lexicon very large and no one is disturbed by the idea of storing tens of thousands of words. What is wrong with the theory of context-sensitive allophones is more obliquely related to the issue of the number of allophones that would be required.

In my view, Wickelgren's theory is falsified by evidence that segment production is generative—that is, it is falsified by the same kind of evidence that falsifies a theory that all possible sentences are stored. Generativity in segment production, as in sentence production, implies procedures for generating appropriate instances of segments in any novel context in which they might appear.

Talkers can produce acceptable versions of phonological segments in ways they never have before. For example, talkers produce normal or near-normal vowels with a bite block clenched between their teeth that fixes the postiion of the jaw (e.g., Lindblom, Lubker, and Gay, 1979). Vowels produced in this way show only minor effects of practice; they are nearly as close to normal as they ever will be from the first pitch pulse of the first vowel produced under bite-block conditions. This observation holds even when the vowels are produced under fairly severe time pressure (Fowler and Turvey, 1980). The limited effects of practice suggest that the small departures from normality of early productions are largely due to consequences of the bite block that physically *cannot* be compensated for.

Even more impressive, perhaps, are talkers' immediate ("on-line") compensations for unpredictable perturbations in movement of an articulator (e.g.) Folkins and Abbs, 1975, 1976; Kelso, Tuller, and Fowler, 1982). Talkers achieve bilabial closure for a /p/ or /b/ when the jaw is unpredictably loaded during its closing gesture. Closure is in part achieved by a short-latency compensatory activation of the upper lip (e.g., Folkins and Abbs, 1976). Under these novel conditions, a talker would be helpless if he or she had only a lexicon of context-sensitive allophones from which to select an allophone.

Speech researchers have been negatively inclined toward Wickelgren's theory for other reasons too, however. One reason is, again, obliquely related to the number of context-sensitive allophones required to cover the different contexts affecting segment production: by assigning the context sensitivity to the stored segments individually rather than to context-sensitizing procedures, the theory of context-sensitive allophones obscures the general character of coarticulation that may explain the *raisons d'être* of context sensitivity. For example (Kent and Minifie, 1977), in English all vowels are nasalized before a nasal consonant. In Wickelgren's descriptive system, this generalization is missed; it is as if coincidental that in the context $_xV_n$ (where "x" stands for any preceding context and "n" stands for any nasal consonant), all Vs are Ṽs.

At the other extreme, in some ways the scheme is insufficiently detailed. In particular, the subscripts surrounding each context-sensitive segment do not really specify the kinds of context effects that will be found. Obviously, not all properties of a segment are shared with neighbors. For example, in the context of a nasal consonant, vowels become nasalized, but they do not become obstruents or take on the nasal's place of articulation. A theory has to specify which properties of a segment will spread, and to what degree. The job of doing so is complicated by the fact that a given segment may share different properties with different neighbors. For example, whereas vowels become nasalized before nasal consonants, oral consonants do not. There is no way to represent that difference in Wickelgren's allophone scheme because vowels and oral consonants before a nasal have the same subscript.

In short, even if the theory of context-sensitive allophones were not falsified by evidence of generativity in segment production, it would need to be supplemented in two ways: (1) by a listing of the general principles of coarticulatory spreading (for example, the principle that nasalization spreads anticipatorily to vocalic segments), and (2) a specification for each kind of segment in the inventory, which of its properties will spread in which contexts. But these supplements to the theory of context-sensitive allophones themselves would constitute a set of procedures for generating coarticulatory effects and would, then, obviate the inventory of allophones.

292	Fowler

Coarticulation as Feature Spreading. The next account of coarticulation (Daniloff and Hammarberg, 1973; Hammarberg, 1982; Henke, 1966) constitutes a sort of compromise between Wickelgren's view that there is no coarticulation and the view that is considered last, of coarticulation as coproduction. In this second view, talkers store phonemes (or perhaps a few extrinsic allophones) rather than context-sensitive allophones. Each stored segment is specified as a bundle of features constituting the segment's "canonical form" (Daniloff and Hammarberg, 1973). Canonical segments influence one another by sharing features. In one account (Daniloff and Hammarberg) assimilation by feature is considered sometimes necessary to avoid production of transitional sounds between two planned phonemes.

Some coarticulatory effects—in particular, those involving anticipatory lip rounding and nasalization—range too far for the explanation in terms of transitional sounds to be plausible. Henke (1966) proposed that features tend to spread in an anticipatory direction so long as segments preceding the segment from which the features originate are unspecified for them. So, for example, a rounding feature can spread from a rounded vowel to any preceding and following consonants, because consonants are not specified on a dimension of lip rounding. Similarly, in English, the nasal feature can spread from a nasal consonant to any vowel because vowels are unspecified for nasality. Spread of the nasal feature will be halted by any oral consonant. This proposal handles gross characteristics of the data on rounding reported by Benguerel and Cowan and on nasalization by Moll and Daniloff (1971), but it fails on closer inspection.

First, segments with incompatible feature specifications do coarticulate. For example, Benguerel and Cowan find a small amount of rounding of /i/ by an upcoming rounded vowel. But /i/ contrasts with the vowel /y/ in French and hence must be specified [—round]. Second, Sussman and Westbury (1981) find earlier rounding activity of the orbicularis oris muscle in an $iC_i^j u$ context than in an aC_i^j context. This is unexpected in Henke's scheme because /i/ is positively specified for a spreading feature antagonistic to rounding, whereas /a/ is simply [—round]. At best, there should be no difference in onset of rounding in these two contexts, according to Henke's theory, because both vowels have rounding specifications. In Sussman and Westbury's view the theory should predict later onset of rounding in the context of /i/ because /i/'s spreading gesture is more antagonistic to rounding than is /a/'s absence of a rounding gesture. Presumably, the earlier orbicularis oris muscle activity occurred precisely because spreading has to be overcome in the context of /i/ and not in the context of /a/.

A second possible difficulty was alluded to earlier. Bell-Berti's data on velar height in oral consonants and vowels suggest the possibility that segments are not really "unspecified" on some feature dimensions (or at least on certain articulatory dimensions) that are not defining for the segments. Rather, in some cases, effects of different segments on the same articulator may combine in some way (see also Perkell, 1980). This does seem to describe what happens in respect to tongue body movement during CV syllables in which the consonant is velar (e.g., Kent, 1983; Perkell, 1969).

Other data and considerations are also hostile to the more general view that coarticulation is feature spreading. Carney and Moll (1971) provide cineradiographic evidence already described of tongue body configurations during closure for a fricative. The evidence shows configurations intermediate between the steady state configuration for the vowel preceding the fricative and that for the following vowel. Evidently, the tongue body moves smoothly from its shape for the first vowel to its shape for the second. An account of this phenomenon as feature spreading is strained, and, in any case, appears to overlook what is really going on.

An account in terms of feature spreading would have to allow the *different* feature specifications for the two vowels' front–back and height dimensions all to spread to the intervening consonant and then for the specifications from the different vowels on each dimension be averaged in a way that weights the first vowel more than the second at the beginning of the consonant with second vowel weighted increasingly throughout the consonant. However, clearly, that is not what is going on; rather, vowel-to-vowel articulatory gestures occur during closure for the fricative.

A second data-based objection to the feature-spreading account is related to the first. It is that coarticulatory gestures are not as neatly timed as the feature-spreading view seems to suggest. Sussman and Westbury point out that, in contrast to Bell-Berti's data on anticipatory lip rounding, their own data show no time-locking of rounding to the measured onset of /u/. Instead, lip rounding anticipates the measured /u/ onset more as the number of preceding consonants increases. Their data also show that onset of lip rounding is time-locked to *no* acoustic marker (see Sussman and Westbury, 1981, Figure 2). In some cases rounding begins well within the initial vowel in the VC_i^jV sequence. But if lip rounding were a feature that had been spread to the first vowel, it should have been realized along with the other features of the vowel and should have appeared at vowel onset. Alternatively, if lip rounding had spread only as far as the first consonant in the intervocalic sequence of consonants, rounding should not have appeared within the first vowel at all.

A difficulty with the theory of feature spreading brought out by these data is its proposal that a segment is *intended* to occupy a discrete interval of time during which its features are realized. It is my belief this idea derives from an overinterpretation of linguistic notational devices (see also Fowler, 1980; Fowler, Rubin, Remez, and Turvey, 1980).

When a linguist chooses a notational device, such as one of representing sequences of segments to be uttered as a left-to-right array of discrete feature columns, his or her choice reflects a convergence of considerations and constraints. One constraint is that the device must reveal clearly the critical properties of the phenomena being represented— here, the distinctive attributes of phonological segments, the coherence of the features of a given segment, the separation of phonological segments in a sequence one from the other, and their ordering in words. Other constraints, however, are more mundane ones—for example, that the device be visible and be conveniently reproducible on paper. These latter constraints, as well as the theoretically interesting ones, guide the selection of a column to represent the coherence of the distinctive attributes of a phonological segment and the selection of a left-to-right array of discrete columns to represent the separation and ordering of phonological segments in a sequence.

As researchers attempting to use the fruits of linguistic analyses, we have to distinguish the essential properties of notational devices such as this one from the properties that are either accidental (for example, that the columns, meant to reveal the grouping of features into segments, make it look—if the order axis is confused with the time axis—as if segments should be temporally discrete and have simultaneous onset of all of their features after spreading) or are promoted by the special physical medium in which the device is realized. A speech plan will not turn out literally to be a buffer consisting of an array of feature columns unless nervous systems and vocal tracts share critical properties with marks that pens make on pieces of paper. The means of realizing the speech plan and the utterance will be a means that preserves the critical linguistic properties of phono-logical segments in the medium in which they are instantiated.

Coarticulation as Coproduction. In a view of coarticulation as feature spreading, segments ideally are temporally extended in a simple way. Features within a column are turned on at some point in time, and then later are turned off. A segment extends in time from activation to deactivation of its features. In this way, segments are discrete one from the other.

In contrast, in a view of coarticulation as coproduction, segments are temporally extended in more complex ways. Their constituent gestures are not initiated concurrently and they typically overlap with gestures for neighboring segments. In this way, segments literally are coarticulated (Fujimura, 1981). For example, onset of lip rounding for a rounded vowel generally precedes onset of gestures of the jaw and tongue body for the same segment and it overlaps with gestures for preceding segments. In a view of coarticulation as coproduction, despite its temporal precession of jaw and tongue body movement, the lip rounding gesture is tied to the other gestures producing the rounded vowel and not with gestures for the earlier segments with which it overlaps.

Evidence that coarticulation is, at least in part, coproduction of neighboring segments is perhaps strongest in respect to movements of the tongue body and jaw for vowels. In VCVs, gestures for the first vowel overlap with those for the following consonant so that, for example, a bilabial consonant has a lower jaw position during closure if the vowel is /ae/ than if it is /ɛ/ and lower if /ɛ/ than /i/. Likewise, the jaw shows less elevation in the closing gesture for the bilabial consonant if the second vowel is /ae/ than if it is /ɛ/ and less if it is /ɛ/ than /i/ (Sussman, MacNeilage, and Hanson, 1973). Data from three studies already described (Carney and Moll, 1971; Kent and Moll, 1971; Ohman, 1966) suggest that during consonant closure in a VCV, gestures of the tongue body are smooth gestures from V_1 and V_2. Ohman's proposal that vowels are produced as diphthongal gestures with consonants superimposed seems to fit the extant data on VCVs more naturally than a proposal that tongue body positions are features spread from both vowels to the consonant and given differential weightings throughout the consonantal closure.

The specific proposal that vowels are partially coproduced with consonants appears to have independent support from the data on durational shortening described earlier. Vowels in a syllable are measured to shorten as consonants are added to the syllable. However, although they are measured to shorten, in fact they may not shorten at all in their articulatory extents; indeed, they may even lengthen a little. Measuring conventions select as measured onset of a segment a point where the segment begins to predominate over neighbors in an acoustic signal; they do not include the whole extent of a segment's influence on the acoustic signal. If consonants overlap with vowels, then even were the vowels' articulatory extents invariant in isolation and in the context of a consonant, they would be measured to shorten in the second context. Figure 6–11 illustrates this idea.

In the figure, the horizontal axis represents time and the vertical axis an abstract dimension of "prominence." This refers to the extent to which relevant articulators are given over to the production of a particular segment and similarly to the extent that the acoustic signal's dominant character is that of the segment. Dashed lines in the figure represent places in an acoustic signal where a given segment begins or ends its phase of predominance. If a vowel is produced in isolation, as in Figure 6–11a, the

Figure 6–11. Schematic view of syllable production in which vowel and consonant production overlap.

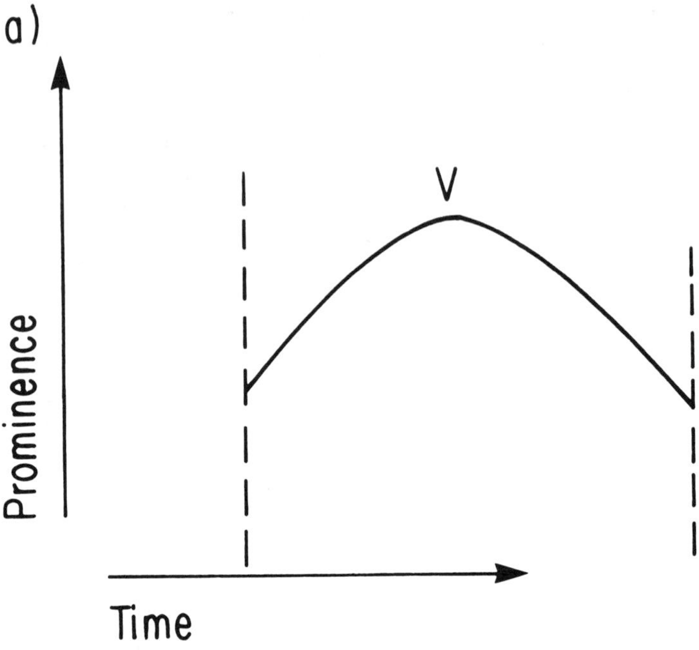

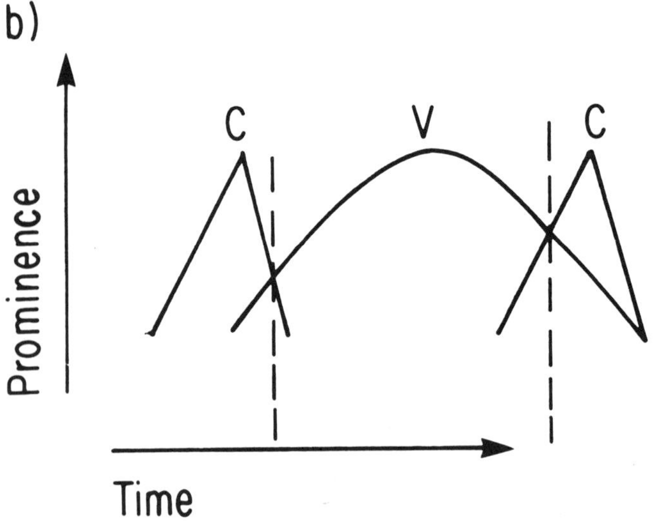

dashed lines will be at onset and offset of voicing. For a vowel in a CVC, however, one line will be drawn where the constriction for the first consonant has given way sufficiently for the vowel's formant pattern to begin to dominate in the acoustic signal; another line will be drawn at closure for the final consonant. In a CVC, then, the vowel's produced extent is greater than its measured extent. This is less true in an isolated vowel.

The measured shortening of a vowel when a consonant is added to a syllable is less than the duration of the added consonant. This may be (as Figure 6–11 indicates) that the vowel's articulatory extent does not span the whole syllable, or it may be because the vowel in fact lengthens.

Shortening at the foot or word level has a similar explanation within a view of coarticulation as coproduction. Figure 6–12 illustrates coarticulatory effects of preceding and following stressed /i/, /a/, and /u/ on a medial unstressed schwa (data from Fowler, 1981b). The figure shows substantial carrry-over influences on schwa and lesser anticipatory effects. On a coproduction view, the medial unstressed vowel is produced as a brief deflection of gestures of the tongue body and jaw from their stressed-vowel to stressed-vowel trajectory. That is, the medial unstressed vowel is coproduced with both stressed vowels, but it overlaps with the first one more than with the second.

Figure 6–13 depicts the asymmetry schematically. It appears to reflect the foot structure of English reported by linguists (Abercrombie, 1964; Catford, 1977; Selkirk, 1980a) and encountered earlier in this manuscript as a production unit proposed by Sternberg and associates (1978). In the linguistics literature, the foot emerges from analyses of the metrics of English and other languages as a structure superordinate to the syllable that organizes the placement of strong and weak syllables in words. It consists of a strong (stressed) syllable followed by any weak syllables up to the next strong one. That is, in a foot, weak syllables cohere more with preceding than with following strong syllables. Figure 6–12 shows that this coherence pattern is also reflected in coarticulatory relationships between stressed and unstressed syllables and Figure 6–10 shows that it is reflected in shortening patterns at the foot or word level. Figure 6–13 illustrates why coarticulation and shortening patterns are similar.

The dashed lines in Figure 6–13 represent segmentation lines that would be drawn if the syllables in the figure were to be measured. If the utterance were a disyllable VV (the presence of any consonants in the sequence will be ignored here), measurement lines would be drawn at points a, c, and e in the figure. The measured duration of the first vowel, then, would be c–a and of the second e–c. In a VvV utterance (where V is stressed and v unstressed), however, segmentation lines are drawn at a, b, d, and e and

Figure 6–12. Coarticulatory effects of a stressed vowel on unstressed schwa. The plot on the right gives F1 and F2 values for preceding and following /i/, /a/ or /u/. The plot on the left gives the F1 and F2 values for schwas in the context of preceding or following /i/, /a/, or /u/.

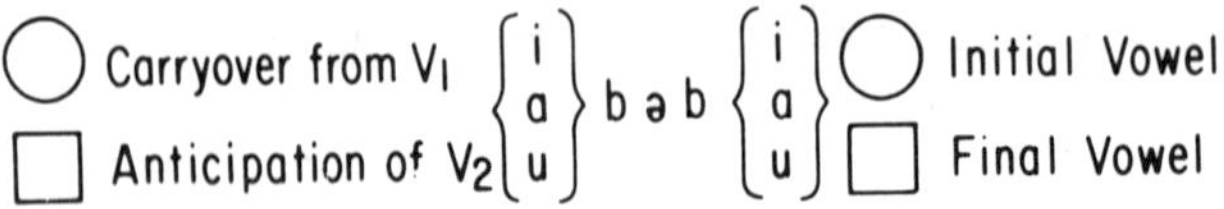

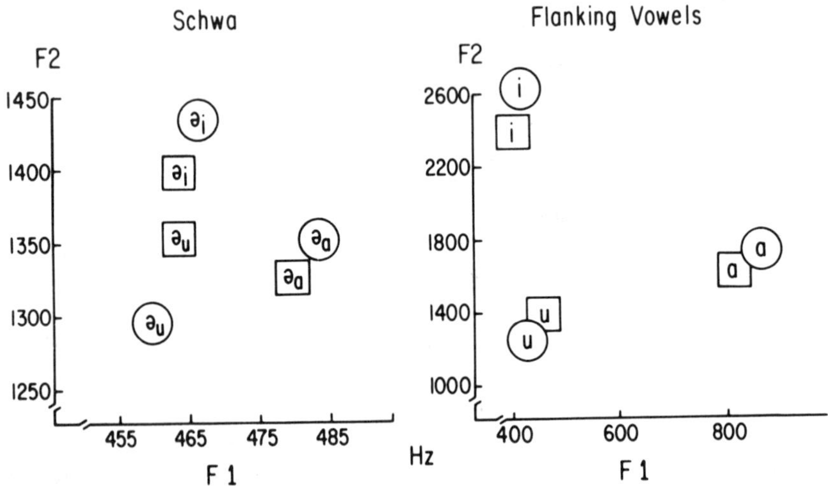

the measured durations for the stressed vowels are b–a and e–d, respectively.

Just as a vowel in a CVC is measured to shorten by its extent of coproduction, so is a stressed vowel in a VvV utterance. The measurement lines in Figure 6–13 also show that the first vowel shortens more than the second because, as the coarticulation data reveal, the overlap between a weak syllable and a strong syllable in the same foot is greater than cross-foot overlap.

Recent research of my own (Fowler, 1981a) directly compares coarticulation and shortening effects in sequences of stressed and unstressed syllables. The research shows that measures of the two effects are correlated, and that a version of Lindblom, Lyberg, and Holmgren's equation given above, which was designed to predict shortening effects, does a good job of predicting coarticulatory variability of F_2 in an unstressed vowel as a function of its context of stressed vowels.

The view of coarticulation as coproduction probably does not cover all instances of contextual influence in speech. For example, it may not

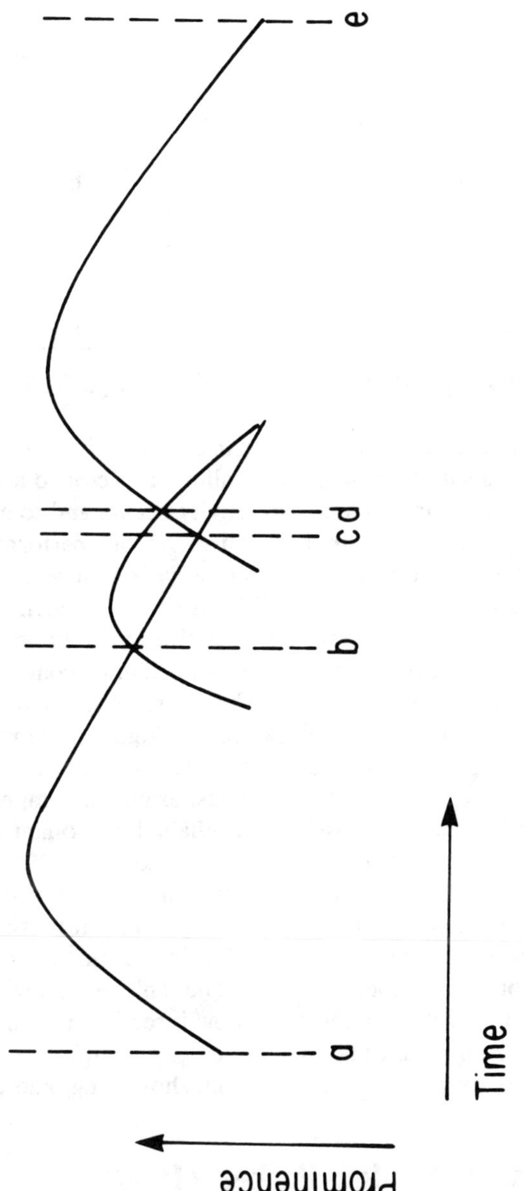

Figure 6–13. Schematic representation of foot production in English showing putative overlap of stressed by unstressed syllables.

explain the shift in place of articulation of /d/ in "width" (Daniloff and Hammarberg, 1973). It does not immediately explain why lip rounding and velum lowering migrate as far as they do. However, the explanation has several strong points in its favor.

1. It provides a more natural account of data on vowel production in VCVs than do other accounts.

2. It provides a unified account of these coarticulation effects and a foot- and syllable-level shortening.

3. It is the only account of the three reviewed here that provides any sort of connection to evidence from language production research that the metrical structure of language organizes speech output.

How Vocal Structures are Regulated to Realize Phonological Segments: Motor Equivalence

Motor equivalence is a flexibility in skilled activity so that a goal may be reached in a variety of ways. This allows an actor to accommodate to the different contexts in which the activity occurs and to compensate for unforeseen perturbations in the course of his performance. Uttered segments exhibit motor equivalence in a variety of ways.

First, uttered segments exhibit motor equivalence in ongoing, unperturbed speech. For example, the relative contributions of the jaw and the lips to bilabial closure varies with the height of coarticulating vowels (Sussman et al., 1973). Second, they show compensation for perturbations both foreseen, as in the bite-block studies (e.g., Lindblom et al., 1979), and unforeseen, as in studies of resistive jaw loading (Folkins and Abbs, 1975; 1976; Kelso et al., 1982). In the last example, compensation by the upper lip to jaw loading closing for a bilabial consonant begins only 15 to 30 ms after onset of a perturbation (Kelso et al., 1982).

Motor equivalence provides a strong hint concerning regulation of vocal structures that realizes phonetic segments. In particular, it reveals that vocal structures are coordinated. The implications of this observation for theories of speech motor control will be explained below. First, however, let us look at Perkell's model to see how it realizes the characteristics of articulated speech outlined above: phonological segments realized as targets or movements toward targets, durational shortening, and coarticulation.

A Summary Model: Perkell (1980)

Perkell (1980) intended his model to provide a heuristic framework for discussion and research rather than to serve as a detailed simulation of processes supporting speech production. The model has three broad phases, depicted in Figure 6-1*b*: preplanning, determination of motor commands, and realization of commands as peripheral vocal tract activity. The first two phases are elaborated further.

In the model, planning for speech production starts with a sequence of phonetic segments. Each consists of a column of features specified as "orosensory goals." Planning provides timing specifications based on several different properties of the sequence of segments. First, each segment has a stored intrinsic duration. This duration is modified by the context in which the segment is produced. For example, research reveals trading relations among velocity of movement, the distance that the articulator has to move (with more extensive movements generally faster than shorter movements, e.g., Kuehn and Moll, 1976), and the required precision of movement. Mechanical interactions among articulators involved in realizing different goals may also affect timing.

The output of the timing component of the model is a temporally specified sequence of orosensory goals. In the model, the temporal regularities described earlier under Duration would arise here along with others, for example, the increased duration of a segment before a voiced consonant.

Next, orosensory goals are converted to motor goals. The strategy incorporates knowledge of the relationships between sensory goals and the patterns of muscle activations required to realize the goals. The conversion is complicated by the fact that orosensory goals having overlapping temporal specifications may make demands on the same articulator. The strategy implemented here "sums," as it were, the different requirements of different orosensory goals to create one composite motor goal.

According to Perkell, it is this strategy that, with minor adjustments, enables compensation for bite blocks or artificial palates (e.g., Hamlet and Stone, 1976). However, because this phase is still in the planning realm, it cannot generate the on-line compensations; these must occur during execution.

A final aspect of planning introduces coarticulatory influences. Presumably, this strategy adjusts the timing specifications determined earlier to accomplish anticipatory look-ahead of "noncompeting aspects of articulation." A reason for look-ahead is to prevent abrupt, and hence needlessly effortful, gestures. "Urgencies," which specify how soon a motor goal has to be reached, are assigned to motor goals during this planning phase.

In the final planning phase of speech production, motor goals are transformed into motor commands. Perkell rejects the idea that the commands selected based on motor goals are fully elaborated, as they would be if speech were fully regulated centrally. Instead he proposes that the strategy for converting motor goals to commands involves internal feedback (that is, feedback entirely within the central nervous system) and possibly peripheral feedback as well. Internal feedback is used in something like a predictive simulation (Lindblom et al., 1979) that enables appropriate motor commands to be computed. A hypothetical "higher motor center" (see Figure 6-1*b*) receives moment-to-moment information via internal feedback about the state of the vocal tract. This is necessary to compute motor commands that will realize motor goals. The internal feedback is supplied by a "lower motor center" that represents the state of the vocal tract to the nervous system. Premotor commands are selected based on the discrepancy between the state of the vocal tract and the state required by the next motor goal. The lower motor center then translates premotor commands into commands to individual muscles. Presumably it is at this stage that on-line compensations occur.

Evaluation

The model is useful in offering an account of most of what a speech production theory must handle. In particular, it provides an account of the three phenomena identified earlier as central: durational patternings, coarticulation, and motor equivalence. The model requires revision or elaboration along three lines.

First, the planning component of the model clearly was not offered as a *minimal* specification of what must be "computed" during speech planning. The planning components of the present model overlap little or not at all with the planning specified in language production models, yet they are complex and include several stages. A job for future theoretical efforts will be to reduce the hypothetical computational component of speech production.

Second, and perhaps relatedly, the concept of coordination—in particular, the observation that speech is a highly coordinated activity— has little significance in the model. Yet (as is argued later), it may be the most important fact of activity on which researchers should focus their efforts; indeed, incorporating coordination into a speech production model may enable substantial reduction of the computational component. In particular, it can help to explain in one stroke how it is possible for talkers to regulate as many separate vocal structures and muscles as they can (the "degrees of freedom" problem; Bernstein, 1967; Turvey, 1977), how talkers can restrict themselves only to performance of coordinated vocal activity (Weiss, 1941), and concomitantly, how talkers can engage in performances that are at once physical (activities of the vocal tract) and "cognitive" or "mental" (utterance of linguistic units). This last question is the problem with which the chapter was introduced and which is addressed in the present subsection on speech production. The concept of coordination is further in the section that follows.

Third, the model does not address the distinction between linguistic units and metrical structures that emerges both in research on language production and from linguistic analysis. It was proposed earlier that metrical structures may require explanation in a theory of speech production more than in one of language production. An explanation is not yet at hand, but one direction in which to search is proposed in the section entitled Cyclicity in Behavior later in this chapter.

Coordination

Coordination is a fundamental property of speech and other biological activities. Understanding what coordination is and how it is achieved may be essential to understanding both the regulation of speech production specifically and, more generally, the sense in which vocal structures can be said to realize linguistic units.

Coordination is not well understood, however. According to Weiss (1941), nearly exclusive focusing on the properties of individual neurons and neural transmission has led to

> the neglect of the problem of how transmission has come to be so discriminatory and selective as to lead to coordinated responses rather than to unorganized convulsions. (p. 3)

More recently, and speaking more generally about biological organization, Pattee (1976) remarked:

> However, in spite of our knowledge of the "palpable detail" which is said to be normal chemistry for all known cellular reactions, the origin and nature of the *coordination* of these reactions remains an obscure and evasive question.

That biological activity is coordinated implies two related consequences for activity and its regulation. First there is a selective loss of degrees of freedom in the regulated physical system. If two variables of a system are coordinated, then they are not independent; changes in the value of one variable imply corresponding changes in the value of the other. Therefore, only some of the conceivable pairings of values of the coordinated variables wil occur—namely, only those compatible with the nature of the coordinative relations between them. For example, if the variables in question are the positions of the two front wheels of a car, then the only pairings of values of the variables that will occur are pairings in which the values are the same. In the example, and generally, loss in the number of possible outcomes in a system owing to coordinative relations among variables is advantageous. The driver happily gives up independent control over the front wheels of a car because he or she never wants to turn the wheels in different directions. Moreover, turning them in the same direction to the same degree is easier if the wheels are coordinated by an axle than if they require separate control.

Coordination, then, is selective loss of independence of the parts of a system, with the result that unwanted outcomes are avoided. At the same time, the task of regulation is made easier because fewer independent choices need to be made and enforced.

A corollary of this may be that coordination enables avoidance of certain errors. In the introduction to this chapter, it was pointed out that walkers do not make global ordering errors. For example, they never take two steps with the right foot without stepping with the left foot in between. Errors *do* occur in nonverbal activities, however (e.g., Norman, 1981). Errors are avoided in locomotion because functional and physical linkages essentially enforce the intended orderings of events. Errors arise, it seems, where sequences of actions are not physically coordinated, or, perhaps equivalently, where the intended sequencing of actions is arbitrary with respect to the system that realizes it.

If misorderings of phonological segments occur during "planning" rather than during execution of speech, as most speech-errors researchers claim, perhaps that is because during planning the ordering of segments *is* arbitrary with respect to the implementing physical (neural) system, whereas it is no longer arbitrary when the vocal tract becomes organized to implement the segments.

Coordination has another consequence that is implied in the quotation from Weiss and that is explicitly studied by Pattee (1973; 1976; 1977; see also Polanyi, 1962). Coordination gives rise to an abstact level of description and functioning in the coordinated system. If there were no coordination in the motor system, then Weiss's unorganized convulsions would be a probable outcome of motor activity. In addition, such an outcome would not be distinguished from any apparently "coordinated" gestures that might occasionally eventuate. (Compare the monkey at the typewriter who occasionally types a letter sequence that people recognize as a word; from the monkey's perspective, there is nothing special about the word.) In another example, if there were no grammatical constraints on word order in English, then no sequence of words in the language would be special or distinguished from others and no sequence would have the superordinate meaning that sentences have as compared to random word strings (Pattee, 1976). By restricting the outcomes of a system to a principled subset of all conceivable ones, coordination creates a new, more abstract level of functioning in the system embodying it. The result is functional activity if the system is a motor system and meaningful sentences if it is also linguistic.

This consequence of coordination—that of creating what Pattee (1973) calls an "alternative description" of a biological system—is exactly what is needed if populations of neurons or if vocal tracts are to realize linguistic units in the way depicted in Figure 6–8*b*. Linguistic units are the alternative, more abstract, description of the vocal tract producing speech. The problems for a theory of speech production, from this perspective, are to identify the coordinations involved in speech and thereby explain in part, how alternative descriptions can be planned and realized in a vocal tract.

Coordinative Structures and Their Properties

"Coordinative structures" are functionally specific units of action defined over groups of muscles and articulator degrees of freedom. Their components are constrained to effect coherent activity. Activities characteristic of coordinative structure regulation have two general characteristics by which they can be identified (Kelso, Tuller, and Harris, 1983). First, their constituent muscle activity or articulator-joint movement exhibits both invariant and variable properties. In particular, over changes in rate of production, or sometimes amplitude of movement, the relative timing of muscle activations remains invariant while the magnitude of muscle activity varies. This means of changing rate is characteristic of locomotion (e.g., Grillner, 1975), handwriting (Viviani and Terzuolo, 1980), and typing (Terzuolo and Viviani, 1979). It may be characteristic of speech as well. Tuller, Kelso, and Harris (1982) reported invariant relative timing of V_1 and C_2 related muscle activity in $C_1V_1C_2V_2C_3$ sequences varying in both rate and stress pattern.

The separation of invariant and variant properties of the coordinative structure suggests a separation of "coordination," responsible for the global form that an activity will take, and "control," responsible for its specific character (Kugler, Kelso, and Turvey, 1980).

A second property of coordinative structure regulated activities is that they interact in various ways with other such activities to form larger functional systems. This is clearly evident in von Holst's classic studies of fish fin activity (1973). It is also characteristic of the limbs in locomotion (Shik and Orlovskii, 1965). Again, it may be characteristic of speech as well. Kelso, Tuller, and Harris (1983) report that production of a repeated syllable interacts with concurrent finger tapping. A talker is asked to produce syllables at a constant amplitude and rate, but to tap his or her finger with alternating long and short finger excursions. The result is an apparent coupling of the two activities—long finger movements are accompanied by higher amplitude syllables than short movements of the finger. Similarly, asked to produce alternating stressed and unstressed versions of a syllable, but to tap evenly, taps accompanying a stressed syllable have a greater amplitude than those accompanying an unstressed syllable. This outcome, it seems to me, it is not predicted by a theory of speech production in which muscles are controlled by independent motor commands.

How is Coordination Achieved?

The example of a car and its axle was used earlier to illustrate a benefit of selective degrees of freedom loss. The example is misleading, however, because in speech activity, coordinative coupling of vocal structures is transient.

How is activity coordinated when the particulars of the coordinations apparently undergo moment-to-moment revision? One possibility is that peripheral reflexes are selectively potentiated and disabled in the course of talking. There is evidence of this in regulation of activities other than speech (Fukuda, 1961; Gottlieb, Agawarl, and Stark, 1970; Grillner, 1975) and some in the speech domain as well.

McClean, Folkins, and Larson (1979) have studied a possible role of the perioral reflex in speech. The perioral reflex is elicited in the laboratory by stretch of the lip or by electrical stimulation. It has a short latency response (10 to 15 ms) and a longer latency response (35 ms). Both McClean (1978) and Netsell and Abbs (1975) have shown an increase in the amplitude of the perioral reflex recorded from the orbicularis oris muscle in the latent interval before muscle activation for a bilabial consonant. In addition, Netsell and Abbs reported a suppression of the reflex during production of /a/ in /pa/. This outcome is similar to outcomes reported for other skilled activities. As reported in this literature, reflexes are potentiated when their action will promote a voluntary movement. Activating reflex has the consequence, in addition, of suppressing excitability of reflexes with action antagonistic to the intended movement. That the perioral reflex itself is inhibited during /a/ would seem to imply a reciprocal relationship between it and antagonistic reflexes.

However, there is reason to doubt that these data should be read in this way. Recently Abbs and Cole (1982) have expressed strong doubt that brainstem reflexes (having latencies in the range of that of the perioral reflex) play an important role in speech. They point out that if the perioral reflex were recruited for speech, several consequences should be realized:

it should inhibit its antagonists; effects of stimulating it should be local; and the reflex itself should be responsive only to stimuli generating local movement. According to Abbs and Cole, none of these outcomes is obtained. Actions antagonistic to those promoted by the perioral reflex are excited by stimuli eliciting the reflex. Loading and unloading the orbicularis oris muscle both give the same excitatory response. In addition, the lip stretch that elicits the perioral reflex also gives rise to responses in distant facial and neck muscles. Finally, excitatory oris responses can be elicited by distant stimuli.

Most telling, perhaps, according to Abbs and Cole, the perioral reflex is not very sensitive to movement velocities in the speech range. They propose that the reflex is part of a generalized response to aversive or potentially injurious stimuli.

A more promising source of information concerning coordination in speech may be offered by studies of temporary, functional coordinations among articulators as studied by Abbs and his colleagues (Folkins and Abbs, 1975, 1976; see also Kelso et al., 1982). Specifically, a talker can achieve the "orosensory goal" of bilabial closure in a variety of ways involving different contributions of the jaw and the two lips. Indeed, in different syllable contexts, talkers will exhibit different relative contributions of these three structures (Sussman et al., 1973). For example, in the context of a high vowel, the jaw will contribute relatively more to closure of a bilabial consonant than in the context of a low vowel. This "context-conditioned variability" can be viewed in a variety of ways, as discussed earlier, but so far as efficiency of regulation is concerned, an efficient way to ensure bilabial closure but allow contextual influences would be to establish a coordinated relationship among the articulators so that they bear, in effect, a negative relationship to each other. Any decrease in the contribution of the jaw, then, by virtue of the jaw's relationship to the lips would give rise to a corresponding increase in the contribution of the upper or lower lip, or both.

This, in fact, appears to characterize the jaw–lip relationship during bilabial consonant production (Folkins and Abbs, 1975, 1976; Kelso et al., 1982). Unexpected jaw loading during closing for a bilabial stop gives rise to compensatory lip movement so that closure is achieved. The same compensatory relationship is observed both during unperturbed repeated productions of bilabial consonants in a vocalic context (Hughes and Abbs, 1976; but see Sussman, 1980), and, as already noted, during production of bilabial consonants in the context of vowels varying in height.

In contrast to the general excitability of the perioral reflex, excitatory lip activity is not observed to the same degree if jaw closing is impeded during production of a nonlabial consonant (Kelso, Tuller, and Fowler, 1982). That is, for example, if jaw closing for /z/ in /baez/ is impeded, the upper lip does not show the same magnitude of increase in excitation that it shows when jaw closing for final /b/ in /baeb/ is impeded. This suggests a temporary coupling of jaw and lips established only when bilabial closure is a goal of articulatory gestures.

Abbs and Kennedy (1982) refer to this mode of control as "open-loop, feed-forward" control. It is open loop in the sense that afferent information about jaw postion appears not to feed back to jaw closing muscles as it would if the system were "closed loop." Instead, it feeds "forward" to other articulators—here, the lips—thereby coordinating the activities of the different articulators for the achievement of an articulatory goal.

Similar couplings between jaw and tongue for vowels and lingual consonants have not been studied systematically. However, Chuang, Abbs, and Netsell (1978) find negative correlations between jaw and tongue positions in repeated productions of some vowels. As for lingual consonants, Kelso and colleagues (1982) find on-line compensatory activity of the genioglossus to unpredicted jaw perturbations during closure for /z/ in /baez/, but not during closing for final /b/ in /baeb/.

These coordinations of articulators to achieve a common outcome also achieve the selective loss of degrees of freedom characteristic of a coordinated system. Moreover, by interacting, the jaw–lip and jaw–tongue systems may further reduce controlled degrees of freedom. Figure 6–14 is a schematic illustration of this idea. It plots the jaw–lip–tongue relationship suggested by the study of Sussman and colleagues (1973) and by the studies of compensatory behavior just described. The figure indicates that jaw height during bilabial closure varies due to vocalic context. This implies that neighboring (coarticulated) segments help to choose which particular values of jaw height and lip positions will occur in production of a particular bilabial-consonant token. In addition, however, the jaw-height requirements of the consonant will help to select the relative contribution of the jaw and tongue movements to vowel production. It is as if the bilabial consonant coordinate structure and the vowel coordinative structure share control for a period of time over a common set of articulatory variables. Because both sets of functional coordinative relationships must hold during overlapping time slots, each constrains the values that the shared variables will take. To the extent that there is a unique or nearly unique value of the shared variables that allow both coordinative relationships to hold, the number of controlled degrees of freedom in the system is further reduced.

Cyclicity in Behavior

Research on language production and that on systematic properties of linguistic utterances both uncover "metrical structures." These are

Figure 6–14. Schematic illustration of jaw, lip and tongue coordination for production of a bilabial consonant/vowel syllable, and for production of bite-block speech. See the text for elaboration.

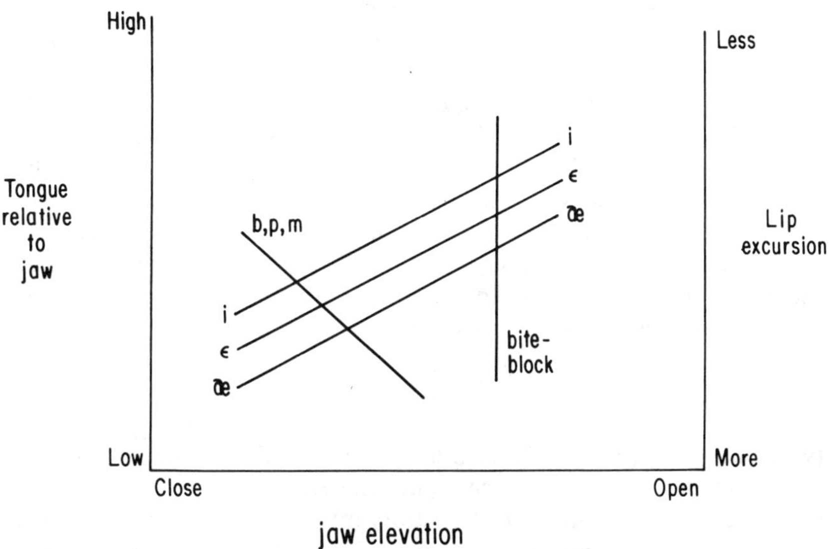

remarkable in two respects as already discussed. They are not necessarily coextensive with linguistic units, and they suggest underlying cyclicity in talking.

I have not found any rationale for these structures in language itself; yet the literature on speech production has suffered no insights, either. In this final section of the paper, the question is asked whether a rationale could be developed within the study of speech production.

Research findings on performance of cyclic motor skills other than speech recently have been interpreted in the light of the physical theory of the dynamics of "open" physical systems (e.g., Kugler, Kelso, and Turvey, 1982). For reasons to be discussed shortly, such physical systems—which include biological ones—are inherently cyclical in nature. The following section examines this view of physical systems in relation to the performance of skilled activity. (The discussion is taken from Kelso, Tuller, and Harris [1983] and Kelso, Holt, Rubin, and Kugler (1981), who provide more detail.) Next the relevance that this theory may have for understanding metrical structures in speech is considered.

According to Kelso and associates (1981), until recently, the physical theory of dynamics has had little to offer in the way of explaining biological activity because it has dealt largely with "closed" physical systems. Closed systems do not exchange energy and matter with their environments. Whereas closed systems very evidently "obey" the second law of thermodynamics—that is, they move toward states of decreasing organization—open systems, including biological systems, "accumulate negentropy" (Schrodinger, 1945). Thereby they are able to develop and maintain their organized forms and functions over long periods of time.

Open systems maintain their forms and functions by offsetting energy losses with periodic energy gains. Energy flow into and out of the system is a chief organizing property of living systems; moreover, tracking the flow of energy from "source" to "sink" identifies one cycle in a necessarily cyclic life style of the system (Morowitz, 1978, cited in Kelso et al., 1981). How is the cyclicity realized? To illustrate cyclicity in living systems, Kelso and associates (1981; see also Kelso et al., 1983) begin by describing a familiar oscillatory system: a linear damped mass-spring system. This system is described by the following equation:

$$m\ddot{x} + c\dot{x} + k\dot{x} = 0$$

(where m is mass, k is stiffness, and c is a frictional component; x, $\dot{x}$, and $\ddot{x}$, refer to displacement, velocity, and acceleration, respectively). Set in motion by a displacement, its oscillatory motion decays over time as the second law of thermodynamics predicts. To prevent decay, the system has to be supplied with an energy source:

$m\ddot{x} + cx + k\dot{x} = F(\Theta)$ (where k is stiffness, F is force, $F(\Theta)$ is a forcing function, and other variables are as above).

To be usable, the energy source has to be tapped by the system at the proper phase in the cycle. In living systems, and in some nonliving systems, this requirement is met by an "escapement"—a nonlinear element that taps an energy source and injects it into the system at the proper phase in its cycle. (Pendulum clocks have escapements which ensure that potential energy from a hanging weight is delivered to the swinging pendulum only in the middle of its arc where the pendulum is most effectively influenced by outside forces; see Fitch, Tuller, and Turvey, 1982.) An example of the escapement principle in skilled activity is provided by research or Orlovskii (1972). Orlovskii found that stimulation of the red nucleus of the cat excited flexion in the resting limb. Stimulation of Deiter's nucleus excited extension. During locomotion, however, continuous stimulation of the red (Deiter's) nucleus energized flexion (extension) only during the swing (stance) phase of the stepping cycle. In short, the supraspinal "energy source" supplied by stimulation of the red and Deiter's nuclei was tapped by the spinal locomotion system only during appropriate phases of the stepping cycle.

Nonlinear oscillators with the escapement property are called "limit cycle oscillators" and they are believed to characterize systems such as living ones that maintain themselves consistently far from thermodynamic equilibrium (e.g., Yates, 1980; Yates and Iberall, 1973; and others cited in Kelso et al., 1981).

According to Kelso and associates, limit cycle oscillators have at least some of the characteristics exhibited by muscle systems engaged in functional activity. In addition to their cyclicity and the escapement property already discussed, two other characteristics are salient. First, because of the escapement feature, "power" and timing are independent. That is, for example, in a pendulum clock, increasing the amount of energy that is injected into the system in the middle of a pendulum swing does not affect *when* in the cycle the injection occurs. The same feature, invariant relative timing, over changes in amplitude of muscle activation has already been described for speech and other activities. Second, limit cycles exhibit at least some varieties of "equifinality." Their cycles are stable and return to normal very soon after perturbation.

What, if anything, can the concept of limit cycle contribute to understanding metrical structures in speech? An answer will have to await more careful study and investigation. However, the concept is promising because it rationalizes cyclicity in activity and that is partly the aspect of metrical structures that needs understanding.

The "breath group," and ideally, the domain of declination, appear to be natural "cyclers" of the limit cycle variety. From this perspective, inspiration provides a source of potential energy used during utterance production. For different reasons, a syllable also appears subsumable under the idea of a limit cycle mode of functioning (see Kelso and Bateson, 1983, for an elaboration of this idea). Finally, stressing may be a reflection of energy injection into the articulators. An idea compatible with this concept is that of Catford (1977), who has suggested that "isochrony" of the stress foot may not be isochrony in fact, but rather "isodynamism"—an injection of about the same amount of "initiator power" (that is, work done per unit time by a pulmonic pressure pulse) for each foot. This idea does not shed light on why the foot is the domain of the pressure pulses. Conceivably, the principle is simply one of alternation—one pulse approximately every other syllable.

CONCLUDING REMARKS

The intent of this chapter was to review most of what researchers are researching and writing about language and speech production. Several concluding observations are suggested by the review.

1. Researchers have devoted little attention to the relation of speech to language. This has allowed models of each to be developed that have limited bearing one on the other and that together posit, in my view, implausibly many computational planning and execution stages of production. In addition, the default view of the relation of speech to language suggested by researchers—namely, that planned linguistic units are *translated* into articulatory gestures—raises what seem to be insurmountable difficulties that can be avoided if the view of the relationship of speech to language depicted in Figure 6-8*b* is adopted.

2. Figure 6-8*b* allows for physical systems, by virtue of their superordinate organization, to embody psychological (cognitive, mental) functions. In my view, an important avenue for future research is one of understanding this characteristic of complex living systems, and of seeing how it is exploited to reduce the number of computationally or representationally controlled aspects of talking.

3. Research, theorizing, and modeling in speech and language production have been somewhat narrow in scope. If a language production researcher studies and models the structure of pausing in language production, he or she is unlikely to constrain theorizing and modeling by reference to data on spontaneous errors of speech, for example, or even to data on durational shortening in speech production. Collectively, researchers in the fields of language and speech production know a great deal about the superficial systematic properties of utterances. It becomes important now to attempt a realistic comprehensive theory of their underlying causes.[1]

FOOTNOTES

[1]This research was supported by NSF Grant BNS 8111470 and by NICHD Grant HD 16591-01 to Haskins Laboratories. I thank Elliot Saltzman and George Wolford for their comments on parts of the manuscript.

REFERENCES

Abbs, J., and Cole, K. (1982). Considerations of bulbar and suprabulbar afferent influences upon speech motor coordination and programming. In S. Grillner, B. Lindblom, J. Lubker, and A. Persson (Eds.), *Speech motor control.* Oxford: Pergamon.

Abbs, J., and Kennedy, J. (1982). Neurophysiological processes of speech movement control. In N. Lass (Ed.), *Speech, language and hearing* (Vol. 1). Philadelphia: Saunders.

Abercrombie, D. (1964). Syllable quantity and enclitics in English. In D. Abercrombie, D. Fry, P. MacCarthy, N. Scott, and J. Trim (Eds.), *In honour of Daniel Jones.* London: Longman.

Baars, B. (1980). On eliciting predictable speech errors in the laboratory. In V. Fromkin (Ed.), *Errors in linguistic performance: Slips of the tongue, ear, pen and hand.* New York: Academic Press.

Baars, B., Motley, M., and MacKay, D. (1975). Output editing for lexical access in artificially elicited slips of the tongue. *Journal of Verbal Learning and Verbal Behavior, 14,* 382–391.

Barry, W., and Kuenzel, H. (1975). Co-articulatory airflow characteristics of intervocalic voiceless plosives. *Journal of Phonetics, 3,* 263–282.

Bell-Berti, F. (1980). Velopharyngeal function: A spatial–temporal model. In N. Lass (Ed.), *Advances in basic research and practice.* New York: Academic Press.

Bell-Berti, F., and Harris, K. (1976). Some aspects of coarticulation. *Haskins Laboratories Status Report on Speech Research, SR 45/46,* 197–204.

Bell-Berti, F., and Harris, K. (1979). Anticipatory coarticulation: Some implications from a study of lip rounding. *Journal of the Acoustical Society of America,* 1268–1270.

Bell-Berti, F., and Harris, K. (1981). A temporal model of speech production. *Phonetica, 38,* 9–20.

Benguerel, A. P., and Cowan, H. A. (1974). Coarticulation of upper lip protrusion in French. *Phonetica, 30,* 41–55.

Bernstein, N. (1967). *The coordination and regulation of movement.* London: Pergamon.

Bladon, A., and Al-Bamerni, A. (1982a). One-stage and two-stage temporal patterns of velar coarticulation. Paper presented to the Acoustical Society of America, Orlando, FL.

Bladon, A., and Al-Bamerni, A. (1982b). Nasal coarticulation of pharyngeal and glottal consonants: A deductive account. Paper presented to the Acoustical Society of America, Orlando, FL.

Bolinger, D. (1963). Length, vowel, juncture. *Linguistics, 1,* 1–29.

Breckenridge, J. (1977). Declination as a phonological process. Bell Laboratories Technological Memo. Murray Hill, NJ.

Butcher, A., and Weiher, E. (1976). An electropalatographic investigation of coarticulation in VCV sequences. *Journal of Phonetics, 4,* 59–74.

Carney, P., and Moll, K. (1971). A cinefluorographic investigation of fricative-consonant vowel coarticulation. *Phonetica, 23,* 193–201.

Catford, J. C. (1977). *Fundamental problems in phonetics.* Bloomington, IN: Indiana Univ. Press.

Chuang, C. K., Abbs, J., and Netsell, R. (1978). Possible role of tongue–hard palate contact in vowel production. *Journal of the Acoustical Society of America, 63,* Supplement 1.

Cohen, A., Collier, R., and t'Hart, J. (1982). Declination: Construct or intrinsic feature of speech pitch? *Phonetica, 39,* 254–273.

Cooper, W., and Paccia-Cooper, J. (1980). *Syntax and speech.* Cambridge, MA: Harvard University Press.

Cooper, W., and Sorenson, J. (1981). *Fundamental frequency in sentence production.* New York: Springer-Verlag.

Cutler, A. (Ed.) (1982). *Slips of the tongue.* The Hague: Mouton.

Daniloff, R., and Hammarberg, R. (1973). On defining coarticulation. *Journal of Phonetics, 1,* 239–248.

Dell, G. (1980). *Phonological and lexical encoding in speech production: An analysis of naturally occurring and experimentally elicited slips of the tongue.* PhD thesis, University of Toronto.

Dell, G., and Reich, P. (1980). Toward a unified model of slips of the tongue. In V. Fromkin (Ed.), *Errors in linguistic performance: Slips of the tongue, ear, pen and hand.* New York: Academic Press.

Dell, G., and Reich, P. (1981). Stages in speech production: An analysis of speech error data. *Journal of Verbal Learning and Verbal Behavior, 20,* 611–629.

Donegan, P., and Stampe, D. (1979). The study of natural phonology. In D. Dinnsen (Ed.), *Current approaches to phonological theory.* Bloomington, IN: Indiana University Press.

Fant, G. (1962). Descriptive analysis of the acoustic aspects of speech. *Logos, 5,* 3–17.

Fay, D., and Cutler, A. (1977). Malapropisms and the structure of the mental lexicon. *Linguistic Inquiry, 8,* 505–520.

Fitch, H., Tuller, B., and Turvey, M. T. (1982). The Bernstein perspective. III. Tuning of coordinative structures with special reference to perception. In J. A. S. Kelso (Ed.), *Human motor behavior: An introduction.* Hillsdale, NJ: Lawrence Erlbaum Associates.

Folkins, J., and Abbs, J. (1975). Lip and jaw motor control during speech: Responses to resistive loading of the jaw. *Journal of Speech and Hearing Research, 18,* 207–220.

Folkins, J., and Abbs, J. (1976). Additional observations on responses to resistive loading of the jaw. *Journal of Speech and Hearing Research, 19,* 820–821.

Fowler, C. (1977). *Timing control in speech production.* Bloomington, IN: Indiana University Linguistics Club.

Fowler, C. (1980). Coarticulation and theories of extrinsic timing. *Journal of Phonetics, 8,* 113–133.

Fowler, C. (1981a). A relationship between coarticulation and compensatory shortening. *Phonetica, 38,* 35–50.

Fowler, C. (1981b). Production and perception of coarticulation among stressed and unstressed vowels. *Journal of Speech and Hearing Research,* 127–139.

Fowler, C., Rubin, P., Remez, R., and Turvey, M. T. (1980). Implications for speech production of a general theory of action. In B. Butterworth (Ed.), *Language production,* Vol. 1. London: Academic Press.

Fowler, C., and Turvey, M. T. (1980). Immediate compensation for biteblock speech. *Phonetica, 37,* 306–326.

Freud, S. (1958). *The psychopathology of everyday life.* New York: New American Library [1901].

Fromkin, V. (Ed.) (1973). *Speech errors as linguistic evidence.* The Hague: Mouton.

Fromkin, V. (Ed.) (1980). *Errors in linguistic performance: Slips of the tongue, ear, pen and hand.* London: Academic Press.

Fujimura, O. (1980). Elementary gestures and temporal organization: What does articulatory constraint mean? In T. Myers, J. Laver, and J. Anderson (Eds.), *The cognitive representation of speech.* Amsterdam: North-Holland.

Fujimura, O. (1981). Temporal organization of articulatory movements as multidimensional phrasal structures. *Phonetica, 38,* 66–83.

Fukuda, T. (1961). Studies on human dynamic postures from the viewpoint of postural reflexes. *Acta Otolaryngologica* Supplement 161.

Garding, E. (1979). Sentence intonation in Swedish. *Phonetica, 36,* 207–215.

Garrett, M. (1975). The analysis of sentence production. In G. Bower (Ed.), *The psychology of learning and motivation,* Vol. 9. New York: Academic Press.

Garrett, M. (1976). Syntactic processes in sentence production. In R. J. Wales and E. Walker (Eds.), *New approaches to language mechanisms.* Amsterdam: North-Holland.

Garrett, M. (1980a). Levels of processing in sentence production. In B. Butterworth (Ed.), *Language production,* Vol. I. London: Academic Press.

Garrett, M. (1980b). The limits of accommodation: Arguments for independent levels in sentence production. In V. Fromkin (Ed.), *Errors in linguistic performance: Slips of the tongue, ear, pen and hand.* London: Academic Press.

Gee, P., and Grosjean, G. (1983). Performance structures: A psycholinguistic and linguistic appraisal. *Cognitive Psychology, 15,* 411–458.

Gottleib, G., Agawarl, G., and Stark, L. (1970). Interactions between voluntary and postural mechanisms of the human motor system. *Journal of Neurophysiology. 33,* 365–381.

Grillner, S. (1975). Locomotion in vertebrates. *Physiological Reviews, 55,* 247–304.

Grosjean, F., Grosjean, L., and Lane, H. (1979). The patterns of silence: Performance structures in sentence production. *Cognition, 11,* 58–81.

Hamlet, S., and Stone, M. (1976). Compensatory vowel characteristics resulting from the presence of different types of experimental dental prostheses. *Journal of Phonetics, 4,* 199–218.

Hammarberg, R. (1976). The metaphysics of coarticulation. *Journal of Phonetics, 4,* 353–363.

Hammarberg, R. (1982). On redefining coarticulation. *Journal of Phonetics, 10,* 123–137.

Henke, W. (1966). *Dynamic articulatory model of speech production using computer simulation.* PhD thesis, Massachusetts Institute of Technology, Cambridge.

Hockett, C. (1960). The origin of speech. *Scientific American, 203,* 89–96.

Huggins, A. W. F. (1975). On isochrony and speech. In G. Fant and M. Tatham (Eds.), *Auditory analysis and perception of speech.* London: Academic Press.

Huggins, A. W. F. (1978). Speech timing and intelligibility. In J. Requin (Ed.), *Attention and performance,* Vol 7. Hillsdale, NJ: Lawrence Erlbaum Associates.

Hughes, O., and Abbs, J. (1976). Labial mandibular coordination in the production of speech: Implications for motor equivalence. *Phonetica, 33,* 199–221.

Kelso, J. A. S., and Bateson, E. (1983). On the cyclical basis of speech production. *Journal of the Acoustical Society of America, 73,* Supplement 1, S67.

Kelso, J. A. S., Holt, K., Rubin, P., and Kugler, P. (1981). Patterns of human interlimb coordination emerge from the properties of nonlinear oscillators: Theory and data. *Journal of Motor Behavior. 13,* 226–261.

Kelso, J. A. S., Tuller, B., and Fowler, C. (1982). The functional specificity of articulatory control and coordination. *Journal of the Acoustical Society of America, 72,* S103.

Kelso, J. A. S., Tuller, B., and Harris, K. (1983). A "dynamic pattern" perspective on the control and coordination of movement. In P. MacNeilage (Ed.), *The production of speech.* New York: Springer-Verlag.

Kent, R. (1983). The segmental organization of speech. In P. MacNeilage (Ed.), *The production of speech.* New York: Springer-Verlag.

Kent, R., Carney, P., and Severeid, L. (1974). Velar movement and timing: Evaluation of a model for binary control. *Journal of Speech and Hearing Research, 17,* 470–488.

Kent, R., and Minifie, F. (1977). Coarticulation in recent speech production models. *Journal of Phonetics, 5,* 115–117.

Kent, R, and Moll, K. (1972). Tongue body articulation during vowel and diphthong gestures. *Folia Phoniatrica, 24,* 286–300.

Kenstowicz, M., and Kisseberth, C. (1979). *Generative phonology: Description and theory.* New York: Academic Press.

Klatt, D. (1976). Linguistic uses of segment duration in English: Acoustic and perceptual evidence. *Journal of the Acoustical Society of America, 1976, 59,* 1208–1221.

Klatt, D. (1980). Speech perception: A model of acoustic–perceptual analysis and lexical access. In R. Cole (Ed.), *Perception and production of fluent speech.* Hillsdale, NJ: Lawrence Erlbaum Associates.

Klima, E., and Bellugi, U. (1979). *The signs of language.* Cambridge, MA: Harvard University Press.

Kuehn, D., and Moll, K. (1976). A cineradiographic study of VC and CV articulatory velocities. *Journal of Phonetics, 4,* 303–320.

Kugler, P., Kelso, J. A. S., and Turvey, M. T. (1980). On the concept of coordination as dissipative structure. I. Theoretical lines of convergence. In G. Stelmach and J. Requin (Eds.), *Tutorials in motor behavior.* Amsterdam: Elsevier/North-Holland.

Kugler, P., Kelso, J. A. S., and Turvey, M. T. (1982). On the control and coordination of naturally developing systems. In J. A. S. Kelso and J. Clark (Eds.), *The development of movement control and coordination.* New York: Wiley.

Kupin, J. (1979). *Tongue twisters as a source of information about speech production.* PhD thesis, University of Connecticut, Storrs.

Lamb, S. (1966). *Outline of stratificational grammar.* Washington, DC: Georgetown University Press, 1966.

Lass, N., and Davis, M. (1976). An investigation of speaker height and weight identification. *Journal of the Acoustical Society of America, 60,* 700–703.

Lehiste, I. (1980). Phonetic manifestations of syntactic structure in English. *Bulletin of the Research Institute of Logopedics and Phoniatrics, 14,* 1–27.

Liberman, M., & Prince, A. (1977). On stress and linguistic rhythm. *Linguistic Inguiry, 8,* 249–336.

Lindblom, B. (1971). Phonetics and the description of language. *Seventh International Congress of Phonetic Sciences.* The Hague: Mouton.

Lindblom, B., Lubker, J., & Gay, T. (1979). Formant frequencies of some fixed-mandible vowels and a model of speech motor programming by predictive simulation. *Journal of Phonetics, 7,* 147–161.

Lindblom, B., Lyberg, B., & Holmgren K. (1981). *Durational patterns of Swedish phonology: Do they reflect short-term memory processes?* Bloomington, IN: Indiana University Linguistics Club.

Lindblom, B., & Rapp, K. (1973). Some temporal regularities of spoken Swedish. *Papers in Linguistics from the University of Stockholm, 21,* 1–59.

Lockwood, D. (1972). *Introduction to stratificational linguistics.* New York: Harcourt, Brace, Jovanovich.

Lyberg, B. (1979). Final lengthening—partly a consequence of restrictions on the speech of fundamental frequency change? *Journal of Phonetics, 7,* 187–196.

Lyberg, B. (1981). Temporal properties of spoken Swedish. *Monographs in linguistics from the University of Stockholm,* Vol. 6.

MacKay, D. (1982). The problems of flexibility, fluency and speed–accuracy tradeoff. *Psychological Review, 89,* 483–506.

MacNeilage, P. (1970). Motor control of serial ordering in speech. *Psychological Review, 77,* 182–196.

MacNeilage, P., & DeClerk, J. (1969). On the motor control of coarticulation in CVC monosyllables. *Journal of the Acoustical Society of America, 45,* 1217–1233.

MacNeilage, P., & Ladefoged, P. (1976). The production of speech and language. In E. C. Carterette & M. Friedman (Eds.), *Handbook of perception: Language and speech.* New York: Academic Press.

Maeda, S. (1976). *A characterization of American English intonation.* PhD thesis, Massachusetts Institute of Technology, Cambridge.

McClean, M. (1978). Variation in the perioral reflex amplitude prior to lip muscle contraction for speech. *Journal of Speech and Hearing Research, 21,* 276–284.

McClean, M., Folkins, J., and Larson, C. (1979). The role of the perioral reflex in lip motor control. *Brain and Language, 7,* 42–61.

McClelland, J., and Rumelhart, D. (1981). An interactive activation model of context effects in letter perception. *Psychological Review, 88,* 375–407.

Merringer, R., and Meyer, K. (1895). *Versprechen und Verlesen: Eine Psycholigisch–Linguistiche Studie.* Stuttgart: Goschensche Verlagsbuchhandlung. (Reissued: Amsterdam: John Benjamin, 1978).

Moll, K., and Daniloff, R. (1971). Investigation of the timing of velar movements during speech. *Journal of the Acoustical Society of America, 50,* 678–684.

Morowitz, H. J. (1978). *Foundations of bioenergetics.* New York: Academic Press.

Netsell, R., & Abbs, J. (1975). Modulations of perioral sensitivity during speech movements. Paper presented to the Acoustical Society of America, San Francisco.

Norman, D. (1980). Copycat science or Does the mind really work by table look-up? In R. Cole (Ed.), *Perception and production of fluent speech.* Hillsdale, NJ: Lawrence Erlbaum Associates.

Norman, D. (1981). Categorization of action slips. *Psychological Review, 88,* 1–15.

Ohala, J. (1971). Monitoring soft palate movements in speech. *Project on linguistic analysis reports.* (Phonology Laboratory, Department of Linguistics, University of California, Berkeley), 13, JO1–J05.

Ohala, J. (1981). The listener as a source of sound change. In M. F. Miller (Ed.), *Papers from the parasession on language behavior.* Chicago: Chicago Linguistic Association.

Ohala, J., & Ewan, W. (1973). Speed of pitch change. *Journal of the Acoustical Society of America, 53,* 345(A).

Ohman, S. (1966). Coarticulation in VCV utterances: Spectrographic measures. *Journal of the Acoustical Society of America, 39,* 151–168.

Orlovskii, G. (1972). The effect of different descending systems on flexion and extensor activity during locomotion. *Brain Research, 40,* 359–371.

Pattee, H. H. (1973). The physical bases and origin of hierarchical control. In H. H. Pattee (Ed.), *Hierarchy theory: The challenge of complex systems.* New York: Braziller.

Pattee, H. H. (1976). Physical theories of biological coordination. In M. Grene and E. Mendelsohn (Eds.), *Topics in the philosophy of biology.* Dordrecht, Holland: Reidel.

Pattee, H. H. (1977). Dynamic and linguistic modes of complex systems. *International Journal of Complex Systems, 3,* 259–266.

Perkell, J. (1969). *Physiology of speech production: Results and implications of a quantitative cineradiographic study.* Cambridge, MA: MIT Press.

Perkell, J. (1980). Phonetic features and the physiology of speech production. In B. Butterworth (Ed.), *Language production,* Vol. I. London: Academic Press.

Polanyi, M. (1962). *Personal knowledge.* Chicago: University of Chicago Press.

Prince, A. (1983). Relating to the grid. *Linguistic Inquiry, 19–100.*

Reich, P. (1970). *A relational-network model of language behavior.* PhD thesis, University of Michigan, Ann Arbor.

Repp, B. (1981). On levels of description in speech research. *Journal of the Acoustical Society of America, 69,* 1462–1464.

Ryle, G. (1949). *The concept of mind.* New York: Barnes & Noble.

Sampson, G. (1980). *Schools of linguistics.* Stanford, CA: Stanford University Press.

Scherer, K. (1981). Speech and emotional states. In J. Darley (Ed.), *The evaluation of speech in psychiatry.* New York: Grune & Stratton.

Scherer, K. (1982). Methods of research on vocal communication: Paradigms and parameters. In K. Scherer and P. Ekman (Eds.), *Handbook of methods in nonverbal behavior research.* Cambridge: Cambridge University Press.

Selkirk, E. (1980a). The role of prosodic categories in English word stress. *Linguistic Inquiry, 11,* 563–605.

Selkirk, E. (1980b). *On prosodic structure and its relation to syntactic structure.* Bloomington, IN: Indiana University Linguistics Club.

Shattuck-Hufnagel, S. (1979). Speech errors as evidence for a serial-ordering mechanism in sentence production. In Cooper, W. and Walker, E. (Eds.), *Sentence processing.* Hillsdale, NJ: Lawrence Erlbaum Associates.

Shik, M., and Orlovskii, G. (1965). Coordination of the limbs during running of the dog. *Biophysics, 10,* 1148–1159.

Shrodinger, E. (1945). *What is life?* London: Cambridge University Press.

Simon, H. (1980). How to win at twenty questions with nature. In R. Cole (Ed.), *Perception and production of fluent speech.* Hillsdale, NJ: Lawrence Erlbaum Associates.

Smith, E., & Medin, D. (1981). *Categories and concepts.* Cambridge, MA: Harvard University Press, 1981.

Sorenson, J., & Cooper, W. (1980). Syntactic coding of fundamental frequency in speech production. In R. Cole (Ed.), *Perception and production of fluent speech.* Hillsdale, NJ: Lawrence Erlbaum Associates.

Stemberger, J. (1982). *The lexicon in model of language production.* PhD thesis, University of California, San Diego.

Sternberg, S., Monsell, S., Knoll, R., and Wright, C. (1978). The latency and duration of rapid movement sequences: Comparison of speech and typewriting. In G. Stelmach (Ed.), *Information processing in motor control and learning.* New York: Academic Press.

Sternberg, S., Wright, C., Knoll, R., and Monsell, S. (1980). Motor programs in rapid speech: Additional evidence. In R. Cole (Ed.), *Perception and production of fluent speech.* Hillsdale, NJ: Lawrence Erlbaum Associates.

Stevens, K., & Blumstein, S. (1981). The search for invariant correlates of phonetic features. In P. Eimas and J. Miller (Eds.), *Perspectives on the study of speech.* Hillsdale, NJ: Lawrence Erlbaum Associates.

Studdert-Kennedy, M. (1980). Language by hand and by eye: A review of Edward S. Klima and Ursula Bellugi's *The signs of language. Cognition, 8,* 93–108.

Sundberg, J. (1979). Maximum speed of pitch changes in singers and untrained subjects. *Journal of Phonetics, 7,* 71–79.

Sussman, H. (1980). Methodological problems in evaluating lip–jaw reciprocity as an index of motor equivalence. *Journal of Speech and Hearing Research, 23,* 699–702.

Sussman, H., MacNeilage, P., & Hanson, R. (1973). Labial and mandibular dynamics during the production of bilabial consonants: Preliminary observations. *Journal of Speech and Hearing Research, 16,* 397–420.

Sussman, H., and Westbury, J. (1981). The effects of antagonistic gestures on temporal and amplitude parameters of anticipatory labial coarticulation. *Journal of the Acoustical Society of America, 46,* 16–24.

Tarttar, V. (1980). Happy talk: Perceptual and acoustic effects of smiling on speech. *Perception and Psychophysics, 27,* 24–27.

Terzuolo, C., and Viviani, P. (1979). The central representation of learned motor patterns. In R. Talbott and D. Humphrey (Eds.), *Posture and movement.* New York: Raven Press.

Tuller, B., Kelso, J. A. S., and Harris, K. (1982). Interarticulator phasing as an index of temporal regularity in speech. *Journal of Experimental Psychology: Human Perception and Performance, 8,* 460–472.

Turvey, M. T. (1977). Preliminaries to a theory of action with reference to vision. In R. Shaw and J. Bransford (Eds.), *Perceiving, acting and knowing: Toward an ecological psychology.* Hillsdale, NJ: Lawrence Erlbaum Associates.

Viviani, P., & Terzuolo, C. (1980). Space–time invariance in learned motor skills. In G. Stelmach & J. Requin (Eds.), *Tutorials in motor behavior.* Amsterdam: Elsevier/North-Holland.

von Holst, E. (1973). *The behavioral physiology of animals and man: The collected papers of Erich von Holst.* London: Methuen (originally published in 1937).

Weiss, P. (1941). Self-differentiation of the basic pattern of coordination. *Comparative Psychology Monographs, 17,* 21–96.

Wickelgren, W. (1969). Auditory or articulatory coding in verbal short-term memory. *Psychological Review, 76,* 232–235.

Wickelgren, W. (1976). Phonetic coding and serial order. In E. C. Carterette and M. P. Friedman (Eds.), *Handbook of perception: Language and speech.* New York: Academic Press.

Williams, C., and Stevens, K. (1972). Emotions and speech: Acoustical correlates. *Journal of the Acoustical Society of America, 52,* 1238–1250.

Yates, F. (1980). Physical causality and brain theories. *American Journal of Physiology, 238,* R277–R290.

Yates, F., and Iberall, A. (1973). Temporal and hierarchical origin in biosystems. In J. Urquhart and F. Yates (Eds.), *Temporal aspects of therapeutics.* New York: Plenum.

CHAPTER 7
Electromyographic Invariance of Lip Closure for /p/–/b/

Marcel A. A. Tatham
Raymond G. Daniloff
Paul R. Hoffman

This chapter reports the results of a study that continues a line of research (Tatham and Morton, 1968, 1970, 1973) on the use of surface electromyographic (EMG) recordings to make critical inferences about how coarticulatory and distinctive feature effects are manifested in simple articulatory movements. The study is relatively large scale to control as many artifacts as possible.

Above all, our aim has been to cast our study of articulatory invariance in a linguistic context. That is, we are first and foremost linguists, placing our laboratory-derived data in the general framework of the study of language (Tatham, 1980). Our data have little relevance outside of a linguistic context.

As linguists we have adopted the now generally accepted view that language is a means of encoding and decoding thought as sound. The encoding process, at least (since that is the side of the coin that has attracted most research effort in linguistics), proceeds in the model we have of language (which is essentially Chomskyan in origin) in more or less well defined stages beginning with a cognitively placed generation of sentences. We subscribe to the idea that a conditioning or interpreting of these sentences (construed as cognitive objects) occurs prior to the use of the vocal apparatus to produce speech sounds. This interpretation is called phonology, and is active, voluntary, and therefore also cognitively placed. The business of phonology is to interpret sentences according to a language's established rules for doing so, and according to some necessary procedures in such a way as to provide them with a phonetic specification that permits their realization as actual sound. This general position is uncontroversial today, but it has led many researchers to ascribe a noncognitive automatic role to the final phonetic stages of the process. We shall return to this point a little later.

Many of the rules that occur in phonology are idiosyncratic in the sense that no reason connected with, say, encoding efficiency can be found to justify their inclusion. Such, for example, is the distribution of palatalized and velarized /1/ in English. Having two surface [ɫ]'s is not motivated by morphemic considerations (no two morphemes are differentiated by them), nor by articulatory considerations (one is not easier or better than the other in any particular phonetic context), nor by mechanical or other similar considerations (specific groupings of muscles or muscular cooperation do not make either more likely in particular contexts), nor by acoustic or perceptual considerations. There is a simple demonstration of these facts: many languages do not have two [ɫ]'s, and even those that do (where their distribution is not of morphemic importance) the rules can be violated easily both cognitively and physically.

Other rules in the phonology are less easily ascribed to an idiosyncratic role. Aspiration of initial [−voice] stops and the lengthening of vowels before [+voice] consonants are two such rules. It is still arguable whether these phenomena are basically phonetically dominated in the sense that they are phonetically *necessary* or physically *natural,* and that they may somehow or other have become caught up in the cognitive areas of phonology (Tatham, 1984). There has been discussion elsewhere of how a physical tendency might be manipulated cognitively at various levels in the phonological encoding process (Tatham and Morton, 1983).

Much recent work has discussed the extent to which there are low-level combinatorial constraints on what at one time were taken to be independently controllable features of articulation. Those low-level constraints may be essential hardware (Fowler, 1980, 1983; Fowler, Rubin, Remez, and Turvey, 1980) or firmware, or both (Tatham, 1984). *In encoding terms it can be argued convincingly that prephonetic specifications are relatively simple and that some physically dominated articulation generator takes care of specific overall gestures.* Such an image is consistent with the analogy of a matrix printer's or graphics terminal's character generator which is triggered by somewhat "simpler" input than its resultant ouput—rather like the Morse code dot triggering an *e.* Notice that *e* can have many shapes depending on font, and so forth, and that the single dot of the code does not, in a sense, represent any of these, but rather some *e-ness* common to, or dominating all possible physical shape manifestations of the letter.

We concur with this general view, but we believe that it opens up considerable areas for discussion as to the nature and permanence (for want of a better word) of the interpretation of the dot by the articulation generator. Is the generator reprogrammable, for example, or is it fixed by some extralinguistic rules of motor control or articulator functioning? Can the overall articulation so generated be subtly modified by some cognitive intervention, as we have recently argued? In general, the idea of some low-level physical articulation generator seems very plausible and fits the broad picture of the data rather well, but on a detailed inspection certain questions arise regarding the flexibility of the system. This in turn raises questions of cognitive manipulation, at a *phonetic* level, of the system (Tatham and Morton, 1980).

Our study did not set out to answer these questions, which arise because of the philosophy we have adopted. It merely sought to examine the enormous problem of relating a mentally oriented phonology to a physically oriented phonetics. Philosophically we have no answers, of course, but we have tried to clarify some tiny area of what a theory which does link the two must account for.

There are those phonologists who would argue that in the current theory phonology describes, as part of linguistics, a closed system. That is, abstract phonology is not about deriving a phonetics but simply a characterization of a language's sound pattern. That is all well and good, but while acknowledging this position, we prefer to believe that even this phonological isolationism ultimately has to take a close look at phonetics. It is true, of course, that cognitive operations themselves do not depend on real-world considerations, but it is equally true that it is quite ridiculous to imagine that phonology is constrained only by cognitive ability. Such a phonology denies itself a place in general linguistics and as such has no meaning for us. Fortunately, few take this extreme position. Obviously there are real-world constraints on what a phonology does do (although less on what it might, but never does do); consequently, the feature system of phonology is heavily phonetically constrained. As a result there is interaction between the cognitive and the noncognitive; therefore, there is a need to understand the interface.

Interim phonologies wait uneasily, though, for phonetics to catch up. Why else would there have been talk of *independently controllable* features except that there was no theory of the interdependence of the components of complex articulatory gestures? Why else would there be a hypothesis of the mental reality of segments if there is no adequate theory of the interdependence of sequencing gestures (if we may beg the question somewhat)?

Using, then, a phonology that is much more formal than phonetics and much more explicit, we have generated some hypotheses concerning what should be happening at the phonetic level in the system. Some of those hypotheses have been given support, others have been rejected, and a general conclusion has been that, for all its clumsiness, the technique we have been using in this study has been able to throw some light on the theory of the relationship between phonology and phonetics.

BACKGROUND

Two decades ago, Fromkin (1966) and Harris, Lysaught, and Schvey (1965) used EMG to explore the invariance of articulatory gestures for labial "phonemes." Motivation for such research is understandable since one of the key problems in the study of articulation is how the ensemble of muscle commands inherent to a phoneme is transformed into a series of articulatory gestures. Research suggests that invariance is unlikely since coarticulatory perturbation of segmental articulatory commands is the rule, not the exception (see Chapter 6). That being the case, it would be of considerable theoretical interest to minimize the surface phonetic allophonic variation that characterizes contextual, continuous speech in order to gauge the magnitude of coarticulatory perturbation. To avoid complicating the underlying systematic-phonetic level of representation of an utterance, linguists and others have claimed that most allophonic variation occurs because of inherent neuromuscular *processes* or *constraints* of the speech production mechanism (SPM). If such limiting physiological processes are the major source of allophonic variation, it can be but of *minor* linguistic interest.

Electromyographic Recording

Muscle tissues are organized into muscle bodies; each muscle body consists of groups of muscle "motor units" (MUs), the motor unit being the basic controllable *contractile* element of muscle. A motor unit consists of a group of muscle fibrils, all of which are exclusively innervated by the axonal fibril(s) of a single motoneuron, the cell body of which is found in various cranial or spinal nuclei. When excited, an axonal spike traverses the axon of the motoneuron and its fibrils, causing the release of a chemical transmitter at the motor end plates, the point of interface between axon fibrils and muscle fibers. The transmitter elicits a wave of electrical depolarization, the so called motor unit action potential (MUAP), which propagates along the membrane covering the muscle fibers. The MUAP in turn elicits a twitch or contraction from the muscle fiber. If unrestrained, the twitching fibers shorten in length, exerting mechanical force upon their points of attachment. The MUAPs from the simultaneously excited fibers of each MU in turn disperse through the anisotropic medium of surrounding tissue where the MUAPs undergo a complex temporal and spatial summation. If a recording electrode inserted into the muscle body has but a small pick-up surface (such as a needle or fine hooked wire), the electrode will record from a very limited volume of tissue and will reveal the MUAPs from several adjacent or even *one* MU, in such a distinctive fashion that the individual peculiarities of the MUAP wave form for a particular MU can be observed repeatedly during many successive bursts of muscle activity. If the electrode is very large or positioned on the surface of the skin directly above a contracting muscle body, the electrode will pick up a complicated interference pattern consisting of the spatially and temporally integrated, volume conducted MUAPs of many active MUs beneath the electrode. If the muscle beneath is architecturally simple in that its fibers run in only a single general direction or pattern, and if fibers from other muscles are not nearby or do not intermingle with the fibers of the muscle under investigation, then the gross, electromyographic interference pattern (EMG signal, as it is called) is a useful estimate of the level of function of the *entire muscle*, and a good index of the relative force being exerted by that muscle body (Bigland and Lippold, 1954). On the other hand, if the muscle beneath the electrode site is anatomically complex, with fibers running in several directions, and if fibers from other muscles overlap or are interwoven with those of the muscle in question, surface electrodes yield a poor index of muscle function. Instead, needle or hooked wire electrodes capable of recording from a very small number of adjacent MUs should be used.

For the topographically "simple" skeletal muscles, under conditions of slow, steady isometric contraction (no change in muscle length), the integrated EMG signal is linearly related to muscle force over a wide range (Coggshall and Bekey, 1970). When applied muscle force changes rapidly under isotonic conditions, the force versus integrated EMG signal is nonlinear. The muscles of the vocal tract are nonskeletal, often engage in isotonic maneuvers, operate with relatively low force, and are swiftly recruited and released from excitation. In addition, the vocal tract muscles are often topographically complex, having broad insertions and origins, with fibers coursing in diverse directions, often inserting not on bones via tendons but on muscles, fasciae, and other soft tissues; in addition, often in a given locale, fibers from several muscles overlap or overlay each other. As a result, neither surface electromyogram or single unit recording gives an unambiguous estimate of the level of muscle activation.

The motor command to a particular muscle is reflected in two parameters: (1) the number of motor units activated, and (2) the frequency of firing of individual motoneurons. If each of the MUAPs of the active, contracting muscle emerged as a clear, well-differentiated spike of electrical activity, the number of spikes per unit time could be counted as an estimate of muscle activation. The rectified, integrated spike pattern could also be used as an estimate of muscle activation, but this suffers from some inaccuracy because MUs close to the recording site would contribute disproportionately to the integrated activity level, being greater in amplitude. Spike counting would fall into error because individual MUAP spikes overlap and merge into an interference pattern wherein individual spikes may be lost or of such small amplitude as to be below spike detection threshold. Imaizumi and Hiki (1975) demonstrated that with optimum hooked wire electrode placement in vocal tract muscles, pulse counting methods were slightly better (more accurate) than rectifying and averaging the analogue recording of the MUAP spike train. Whether such results would hold for the more complex interference pattern for surface electrodes is problematic. Other things being equal, a surface electrode samples activity from more MUs than do indwelling needle or wire electrodes and therefore offers a better statistical estimate of the whole muscle activation level than do the smaller electrodes. This is not to deny the great usefulness of needle or wire electrodes in detecting MUAPs from fibers of a given muscle when different muscles overlap each other. Indeed, faced with the complex topography of vocal tract muscles, most recent EMG work with speech musculatures involves the use of needle or hooked wire electrodes. Although such electrodes record from a limited population of MUs, Leanderson (1972) argues that such electrodes produce EMG patterns reflective of whole muscle activity, stating that "Edström and Kugelberg (1968) [have shown] that since the fibers of a motor unit are widely dispersed in the cross section of a muscle, the activity sampled can thus be regarded as representative for a significant number of MUs of the small lip muscles." But even hooked wire or needle electrodes may yield varying results, since "it may be that if muscle origin is spatially diffuse with many heads, differing portions have differing functions in a limited area, thus variation in electrode placement would cause variation in EMG signals" (Fritzell, Kotby, and Möller, 1975). Thus, the choice of the type of electrode to be used for EMG work depends on the anatomical complexity of the muscle distribution at the electrode site, the accessibility of the muscle body, and the degree to which it may be assumed that small, indwelling electrodes provide a good estimate of whole muscle body activity level.

The Problem

We wished to determine the degree to which a "simple" articulatory gesture would show significant contextual perturbation as a function of selected contextual variables. By reducing instrumental, training, and performance artifacts to a minimum, we sought to more clearly assess the underlying magnitude and intersubject variability of such perturbation.

Labial closure consists of upper lip depression and lower lip elevation driven primarily by contraction of the musculus orbicularis oris (MOO), with lesser contributions from the mandible, and a variety of upper lip depressors and lower lip elevators among the array of facial muscles. Lip movement is known to be influenced by afferents from the temporomandibular joint (TMJ), tongue and so forth. By placing a pair of simple concentric surface electrodes on the upper lip lateral to the philtrum, we sought to sample the MOO superioris contractions, the prime mover for upper lip closure.

A wide array of contextual factors thought to be likely sources of perturbation for this simple articulatory gesture were chosen. By using /p/b/, the voiced or voiceless (fortes or lentis) featured contrast was free to affect closure. The choice of three vowels /i, u, ʌ/ provided coarticulatory perturbation for labial closure, primarily in terms of lip rounding or spreading and differences in mandibular height. Syllable structure, in terms of a preconsonantal and postconsonantal position for /p/b/, was introduced, as was the suprasegmental factor of stress involved in the prestress and poststress position of C in /'VCV/ and /V'CV/ tokens. Our predictions of possible contextual effects to be observed in the labial closure gesture were as follows:

1. *Consonant voicing:* Longer or stronger closure for /p/ than /b/ was expected, especially in postvocalic position (Ladefoged, 1975).

2. *Vowel context:* Greater perturbation of labial closure might be expected in left-right (carry-over) context in postvocalic position since closure would be initiated during the labial or mandibular postures associated with the preceding vowel.

3. *Syllable position:* Since obstruent duration differences vary most postvocalically, greater /p/b/ differences were expected there.

4. *Stress level:* Prestress position was fully expected to elicit a stronger consonantal closing gesture; furthermore, the symmetrical V-V environment might be expected to yield largest vowel interactions (coarticulation with the closure gesture).

5. *Intersubject differences:* Most important of all, we expected minimal intersubject differences for this simple articulatory gesture since it is mandatory for stop consonants. Thus any intersubject differences found for a contextual effect would suggest a nonobligatory difference in articulatory encoding.

We further sought to assess the magnitude of variability in a series of repeated utterances by analyzing the mean and standard deviation of EMG measures as larger and larger portions of the ensemble of utterances were examined.

Our study of variability focused upon the polar conditions of unanimous group performance versus varying group performance. Specifically, invariance was taken to mean either (1) no context sensitivity of gesture for a contextual factor for any subject, or (2) all subjects evidenced the same context-sensitive change of gesture; whereas variability implied that the group context sensitivity differed significantly among subjects. The implications of these outcomes are important. Uniform group performance implies that a component gesture is strictly, non-idiosyncratically controlled, whereas a variable group performance implies that the component gesture was not crucial to the phonological feature(s) being encoded, and hence it was free to vary in a relatively random fashion.

METHODS OF PROCEDURE

General Procedures

Simultaneous voice signals and electromyographic records were obtained from surface electrodes on the upper lip of each of four speakers as they produced lip closures for bilabial consonants contained within carrier sentences. Data analysis was performed on the smoothed, integrated EMG signals aided by raw and integrated voice signals. Independent parameters manipulated included (1) voicing, (2) syllable position, (3) vowel environment, (4) syllable shape, and (5) stress environment of stop consonants. Control parameters included tempo and effort of utterance.

Statistical analysis consisted of ANOVAs computed for each contextual factor and each subject. The 25 repetitions of each word by each subject were treated as randomly selected replications. Thus, each ANOVA sought to describe the typical performance of an individual subject.

Subjects

Relevant characteristics for the subjects in this study are set forth in Table 7-1. Subjects 1 and 3 were informed of the design of the study, whereas 2 and 4 were kept uninformed. Subjects 1, 2, and 3 were considered to be phonetically sophisticated, whereas subject 4 was phonetically naive. Inspection and analysis of the mean data and variance measures demonstrated to our satisfaction that age, sex, sophistication, and dialect appeared to have little effect, if any, upon the stereotypy of the speakers' labial gesturing. All subjects were made aware, well in advance, that the purpose of the study was to investigate the "accuracy of their optimally normal" speech patterns. Several subjects were rejected because of their

**Table 7–1. Pertinent Distinguishing Characteristics
of Subjects Who Served as Speakers**

Subject	Sex	Age	Occupation	Dialect
(1) RGD	M	38	Phonetician	General American (Pennsylvania)
(2) LS	F	36	Phonologist	General American (Ohio)
(3) MAAT	M	38	Phonologist	Standard Southern British English (Kent)
(4) HR	F	20	Student of phonetics	Standard British English (Northern)

inability to relax between utterances, thus yielding a high level of interutterance residual EMG activity, or because EMG signals were of small amplitude throughout trial runs, thus yielding an unsatisfactory stimulus-noise (S-N) ratio on recordings.

Subject Training—Preparation. Prior to the test session, subjects were asked to enter the laboratory and to practice repeating sentences heard over a loudspeaker, paying special attention to matching the exact tempo, effort, and stress patterns of a tape recorded speaker-prompter. After sufficient trials to ensure that subjects were familiar and comfortable with the task, subjects were prepared for the test sessions.

Preparations involved abrading the subject's upper lip with fine-grain sandpaper to remove dead skin. After washing with methanol to remove oil, a pair of circular silver electrodes were placed on the upper lip just lateral to the philtrum of the lip. Each electrode was greased on its concave inner surface with electrode jelly, spaced one electrode diameter apart, and fixed firmly in place with Blenderm EMG-tape. The temperature of the room was kept low enough to keep the subjects from sweating, which would tend to lift the electrodes and thus degrade the S-N ratio of the EMG signals or introduce artifacts associated with varying contact impedance or low-frequency electrode movements. Subjects were then asked to produce syllable trains of /pʌ/ syllables—if movement artifacts were large, the subject's electrodes were repositioned until electrode movement–induced perturbations of the EMG signal were minimized. Periodic checks were made throughout the 2 hour experimental session to ensure that sweating under the Blenderm tape did not cause an unacceptable worsening of EMG S-N. Electrode lead wires were attached to a headband. Each subject's hand was washed with alcohol before he or she was told to gently grasp a brass doorknob, which served as a ground-electrode for the two active lip electrodes.

Speech Stimuli

Table 7–2 lists the speech stimuli used in this investigation. Inspection of Table 7–2 reveals that for the /cvd-dvc/ stimuli, voicing, syllable position initial versus final, and vowel context, were systematically permuted, with the neutral (vis-a-vis labial closure) alveolar /d/ serving to eliminate possible transvowel labial interaction between the syllabic consonants. The /CVC/

Table 7–2. Speech Stimuli Used in this Investigation

/Cvd-dvC/ stimuli			
pid	dip	bid	dib
pud	dup	bud	dub
pʌd	dʌp	bʌd	dʌb

/CVC/ stimuli	
pip	bib
pup	bub
pʌp	bʌb

Carrier phrase for /cvd-dvc/ and /cvc/ stimuli
"He'll spoof the _________ again."

/VCV/ stimuli			
ʹipi	iʹpi	ʹibi	iʹbi
ʹupu	uʹpu	ʹubu	uʹbu
ʹʌpʌ	ʌʹpʌ	ʹʌpʌ	ʌʹpʌ

Carrier phrase for /VCV/ stimuli
"Smell this poof of _________ again."

stimuli were included to determine the difference, if any, between the neutral /d/ consonant, and the labial consonants with respect to the labial closure gesture. The carrier phrase for the /cvd-dvc/ and /CVC/ stimuli was, "He'll spoof the_________again." This sentence was spoken with sentence level stress on the test word. The test word was flanked by the labially neutral vowels /ə____ə/, which were doubly convenient: acoustically, the consonants of the test word stood out on the oscillogram well for segmentation purposes, and electromyographically, the neutral vowel provided minimal interaction with the labial closure gesture for the labial stop consonants. In addition, the /sp/ consonant cluster provided information on labial closure in another phonetic environment.

For the /VCV/ utterances, inspection of Table 7–2 demonstrates that vowels, voicing, and stress (prestress versus poststress) were the phonetic parameters manipulated in the construction of these stimuli. The carrier sentence, "Smell this poof of_________again," was read with sentence stress on the test word.

Consideration of these stimuli demonstrate that in addition to voicing, vowel environment, syllable position, and stress-position, syllable shape was also an independent factor insofar as the stop consonant could appear in pre- or postvocalic position in /cvd-dvc/ syllables; in pre- or postvocalic position in symmetrical /CVC/ syllables; or intravocalically, prestress or poststress, in /VCV/ syllables, so that syllable shape also constituted a control parameter subject to test.

After careful consideration, we decided to present the stimuli auditorially to the subjects, who would then repeat the test sentence exactly as they heard it.

To prepare the stimulus recording, subject 3 practiced reading the fully randomized set of sentences with as unvarying a tempo and effort as possible; tempo was checked with mingogram recordings, and effort was tested via VU-meter deflections. Special care was taken to see that appropriate intonational stress and articulatory patterns were maintained as exactly as possible. After the practice sessions, subject 3 was presented with a script in which the carrier sentences for /cvc, cvd, dvc/ syllables were fully randomized with 25 repetitions for each. Recording was interrupted and remarks made at any time that the experimenters were aware of any unusual variations. Follwing that, the /VCV/ test sentences, also fully randomized with 25 repetitions for each stimulus, were also recorded. Sentences were spoken at an average tempo of about 2.8 syllables/s, or about 180 words/min, with about 2.5 to 3.0 s pause between sentences during which the subjects repeated the sentence presented.

Data Recording Equipment

Subjects were seated in a sound-treated recording studio used for a language laboratory. The data recording array is shown in Figure 7–1. Electrodes were fabricated of 1/64 inch thick silver sheet, punched with a slightly concave die, and trimmed to a nearly circular 3.5 mm diameter; the electrodes were then soldered to leads of shielded phonograph-cartridge pickup wire. The ground-electrode terminated in a brass doorknob clutched in the subject's left hand. The EMG signals were led to a custom-built, six-channel, differential EMG amplifier with a gain of 1000X. From the EMG preamplifier, the EMG signal was led to one FM-mode channel of an Ampex SP-300 data recorder, set to record at 7½ inches per second (ips) using BASF ¼ inch LP 35 LH tape. The raw EMG and raw voice signals were led to the two inputs of dual channel oscilloscope, where they were constantly monitored by an experimenter throughout the data recording session. Voice signals were recorded with a Shure Model 55 unidirectional microphone placed, via a boom, about 12 inches from the subject's mouth at an angle of 30 degrees to the sagittal plane of his or her head. The voice signal was amplified by the preamplifier of a Tandberg tape recorder before being led to the direct mode voice-edge recording channel of the Ampex data recorder. To help the subject keep his or her articulatory effort relatively constant, the raw voice signal was split after leaving the Tandberg recorder and passed through an integrator circuit with a 20 ms time constant and delivered to the input of an oscilloscope whose horizontal deflection was disabled. As the subject spoke, the integrated voice signal rose and fell on the oscilloscope screen, which was set at the subject's eye level. The gain of this circuit was set so that a 65 to 70 dB voice signal produced 5 cm deflection as signal intensity varied over about a 5 dB range. The subject was instructed to keep his or her vocal intensity sufficiently constant so that the trace of the oscilloscope did not move from between the two horizontal lines marked on the oscilloscope face. The audio gain of this circuit was not altered for any of the subjects.

The prerecorded speech stimuli were played to the subject free field, at a comfortable loudness level sufficiently intense to be picked up by the Shure microphone at a level 5 to 7 dB less intense than the subjects's own speech signal.

Data Processing Equipment

Upon play-back, the EMG and voice signals were led to a custom built, six-channel, rectifier-integration processing circuit. The raw voice signal

Figure 7–1. Block diagram of experimental array.

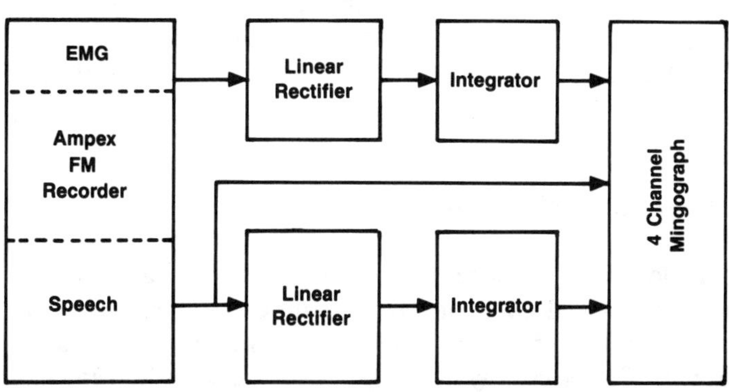

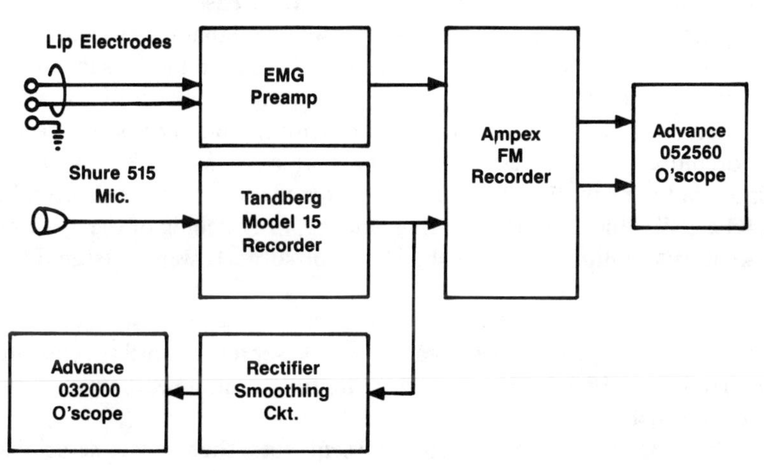

was led directly to one channel of an Elema Schonander EM-347 four channel mingograph set to reproduce at 100 mm/s paper speed. On track two of the mingograph, the rectified, smoothed voice signal (time constant = 6.3 ms) was recorded. With this integration time, plosive releases stood out sharply and conveniently for purposes of segmentation. On track three of the mingograph, the high-pass filtered (33 Hz cutoff frequency), linearly rectified and smoothed (time constant = 22 ms) EMG signal was recorded. On track four was recorded the interval timing signal of the mingograph.

Experimental Session

Following a practice session during which each subject practiced repeating a subselection of the prerecorded test sentences containing all of the stimuli, the subject was seated in a chair in the sound treated room and wired for electromyography, with the electrode being held by clips attached to an elastic headband. With the microphone in position, the subject practiced an additional series of sentences, attempting to keep the dot on the oscilloscope within the circumscribed limits. When the experimenter was satisfied that the subject could easily perform the task, final instructions were given. The speakers were told that they were to repeat the sentences they heard as "exactly as possible," keeping the same tempo and stress patterns as the speaker, and keeping their overall voice level sufficiently constant to remain within the horizontal lines on the face of the oscilloscope set at eye level. They were also instructed that is was important to "relax, as fully as possible, between utterances," so that residual EMG activity due to tonic posturing, tensing, or twitching of the lips could be kept to a minimum. As we shall see, our subjects were outstanding in this regard.

Recording of the /cvd-dvc/ and /cvc/ stimuli began first. Five minute rest periods were given between each set of 90 sentences until these stimuli were recorded; then, in the same way, the fully randomized /vcv/ stimuli were recorded.

During each continuous run of 90 sentences, the text was scrutinized by one experimenter, and *any* articulatory, stress, or intonation errors were noted; these tokens were rerecorded at the end of that session. Errors averaged about two to three per 90 utterances, on the average. As will be seen later, the speakers as a group were remarkably successful in controlling tempo and effort, which contributed substantially to the relatively low variability of the data.

Analysis of the Electromyographic Data

Figure 7-2 presents a tracing of an actual mingographic display of the voice and electromyographic data. We should first remark that the electromyographic data were extraordinarily clean; almost no motional artifacts were observed, and the noise floor of the integrated EMG signal was so low that in up to 80% of cases it appeared as a barely visible ripple. This was convenient because it allowed the single analyst to define unambiguously the onset and offset of the EMG pulse for labial closure as it rose above and then descended to the EMG noise floor.

Explicitly, the measuring procedure proceeded as follows. Each mingogram was placed on a drawing board and a single, best-fitting straight line was drawn across the tops of the ripple in the EMG noise floor preceding and following the subject's utterance. This was easily done in all but 30 of 2800 mingograms. The raw voice signal was inspected for the burst release of the stop consonant, which was invariably detectable (as an initially negative deflection) for voiceless plosives and for the great majority of voiced plosives. If the raw-voice plosive burst was not readily detectable, the integrated voice-signal invariably either revealed a burstlike transient or showed a steep onset into the vowel, either of which served to mark the burst onset. A vertical line was drawn through each burst release and through the EMG trace as well (see line B in Fig. 7-2). The peak of the EMG pulse for the labial closure was located, and vertical line was drawn through the peak down to the noise floor line. The peak EMG amplitude (P) in relative (mV) was measured as the distance from the noise floor to the peak of the EMG amplitude trace. The effective EMG pulse duration (DEL) was measured as the time between the initial rise of the EMG pulse from the noise floor to the onset of the acoustic burst for stop release.

RESULTS

/Cvd/ Syllables

EMG Amplitude

Peak EMG amplitudes for /C/ in /Cvd/ *did not* differ significantly, either as a function of consonant voicing or as a function of vowel environment, for all four subjects. Apparently, in this context the peak

Figure 7-2. A sample mingograph recording showing the criterion measures made on each utterance.

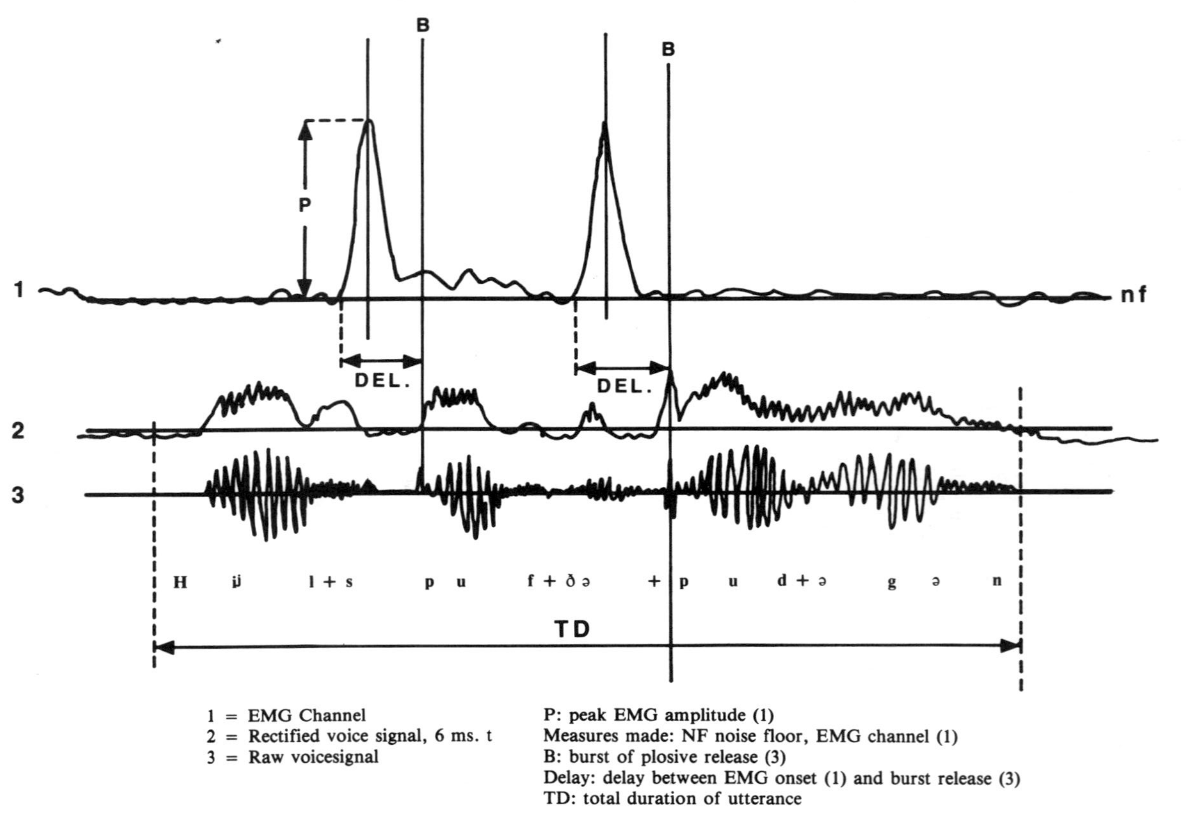

force exerted by the orbicularis oris superioris muscle for labial closure in stop consonants was an invariant gesture for our four subjects. The mean values and standard deviations and summary of statistical testing for differences among criterion measures for /Cvd/ tokens are shown in Tables 7–3 to 7–5.

Duration

The effective duration (DEL) of the EMG pulse (from EMG onset to acoustic release of the stop consonant) was invariant for two subjects (subjects 2 and 3) across vowel and consonant contexts. For subjects 1 and 4, /b/ was significantly longer than /p/ in all vowel contexts, whereas for subject 4, /u/ and /ʌ/ context yielded significantly longer EMG duration than did /i/ (see Table 7–3).

/dvc/ Syllables

EMG Amplitude

Subjects 3 and 4 exhibited no statistically significant differences in peak EMG in any context, whereas for subjects 1 and 2, /p/ elicited greater peak EMG than did /b/. For all subjects, vowels elicited significant differences in peak EMG for labial closure. For three subjects (1, 2 and 4), /i/ and /ʌ/ elicited significantly greater peak EMG than did /u/, whereas for subject 3, /ʌ/ peak EMG was significantly greater than for /i/. Tables 7–6 to 7–8 summarize means, standard deviations, and statistical testing for /dvc/ -syllable criterion measures.

Duration

For three of four subjects (2, 3, 4) consonant type, and for all four subjects, vowel environment produced significant differences in duration of the EMG pulse. In general, /p/ duration exceeded that of /b/. For various subjects, each of the vowels, variously, elicited greatest and least EMG pulse duration (see Table 7–6).

Comparison of Criterion Measures in /cvd/-/dvc/ Syllables

To assess the factor of syllable position, pre- versus postvocalic position of the consonant, analysis of variance was used. Table 7–9 displays a summary of the results of these ANOVAs. For two subjects (1 and 2) peak

Table 7-3. Mean Criterion Measures for Cvd Tokens

	PEAK, mV.										
	pi	pu	pʌ	bi	bu	bʌ	p	b	i	u	ʌ
S1	25.30	22.19	24.20	23.00	23.22	20.92	23.90	22.38	24.15	22.71	22.56
S2	22.96	22.10	20.94	20.40	18.56	22.20	22.00	20.39	21.68	20.33	21.57
S3	32.28	34.00	31.63	31.70	34.98	31.64	32.64	32.77	31.99	34.49	31.63
S4	43.02	45.28	42.94	41.44	41.24	41.12	43.75	41.27	42.23	43.26	42.03
$\overline{X}$	30.89	30.89	29.93	29.13	29.50	28.89	30.57	29.20	30.01	30.20	29.45

	DEL, C.S.										
	pi	pu	pʌ	bi	bu	bʌ	p	b	i	u	ʌ
S1	17.12	17.32	17.50	18.32	18.12	19.59	17.31	18.68	17.72	17.72	18.54
S2	17.29	17.16	17.10	17.55	17.86	17.83	17.18	17.75	17.42	17.51	17.47
S3	17.52	17.52	17.46	16.89	16.96	17.56	17.50	17.14	17.21	17.24	17.51
S4	19.90	20.79	20.34	19.60	22.59	21.78	20.34	21.33	19.75	21.69	21.06
$\overline{X}$	17.96	18.20	18.10	18.09	18.88	19.19	18.08	18.72	18.02	18.54	18.65

EMG discharge was significantly greater in postvocalic position. All subjects revealed a significant vowel × position interaction effect, such that differing vowels elicited greater peak EMG for closure in pre- versus postvocalic, consonantal position. There was no systematic pattern to this interaction.

Results for the pre- and postvocalic comparisons for duration were more complex. For all subjects, the EMG pulse duration was significantly greater in postvocalic than in prevocalic position. The significant consonant × position and vowel × position interactions for all subjects indicate complex interrelations among these phonetic factors. It would appear that the increased duration for final position was somewhat greater for /b/ than for /p/.

CVC Syllables

Data for only three subjects could be reported. In prevocalic position, peak EMG for /p/ was significantly larger than for /b/ for two subjects (1 and 2), whereas vowels elicited no significant differences in EMG amplitude. In postvocalic position, EMG amplitude for /p/ was significantly larger than for /b/ for all three subjects, but in this case, vowels elicited significant differences. For two subjects (1 and 2), /i/ and /ʌ/ exceeded /u/ in peak EMG whereas for subject 3, /i/ context yielded significantly smaller peak EMG amplitude than either /u/ or /ʌ/ context. Mean values and summaries of statistical testing for the CVC tokens are shown in Tables 7-9 to 7-13.

Table7-4. Standard Deviations for Criterion Measures in Cvd Tokens

	PEAK							
	pi	pu	pʌ	bi	bu	bʌ	p	b
S1	8.32	4.91	6.69	5.85	6.05	4.57		
S2	5.78	6.40	4.67	7.50	4.22	6.28		
S3	6.38	7.57	8.79	7.87	7.13	8.87		
S4	7.35	9.29	8.54	9.25	7.47	6.28		
X̄	10.46	11.99	11.17	11.24	11.02	10.50	11.20	10.89

	DEL, C. S.							
	pi	pu	pʌ	bi	bu	bʌ	p	b
S1	2.33	1.35	1.65	2.31	2.16	4.67		
S2	1.16	1.45	1.42	2.07	1.93	3.72		
S3	0.89	1.45	0.92	1.15	1.44	2.07		
S4	1.66	2.87	2.09	1.75	3.87	14.98		
X̄	1.95	2.39	2.03	2.10	3.31	10.99	2.13	2.68

Duration

In prevocalic position, for all three subjects, there were no significant differences in EMG duration, either as a function of vowel or in consonantal context. In postvocalic position (only two subjects could be reported), /p/ duration significantly exceeded /b/ duration, and there were no significant interactions with either vowel or consonant context.

VCV Tokens

VCV tokens were examined primarily to assess the factor of stress, with C in either prestress (V'CV) or poststress ('VCV) position. Mean data and results of statistical testing are shown in Tables 7-14 to 7-17. In /u____u/ context, stress position had no effect upon peak EMG for any of four subjects, and significantly affected peak EMG in /i____i/ context for only one subject (1). In both vowel contexts, stress × consonant interactions were nonsignificant for peak EMG amplitude, indicating that stress position affected both consonantal contexts equally. Not surprisingly, in both /i____i/ and /u____u/ context, two subjects (1 and 2) produced significantly higher peak EMG for /p/ as versus /b/.

The effect of stress position upon EMG pulse duration was more pronounced. In /u____u/ contexts, three of four subjects (1,2,3), and in

Table 7–5. Summary of Statistical Analyses of Cvd Criterion Measures

	PEAK		
	C	V	CV
S1	NS	NS	NS
S2	NS	NS	NS
S3	NS	NS	NS
S4	NS	NS	NS
$\overline{X}$	NS	NS	NS

	DEL		
	C	V	CV
S1	.01	NS	NS
S2	NS	NS	NS
S3	NS	NS	NS
S4	.01	.01	NS
$\overline{X}$	.01	.05	NS

NS, not significant.

/i____i/ context, two subjects (1 and 2), displayed longer EMG pulse duration in prestress environment rather than poststress environments. The consonant × stress interaction was significant for only one subject (1) in both environments. However, for two of four subjects in both vowel environments, the duration (DEL) of P was greater than that for /b/.

Stability of EMG Measures

Our desire to assess the repetition-to-repetition variability of EMG signals led us to compute the mean and standard deviation for all /CVd/ tokens for all subjects based upon sample sizes consisting of the (1) first 5, (2) first 10, (3) first 15, (4) first 20, and (5) entire sample of 25 utterances. These measures were entered into an analysis of variance in which sample size (five levels) served as the independent variable. The results, F = 3.28, yielded a nonsignificant ($\alpha < .01$) effect for sample size. The remarkably invariant mean, SD, and coefficient of variation values shown in Table 7–18 suggest that speakers were remarkably consistent in their articulatory gesturing for stop consonant articulation.

Table 7–6. Mean Criterion Measures for dvC Tokens

	PEAK										
	ip	**up**	**pʌ**	**ib**	**ub**	**bʌ**	**p**	**b**	**i**	**u**	**ʌ**
S1	33.39	25.72	31.64	30.28	20.73	28.56	30.25	26.42	31.83	23.18	30.13
S2	29.80	20.58	32.68	28.00	15.96	29.34	27.69	24.43	28.90	18.27	31.01
S3	29.58	30.81	36.36	29.00	32.30	33.58	32.25	31.63	29.29	31.56	34.97
S4	43.99	38.26	42.96	44.38	35.52	40.26	41.87	40.05	44.18	37.09	41.61
X̄	34.19	28.94	35.91	32.91	26.07	32.98	33.01	30.63	33.55	27.50	34.45

	DEL										
	ip	**up**	**pʌ**	**ib**	**ub**	**bʌ**	**p**	**b**	**i**	**u**	**ʌ**
S1	14.98	16.95	14.99	14.25	17.58	14.49	15.64	15.48	14.62	17.27	14.74
S2	17.13	15.48	16.58	14.52	13.90	13.94	16.40	14.12	15.82	14.69	15.26
S3	15.72	17.39	16.46	13.97	16.09	13.73	16.52	14.60	14.85	16.74	15.09
S4	20.78	18.61	20.53	17.25	18.12	19.13	19.97	18.17	19.01	18.36	19.83
X̄	17.15	17.11	17.14	15.00	16.43	15.33	17.13	15.59	16.08	16.77	16.24

In a final analysis, correlation coefficients were computed to assess the relationship between the two criterion measures: peak EMG − DEL (duration), for /Cvd/, /dvC/, and /CVC/ tokens. The results, shown below,

Token	/Cvd/,	/dvC/,	/CvC/,	/CvC/
	.36	.33	.44	.48

suggest that while the positive correlations were significantly different from zero ($p \geq .05$), they were modest in size, accounting for less than 24% of the variance in the relationship between the two variables.

DISCUSSION

Table 7–19 compactly summarizes the results of statistical testing. In a word, the general tenor of our findings was that lip-closing gesture was relatively invariant, not consistently context sensitive in a singular way to any of the phonetic parameters expected to influence it.

A characteristic example of failure to show consistency is exemplified by the /cvd/ and /cvc/ syllable pair for the prevocalic consonant. In the former syllable, peak EMG is *not* context sensitive, whereas DEL shows significant effects in two of four subjects, which is an anomalous effect at that, insofar as /b/ was longer than /p/. In the latter syllable, peak EMG

Table 7-7. Standard Deviations for Criterion Measures in dvC Tokens

| | **PEAK** | | | | | | | |
	ip	up	p	ib	ub	b	p	b
S1	6.26	6.26	8.39	8.32	6.93	6.85		
S2	5.49	9.91	8.39	6.93	4.46	5.94		
S3	6.52	7.25	7.67	5.48	7.82	7.88		
S4	8.49	8.24	7.66	9.69	6.09	7.94		
$\overline{X}$	8.90	10.37	9.08	10.17	10.27	8.49	9.89	10.18

| | **DEL** | | | | | | | |
	ip	up	p	ib	ub	b	p	b
S1	1.09	3.14	1.61	1.65	3.75	1.46		
S2	1.13	1.28	1.11	0.72	1.57	1.35		
S3	0.84	1.68	1.04	1.11	1.73	1.13		
S4	3.61	2.63	2.13	1.83	2.35	1.97		
$\overline{X}$	2.99	2.53	2.56	1.91	2.97	2.69	2.69	2.63

was significantly different for two of three subjects, whereas for DEL, there were no consistent effects, which is to say, there was no consensual, single characteristic articulatory performance for prevocalic C, even though the two syllable types differed only in the final consonant, which might be predicted at best to amplify, through coarticulation, the articulatory performance on C_1.

One trend that emerged was the tendency for postvocalic stops to experience significant vowel context effects (LR coarticulation), more so than in prevocalic context. This predictable result probably obtains from the fact that postvocalic closure for the consonant is initiated in the midst of the vowel gesture, thus placing the demand for differing closure gestures upon the lip, depending upon lip-jaw posture for the vowel. Indeed, the elevated peak EMG signal for /i/ probably reflects increased work necessary to close spread, opened, slightly stiffened lips. Over all contexts, vowel perturbations were, perhaps, the strongest of contextual effects, but as mentioned, they occurred inconsistently, and the pattern of influence was in most cases, idiosyncratic to particular subjects.

The results of statistical testing of differences in the closure gesture for pre- and postvocalic contexts, /CVd/ versus /dVC/, was interesting. Contrary to expectation (Ladefoged, 1975), peak EMG was greater for two

Table 7–8. Summary of Statistical Analyses of dvC Criterion Measures

	PEAK		
	C	**V**	**CV**
S1	.01	.01	NS
S2	.01	.01	NS
S3	NS	.01	NS
S4	NS	.01	NS
$\overline{X}$	.01	.01	NS

	DEL		
	C	**V**	**CV**
S1	NS	.01	NS
S2	.01	.01	NS
S3	.01	.01	NS
S4	.01	.01	.01
$\overline{X}$	.01	NS	.01

NS, not significant.

of four subjects in postvocalic than in prevocalic position. Complex vowel × position interactions for both criterion measures for all subjects in the /CVd/-/dVC/ comparison suggests that there is differential vowel perturbation of closure in pre- and postvocalic contexts.

In /VCV/ context, for both /i/ and /u/ environments /p/ was greater than /b/ in peak amplitude for two of four subjects, and hence it was inconsistent in effect across the entire group of speakers. Unexpectedly, labial closure in prestress position for /iCi/ context was greater than in poststress position for but a single subject, and not different for any subject in /uCu/ context. For duration (DEL), results were also inconsistent, three of four in /iCi/ context and two of four in /uCu/ context showing *longer* prestress than poststress EMG pulses.

Scanning Table 7–19 for *consistent* subject performance on the two criterion measures as a function of vowel, consonant, or stress, we see the following results:

1. /CVd/—both C and V were nonsignificant for peak EMG
2. /CVC/—both C and V were nonsignificant for DEL
3. /CVC/—both C and V were significant for peak EMG
4. /uCu/—stress had a nonsignificant effect upon peak EMG

Table 7–9. Results of Statistical Analysis of Differences in Criterion Measures in Cvd versus dvC Tokens as a Function of Position, Vowel, and Consonant

	PEAK			
	POS	**C × P**	**V × P**	**CVP**
S1	.01	NS	.01	NS
S2	.01	NS	.01	NS
S3	NS	NS	.01	NS
S4	NS	NS	.01	NS

	DEL			
	POS	**C × P**	**V × P**	**CVP**
S1	.01	.01	.01	NS
S2	.01	.01	.01	NS
S3	.01	.01	.01	.01
S4	.01	.01	.01	NS

POS, position; V, vowel; C, consonant; NS, not significant.

Table 7–10. Mean Criterion Measures for C_1 of C_1VC_2 Tokens

	PEAK										
	pi	**pu**	**pΛ**	**bi**	**bu**	**bΛ**	**p**	**b**	**i**	**u**	**Λ**
S1	23.00	22.40	23.70	21.21	18.20	18.30	23.03	19.24	22.10	20.30	21.00
S2	22.36	24.60	21.67	20.40	19.16	18.98	22.89	19.51	21.38	21.88	20.30
S3	33.54	35.23	34.58	33.92	36.02	30.84	34.45	33.59	33.73	35.62	32.71
S4											
X̄	30.91	31.81	31.35	29.95	28.78	27.80	31.36	28.84	30.34	30.29	29.57

	DEL										
	pi	**pu**	**pΛ**	**bi**	**bu**	**bΛ**	**p**	**b**	**i**	**u**	**Λ**
S1	17.04	15.87	16.61	16.81	17.30	17.68	16.51	17.26	16.92	16.58	17.15
S2	16.99	17.40	16.77	17.27	17.38	17.70	17.06	17.45	17.13	17.39	17.24
S3	17.12	16.89	17.54	16.84	17.09	17.02	17.18	16.98	16.98	16.99	17.28
S4											
X̄	17.90	17.78	17.69	17.73	18.38	18.28	17.79	18.13	17.81	18.08	17.98

Table 7-11. Mean Criterion Measures for C_2 of C_1VC_2 Tokens

	pi	pu	pʌ	bi	bu	bʌ	p	b	i	u	ʌ
PEAK											
S1	30.74	25.14	31.36	28.44	18.68	27.44	29.08	24.85	29.59	21.91	29.40
S2	28.42	20.38	26.90	25.00	13.58	23.60	25.21	20.73	26.71	16.98	25.21
S3	30.66	30.80	35.34	27.70	30.16	29.12	32.27	28.99	29.18	30.48	32.23
S4											
$\overline{X}$	33.76	28.79	34.61	31.55	24.81	31.61	32.38	29.32	32.65	26.80	33.10
DEL											
S1											
S2	16.08	15.66	15.98	13.74	13.15	13.15	15.91	13.35	14.91	14.41	14.54
S3	16.55	16.88	16.92	14.99	16.08	15.22	16.78	15.43	15.77	16.48	16.07
S4											
$\overline{X}$	12.86	13.01	13.04	11.21	11.97	11.42	12.97	11.53	12.04	12.49	12.22

Table 7-12. Summary of Statistical Analyses of C_1VC Criterion Measures

	C	V	CV
PEAK			
S1	.01	NS	NS
S2	.01	NS	NS
S3	NS	NS	NS
S4			
$\overline{X}$	.01	NS	NS
DEL			
S1	NS	NS	NS
S2	NS	NS	NS
S3	NS	NS	NS
S4			
$\overline{X}$	NS	NS	NS

NS, not significant.

Table 7–13. Summary of Statistical Analyses of CVC$_2$ Criterion Measures

	PEAK		
	C	V	CV
S1	.01	.01	NS
S2	.01	.01	NS
S3	.01	NS	NS
S4			
$\overline{X}$	.01	.01	NS

	DEL		
	C	V	CV
S1	—	—	—
S2	.01	NS	NS
S3	.01	NS	NS
S4			
$\overline{X}$	.01	NS	NS

NS, not significant.

Expectations matched experimental outcome for item 3 only, where peak EMG for /p/ exceeded that for /b/ for all subjects and significant vowel perturbation occurred for all subjects. For items 1 and 2, differences in labial closure for /p/b/ were neutralized, as were stress differences for peak EMG in item 4. The slight changes in syllable shape in /CVC/ versus /CVd/ yielded startling differences in labial closure, such as no differences for peak EMG in /CVd/ and two of three subjects showing differences in /CVC/ for peak EMG. Phonetic performance for postvocalic labial closure in /CVC and /dVC/ was not so discrepant, but it still manifested differences.

For a given token type—/CVd/—and a particular criterion measure—peak EMG—results of our tests of response stability were encouraging. Samples of ever increasing size, up to a maximum of 25 responses, proved not to differ significantly in mean values; standard deviations and coefficients of variation were satisfactorily stable for the samples, indicating that well-trained subjects could produce sets of EMG tokens of remarkable stability. As a final comment upon the results, the modest correlations between the peak EMG and DEL criterion measures suggests that control of these two parameters was relatively independent.

Table 7–14. Mean Criterion Measures for Cm /i = i/ Context as a Function of Stress Level

	PEAK							
	ST		UNS		ST	UNS	p	b
	p	b	p	b				
$\overline{X}$	35.50	33.09	38.70	35.39	34.30	37.04	37.10	34.24
S1	36.50	33.42	39.44	33.82	34.96	36.63	37.97	33.62
S2	26.22	21.40	30.94	27.80	23.80	29.40	28.63	24.60
S3	32.98	29.62	34.22	30.92	31.30	32.57	33.60	30.27
S4	45.98	47.90	50.98	49.00	46.92	49.97	48.38	48.45

	DEL							
	ST		UNS		ST	UNS	p	b
	p	b	p	b				
$\overline{X}$	18.46	18.11	17.51	16.33	18.28	16.92	17.98	17.22
S1	18.08	19.70	16.38	15.00	18.89	15.69	17.23	17.35
S2	17.46	17.21	15.98	15.10	17.34	15.55	16.71	16.16
S3	17.30	16.04	17.20	15.95	16.67	16.58	17.25	15.99
S4	20.88	19.48	20.65	19.26	20.20	19.94	20.77	19.37

ST, stressed; UNS, unstressed.

Table 7–15. Mean Criterion Measures for C in /u = u/ Context as a Function of Stress Level

	PEAK							
	ST		UNS		ST	UNS	p	b
	p	b	p	b				
S1	29.66	25.36	28.08	21.76	27.51	24.92	28.87	23.56
S2	19.14	16.80	19.65	15.86	17.97	17.79	19.40	16.33
S3	29.62	26.68	28.48	25.88	28.15	27.18	29.05	26.28
S4	40.30	43.64	40.54	42.34	41.97	41.44	40.42	42.99

	DEL							
	ST		UNS		ST	UNS	p	b
	p	b	p	b				
S1	18.54	21.41	16.72	15.70	19.98	16.21	17.63	18.56
S2	17.76	17.83	16.20	15.40	17.79	15.81	16.96	16.62
S3	18.65	16.96	17.12	14.73	17.81	15.93	17.88	15.85
S4	21.25	20.56	19.72	20.38	20.90	20.05	20.48	20.47

ST, stressed; UNS, unstressed.

Table 7–16. Summary of Statistical Analyses of Criterion Measures in /i = i/ Context as a Function of Stress Level and Consonant

	PEAK		
	S	C	SC
S1	NS	.01	NS
S2	.01	.01	NS
S3	NS	NS	NS
S4	NS	NS	NS

	DEL		
	S	C	SC
S1	.01	NS	.01
S2	.01	NS	NS
S3	NS	.01	NS
S4	NS	.01	NS

S, stress level; C, consonant; NS, not significant.

Ramifications

Except in a few contexts, the pattern of MOO. EMG activity for lip closure *did not* reliably distinguish the following contexts: pre- or poststress, pre- or postvocalic syllable position, and ±voicing for the stop consonant. The expected greater mean values of criterion measures for voiceless, prestress, +syllable inital stops were completely or partially absent. Whereas labial closure does serve to encode the +stop, +labial features, it does not systematically distinguish the voicing contrast, differential stress level, and syllable position.

The voicing contrast is strongly cued by differences in VOT prevocalically, and differential vowel and transition length postvocalically. The generally substantial differences in vowel nuclei found as a function of stress level appear not to be reliably *coproduced* (Chapter 6), with the prevocalic stops. Our results for the comparison of pre- and postvocalic labial closure gestures yielded significantly longer postvocalic consonants for all subjects, and, in two of four cases, higher EMG peak amplitudes postvocalically. Both results are at variance with those of Fromkin (1966). However, the observed lesser peak EMG for closure in /u/ context and

Table 7-17. Summary of Statistical Analyses of Criterion Measures in /u = u/ Context as a Function of Stress Level and Consonant

	PEAK		
	S	C	SC
S1	NS	.01	NS
S2	NS	.01	NS
S3	NS	NS	NS
S4	NS	NS	NS

	DEL		
	S	C	SC
S1	.01	.01	.01
S2	.01	NS	NS
S3	.01	.01	NS
S4	NS	NS	NS

S, stress level; C, consonant; NS, not significant.

greater vowel contexts effects in postvocalic position do agree with Fromkin's results.

We would, therefore, conclude that a differential upper lip closure gesture is not required for the bilabial stops /p/ and /b/. Furthermore, the effective duration and maximum contraction for this closure gesture is not generally systematically different in pre- and postvocalic positions in /i, u, ʌ/ vowel context, nor does it vary systematically in pre- and poststress positions. This gestural invariance may result from use of a single, maximal neuromotor command sufficient to "overdrive" the lip to closure, whatever the biomechanical load offered by the upper lip may be.

Therefore, the articulatory cues for stop voicing, stress level, and C-V coarticulation are systematically encoded with articulatory structures and gestures other than that for upper lip closure. Our results, therefore, confirm and extend those of Lubker and Parris (1970) and Leanderson and Lindblom (1972) concerning the relative invariance of labial closure for /p/ and /b/. The facts that some subjects did produce longer post- than prevocalic stops and that some did produce longer and stronger /p/ than /b/ gestures does not obscure the fact that not all subjects produced these differences. Nonreliable differences, particularly in the case of individual productions of a token, mean that the speaker is not faithfully (obligatorily)

Table 7–18. Means, Standard Deviations, and Coefficients of Variation for Criterion Measures in Samples Ranging from 5 to 25 Tokens

	SAMPLE SIZE				
	5	*10*	*15*	*20*	*25*
$\overline{X}$ *Peak EMG*	*30.35*	*29.40*	*29.55*	*29.70*	*29.89*
SD	*6.75*	*6.76*	*6.89*	*6.86*	*6.89*
SD/$\overline{X}$	*.23*	*.24*	*.24*	*.24*	*.24*

encoding phonological information with that gesture. If the gesture is obligatory but through relaxation or less formal speaking register the speaker's gesture is not distinct, it is possible that the listener can predict, on the basis of other a priori information, what should have been heard had the articulation been slow and careful (Lindblom, 1982). If Lindblom is correct, only in slow, careful, precise speech does full and complete encoding of phonological (nonredundant) information into articulatory gesturing occur. In social situations characterized by more casual, less precise speech, speech reveals a loss of detail and precision that must be added by the predictive ability of the listener.

Since it was the case that three relatively sophisticated speakers attempted, with strenuous practice and strict quality control on the conditions of utterance, to produce the most precise and unvarying tokens possible for *this* investigation,[1] we would argue that speaker precision and care were maximal; therefore, our failure to observe consistent contextual effects suggests that they were absent not because of customary imprecision, but because these contextual factors are not projected by the encoding system upon the labial closure gesture. We might, therefore, conclude that systematic investigations of the encoding of phonological information begin with slow, careful, heavily practiced productions in order to deduce the maximally encoded and cue-rich speech from which speakers derive knowledge of "fully encoded phonological forms" to be used when predicting phonological detail missing in casual, everyday phonetic forms.

---

[1]We might also remark, at this point, that our surface EMGs appear to demonstrate reliability and sensitivity sufficient to make rather refined judgments concerning labial articulations.

Table 7–19. Summary of Statistical Testing of Differences in the Labial Closure Gesture on the Criterion Measures of peak EMG and DEL for the Contextual Factors of Consonant (C), Vowel (V), and Stress (S)

	PEAK					DEL				
	C	V	S	CV	SC	C	V	S	CV	SC
Cvd	NS	NS	—	NS	—	b>p 2/4	1/4	—	NS	—
dvC	p>b 2/4	4/4	—	NS	-	p>b 3/4	4/4	—	1/4	—
CvC	p>b 2/3	NS	—	NS	—	NS	NS	—	NS	—
CvC	p>b 3/3	2/3	—	NS	—	p>b 2/2	NS	—	NS	—
VCV /i___i/	p>b 2/4	—	s>-s 1/4	—	NS	p>b 2/4	—	s>-s 2/4	—	1/4
VCV /u___u/	p>b 2/4	—	NS	—	NS	p>b 2/4	—	s>-s 3/4	—	1/4

CONCLUSION

Models in phonology, whether of the now traditional *Sound Pattern of English* type (Chomsky and Halle, 1968) or of the more recent variants, are essentially descriptive in nature, and are not intended to be recipes for translating the output of a grammar's syntax or semantics into the input of its phonetics. Having said that, the formal stance adopted is nevertheless a *procedural* one, and it has led many a researcher into regarding a set of rules in phonology as an explicit programmable algorithm. Whether this is a proper use of extant phonologies is arguable, but there seems a clear need for just such a phonological procedure when considering from a phonetic viewpoint what it is we want a phonology to do. The interim translation-theory solution adopted over the past two decades is certainly no longer satisfactory (Fowler et al., 1980), but equally unsatisfactory *for linguistics* would be any theory purporting to overthrow such an approach by simply decrying the essentially abstract and mentalistic basis of linguistics by pointing to a few mechanistic "facts" about how the articulatory musculature and other structures might function.

But, referring back to our introductory section, if it is the case that some local hardware or firmware mechanism is responsible for the explanation of many of the findings from laboratory phonetics rather than any higher level intended actions, then, almost in a compensatory fashion, the need to get the cognitively dominated procedures of phonology and phonetics just right is enhanced. These procedures are now going to simplify right down to a very basic programming of the articulatory system (however mechanistically complex this might be). This procedural approach incorporates the notion that much of the detail of what actually happens in speaking is linguistically neither here nor there, and certainly not calling for detailed account all they way through the procedure (a tendency of translation theories).

If the interim translation theories said anything it was to claim the essential dumbness of a procedurally oriented phonology and phonetics. What now is emerging is that, on the contrary, an assumption of smartness is more appropriate. It may well be that a better linguistically motivated model of speech production assumes a rather gross procedure for deriving a base-line articulation from a sentence input by a system cognitively sensitive to all manner of pressures for testing and modifying the anticipated output of that gross procedure and intelligent enough to adjust and tune the output if necessary by appropriately altering the procedure at various points. Such a model accounts for a whole aspect of apparently context-sensitive variability in speech, while preserving both an essentially mentalistic phonology and allowing for low level set-piece effects deriving from actual internally coordinating motor and other mechanisms.

REFERENCES

Bigland, V., and Lippold, O. (1954). The relation between force, velocity and integrated electrical activity in human muscles. *Journal of Physiology, 123,* 214.

Coggshall, J. C., and Bekey, G. A. (1970). EMG-force dynamics in human skeletal muscle. *Medical and Biological Engineering, 8,* 265–270.

Edstrom, L., and Kugelberg, E. (1968). Histochemical composition, distribution of fibers, and fatigability of single motor units. *Journal of Neurology, Neurosurgery, and Psychiatry, 31,* 424.

Fowler, C. A. (1983). Realism and unrealism: A reply. *Journal of Phonetics, 11,* 303–322.

Fowler, C. A. (1980). Coarticulation and theories of extrinsic timing control. *Journal of Phonetics, 8,* 113–134.

Fowler, C. A., Rubin, P., Remez, R. E., and Turvey, M. T. (1980). Implications for speech production of a general theory of action. In B. Butterworth (Ed.), *Language production.* New York: Academic Press.

Fritzell, B., Kotby, M. N., and Möller, B. (1975). Variations in the activity of the palatopharyngeus muscle during speech. In G. Fant (Ed.), *Proceedings of speech communication seminar* (Stockholm, Sweden, 1974). New York: Halstead Press.

Fromkin, V. A. (1966). Neuromuscular specification of linguistic units. *Language and Speech, 9,* 170–199.

Harris, K., Lysaught, G. F., and Schvey, M. W. (1965). Some aspects of the production of *oral* labial and nasal stops. *Language and Speech, 135.*

Imaizumi, S., and Hiki, S. (1975). Extraction of motor command from electromyographic data. In G. Fant (Ed.), *Proceedings of speech communication seminar* (Stockholm, Sweden, 1974) (pp. 14–22). New York: Halstead Press.

Ladefoged, P. (1975). *A course in phonetics.* New York: Harcourt, Brace, Jovanovich.

Leanderson, R. (1972). *On the functional organization of facial muscles in speech.* Stockholm, Sweden: Department of Otolaryngology and Clinical Neurophysiology. Karolinska Sjukhuset.

Leanderson, R., and Lindblom, B.E.F. (1972). Muscle activation for labial speech gestures. *Acta Otolaryngology, 73,* 362–373.

Lindblom, B. (1982). The interdisciplinary challenge of speech motor control. In S. Grillner (Ed.), *Speech motor control.* New York: Pergamon Press.

Lubker, J. F., and Parris, P. (1970). Simultaneous measurements of intraoral pressure, force of the labial contact, and labial electromyographic activity during production of the stop consonant cognates /p/ and /b/. *Journal of the Acoustical Society of America, 47,* 629–633.

Morton, K., and Tatham, M. A. A. (1980). Devoicing, aspiration, and nasality—cases of universal misunderstanding? *Occasional Papers, No. 23.* University of Essex: Department of Language and Linguistics.

Tatham, M. A. A. (1980). The linguistic control of speech production. *Occasional Papers, 23.* University of Essex: Department of Language and Linguistics.

Tatham, M. A. A. (1984). Towards a cognitive phonetics. *Journal of Phonetics, 12.*

Tatham, M. A. A., and Morton, K. (1968). Further electromyography data. *Occasional Papers, 1.* University of Essex: Department of Language and Linguistics.

Tatham, M. A. A., and Morton, K. (1970). Some electromyography data towards a model of speech production. *Language and Speech, 12,* 29–38.

Tatham, M. A. A., and Morton, K. (1973). Electromyographic and intraoral air-pressure studies of bi-labial stops. *Language and Speech, 16,* 336–350.

Tatham, M. A. A., and Morton, K. (1980). Precision. *Occasional Papers, 23.* University of Essex, Department of Language and Linguistics.

Author Index

Subject Index

Italicized page numbers refer to illustrations, (t) refers to a table.

V

VCV tokens, DEL for, 297–298, 305(t)
  peak EMG amplitude of, 297–298, 305(t)
  statistical analyses for, 306(t), 307(t)
Viscous constant, in measurement of canine vocal fold, 29–32, *30, 31, 34*
Vital capacity, restricted, in speech, 50–54
Vocal fold, adjustments in, 36–44
  role of laryngeal muscles in, 37–38, *39*
  animal studies on, 17–23, 18, 19, 20
    cat, 22–23
    dog, 18–21, *18–19*
      viscoelastic measurements in, 24–32
    monkey, 21–22, *20–21*
  changes in structure of, with age, 11–17, *12, 14–16*
  collagenous fibers in, 4–7
  comparative physiology of, 17–23, *18, 19, 20, 21*
  effect of laryngeal adjustment versus vibratory pattern adjustment on, 42, *43*
  effect of longitudinal tension on, 38–40, *41*
  elastic fibers in, 4–7
  fine structure of, 4–7, *5, 6*
  growth of, 11–13, *12*
  histological structure of, 2–4, *3*
    variation in, 7–17, *8,* 9(t), *10, 12, 14–16*
  in vivo measurements of, 34–36
  mechanical properties of, 24–36
    viscosity, 29–32, *30, 31, 34*
    elasticity, 24–29, *26, 27, 28*
    orthotropy, 32–34, *33*
  morphology of, 2–17
    changes in, with aging, 13–17, *14–16*
  of newborn, morphology of, 11, *12*
  orthotropy in, 32–34, *33*
  variation in thickness of, 9(t), *10*
  vibration of, cover-body theory of, 1–44
Vocal models, 88–99
  glottal, 91–95
  subglottal, 89–91
  supraglottal, 96–99

Vocalis Muscle (VOC), role of, in vocal fold adjustment, 37, 38(t), *39*
Voice onset time (VOT), in assessment of speech intelligibility, 117–123
Volume compensation, role of, in speech breathing, 59–60
Vowel identification, age-dependent studies, *132*
Vowel production, phenomenological model of, 73–109

Y

Young's Modulus, in measurement of canine vocal fold, 24–29, *26, 27, 28, 34*